In the Pursuit of Winning

Masood Zangeneh · Alex Blaszczynski ·
Nigel E. Turner
Editors

In the Pursuit of Winning

Problem Gambling Theory, Research
and Treatment

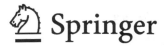 Springer

Masood Zangeneh
Centre for Addiction and Mental Health
Toronto
Canada

Nigel E. Turner
Centre for Addiction and Mental Health
Toronto
Canada

Alex Blaszczynski
The University of Sydney
Sydney
Australia

ISBN-13: 978-0-387-72172-9   e-ISBN-13: 978-0-387-72173-6

Library of Congress Control Number: 2007939286

Printed on acid-free paper.

9 8 7 6 5 4 3 2 1

springer.com

Dedicated to my wife Goli

Contents

Part II

Contributors

Fadi Anjoul
Department of Psychology
University of Sydney
Australia

Malcolm Battersby
Flinders Therapy Service for Problem
Gamblers
Australia

Alex Blaszczynski
School of Psychology
University of Sydney
Australia

Lisa Cavion
Centre for Addiction and Mental Health
Canada

Gary Clifford
Consultant, Responsible Gambling
Consulting International
New Zealand
and private training practice

Emily Cripps
Centre for Addiction and Mental Health
Canada

Ewa Czerny
Centre for Addiction and Mental Health
Canada

Jeffrey Derevensky
Department of Psychiatry
McGill University
Canada

Lea Diakoloukas
Centre for Addiction and Mental Health
Canada

Peter Ferentzy
Centre for Addiction and Mental Health
Canada

Angus Forbes
Flinders Therapy Service for Problem
Gamblers
Australia

Jon E. Grant
University of Minnesota Medical
School
United States of America

Mark Griffiths
Psychology Division
Nottingham Trent University
United Kingdom

Alex Grunfeld
International Journal of Mental Health
and Addiction
Canada

Robert Grunfeld
Professional Advanced Services
in Mental Health and Addiction
Canada

Rina Gupta
School of Applied Child Psychology
McGill University
Canada

Suck Won Kim
Department of Psychiatry
University of Minnesota Medical
School
United States of America

Stephanie Koenig
Centre for Addiction and Mental Health
Canada

Lorne M. Korman
British Columbia Children's Hospital
The Provincial Health Services
Authority of British Columbia
and the University of British Columbia
Canada

G.E. Minchin
Barrister and Solicitor of the High
Court
New Zealand

Gary Nixon
School of Health Sciences
University of Lethbridge
Canada

Jane Oakes
Flinders Therapy Service for Problem
Gamblers
Australia

Jonathan Parke
Psychology Division
Nottingham Trent University
United Kingdom

Rene Pols
Flinders Therapy Service
for Problem Gamblers
Australia

Marc N. Potenza
Department of Psychiatry
Yale University School of Medicine
United States of America

Tony Schellink
Faculty of Management
Dalhousie University
Canada

Wayne Skinner
Centre for Addiction and Mental Health
Canada Toronto
Canada

Jason Solowoniuk
School of Health Sciences
University of Lethbridge
Canada

Amnon Jacob Suissa
Centre de recherche Sur L'itinérance de
L'UQAM
University of Quebec in Ottawa
Canada

Barry Tolchard
Flinders Therapy Service
for Problem Gamblers
Australia

Tony Toneatto
Centre for Addiction and Mental
Health,
and the University of Toronto
Canada

Nigel E. Turner
Centre for Addiction and Mental Health
Canada

Michael Walker
Department of Psychology
University of Sydney
Australia

Carol Wong
Simon Fraser University
Canada

Masood Zangeneh
Centre for Research on Inner City
Health
St. Michael's Hospital
Canada

Chapter 1
Introduction

Masood Zangeneh, Alex Blaszczynski, and Nigel E. Turner

Gambling has been part of the human scene since early recorded history; however, over the last two decades there has been an unprecedented explosion of commercial gambling, and with it, a parallel interest in the impact of this form of entertainment on psychological health and well-being of individuals and specific subpopulations. It is fascinating to observe the growth and development of interest in the psychology of gambling during the last 15 years.

According to prevalence surveys, gambling represents a relatively typical recreational activity for most community members, with more than 80 % of Canadian adults participating to some extent. However, it is relevant to note that, far from being a potential source of revenue, gambling is a losing proposition for the average player simply because the odds are statistically stacked in favor of the house. While most players contain losses to affordable levels, unfortunately, between 1 % and 2 % of the general population report symptoms of a severe gambling problem (Shaffer, Hall, and Vander Bilt, 1999), suggesting that problem gambling affects a relatively small proportion of adults in the community. However, such prevalence statistics are somewhat misleading because most people who gamble do so infrequently. The rates of problem gambling are much higher among "regular gamblers" and, of course, depending on how one defines "regular gambler," the rate in this subpopulation can vary anywhere from 10 % to 80 %.

This book offers one of the first attempts to bring together leading gambling researchers to define collectively what is known in this new area of research. It focuses on both the individual and social levels of analysis to examine risk factors and, even more importantly, to identify and describe the range of personal and social conditions that appear to influence a broad range of health outcomes.

The chapters in this book are divided into two parts. The first part consists of a series of chapters that attempt to understand the reasons why some people develop gambling problems. The second part consists of a number of chapters describing effective forms of treatment for problem gambling.

Masood Zangeneh
Centre for Research on Inner City Health, St. Michael's Hospital, Canada

M. Zangeneh, A. Blaszczynski, N. Turner (eds.), *In the Pursuit of Winning.*
© Springer 2008

Part 1

Chapter 2: Explaining Why People Gamble

The authors of chapter 2 explore why people gamble, even though in gambling an individual is more likely to lose instead of win. The authors assert that gambling cannot be an inherent part of "human nature," as purported by some. Historical and cultural evidence supports that gambling is a learned phenomenon heavily influenced by cultural values.

The authors suggest that problems related to gambling have their genesis in a large number of factors, including the presence of erroneous beliefs contributing to an overestimation of the likelihood of winning, use of gambling to socialize with friends, and use of gambling to escape from home. As the authors note, at the individual level, gamblers may not be aware of factors influencing their gambling activities.

Chapter 3: Games, Gambling, and Gambling Problems

In chapter 3, the author describes the nature of gambling including an examination of the history and economics of gambling, the nature of random chance, the concept of the "house edge," and then offers a detailed exposition of a number of popular games played by gamblers. The main purpose of the chapter is to provide the reader with sufficient information to understand the belief schemas and motivational factors held by gamblers and, for therapists, to facilitate discussions with clients about the nature of erroneous beliefs and expectations.

Chapter 4: Exploring the Mind of the Gambler: Psychological Aspects of Gambling and Problem Gambling

In chapter 4, the authors examine psychological factors that influence the development and maintenance of problem gambling. A number of learning theories are postulated to explain behaviors related to problem gambling: classical conditioning with repeated pairings of wins, arousal and environmental stimuli; and operant conditioning reinforcing continued play all combine to foster rapid learning and persistence in gambling.

Unlike conditioning theories, social learning theory maintains that social facilitation may maintain gambling behaviors. The presence of other individuals through the gambling activity may affect gamblers' behaviors in different ways. On the other hand, implicit learning theory describes gamblers as "absorbing" gambling outcomes, through which some develop erroneous beliefs about the nature of the random events. Irrational thought processes and cognitive distortions of problem gambler are also explored in this chapter. Illusions of control, beliefs in luck, attribution biases, and hindsight biases are aspects of irrational thoughts discussed by the authors.

Chapter 5: Individual Factors in the Development and Maintenance of Problem Gambling

In chapter 5, the authors explore individual factors associated with gambling, such as anxiety and arousal, temperament, attention-deficit/hyperactivity disorder (ADHD), narcissism, and coping skills, as well as their potential relationship to problem gambling. The development and maintenance of problem gambling is likely to be the result of multiple factors, all of which interact in a complex manner. However, it is clear from the chapter that this area of gambling research remains in its infancy and is not sufficiently developed to draw any definitive conclusions about how individual difference factors interact with gambling behavior.

Chapter 6: Gambling: A Sociological Perspective

In chapter 6, the authors examine the development of modern gambling in North America. Through the past 20 years, gambling in North America has been legalized and legitimized both by state sponsorship and commercial interests, as demonstrated in the increased proliferation of gambling and liberalized rules and regulations. Concomitantly, the increased availability, variety, and prevalence of gambling testify to its social acceptance as a legitimate leisure pursuit in North America. For governments and commercial operators, gambling has become established as an excellent revenue source.

The authors also examine the impact of gambling on marginalized and minority groups and on people on low incomes. The authors of this chapter argue that as a stigmatized activity, gambling turns gamblers further away from mainstream society. Within the capitalist society, and for those who are marginalized, gambling is characterized as a means of beating the odds. The beliefs tragically further marginalize and trap individuals into an exploitative system.

Chapter 7: A Critical Perspective on Gambling: A Sociohistorical Analysis

In chapter 7, the author outlines some of the major determinants of gambling. Gambling activities have been traced back to 2000 B.C., with vestiges of dice recently excavated in London. Royal lotteries in France were important sources of revenue, used, for example, to build churches under Louise XIV. In the mid-1600s, rules and regulations for gambling were applied by the Puritans. In the United States, Nevada repealed gaming laws in 1931, with most states still considering gambling as illegal into the 1950s. It is in this context, within the 20th century, that the idea of gambling as a psychopathology emerged. Though one discourse stigmatizes gambling in terms of a pathology, other recent social and institutional processes associated with political and gaming industries have legalized, legitimized, and normalized gambling as a socially acceptable activity.

The author does not consider gambling addiction to be part of a continuum. The author similarly critiques disease dominant definition of addiction referring to the addiction cycle as irreversible as being misguided in its foundation. The author highlights the disagreements between the law and science, with the courts being more apt to define gambling abuse, not as a disease, but as a vice that deserves punishment.

Chapter 8: The Marketing of Gambling

Different forms of gambling in Canada and other countries have been successfully introduced and/or expanded as a result of effective marketing strategies, knowledge of the product, and industry responses to changing customer needs. Casinos, for example, have been successful at performing "situational analyses," interviews or surveys with clients, product assessments, and determining demographics designed to further promote gambling. The authors of chapter 8 examine marketing strategies specific to certain forms of gambling.

The authors note that the working-class are overrepresented among the gambling population and that this may be an indication of the impact of television-based marketing. "Chance ideology," illusion of equal opportunity, "entrapment," and feelings of commitment to a goal that has not yet been achieved (i.e., a person who picks the same lottery numbers every week) operate to popularize gambling. Government backing of lotteries also adds a dimension of credibility, another tactic effectively applied in selling the product.

Chapter 9: Religiosity and Gambling Rituals

In chapter 9, the authors review gambling in the context of religiosity and rituals. Gambling traditionally originated from religious rituals and quests for spiritual experiences. According to the authors, over the past 400 years of social change, the breakdown of traditional, pre-modern society and the rise in individualism has contributed to the loss of individuals' senses of ontological security. Secularization has furthermore contributed to the decontextualization of rituals, also marked by the loss of a sense of community. In other words, the modern gambler has become disconnected from other individuals, unable to meet his or her physical and psychological needs.

The advent of statistics and calculation of probabilities in late 16th century Italy contributed to the secularization of "chance" and determinism lost its religious meaning. Despite mathematical realities, a belief in the supernatural may create a sense of grandeur that leads individuals to make large risks in gambling. In a real sense, casinos are modern cathedrals. This is nowhere more apparent than with the breathtaking displays of wealth and power along the Las Vegas Strip.

Chapter 10: Buying a Risk: An Application of Insurance Law to Legal Gaming

At law, the imposition of novel duties of care may be arrived at by way of analogy with extant obligations. In chapter 10, such an analogy is made between the provision of gambling opportunities and the legal duties that subsist in any contract of insurance. A legal methodology is employed to explicate the core principles that give rise to fiduciary duties resulting from contracts of insurance, and to apply judicial decisions in the area of insurance law to the gambling construct.

Part 2

Chapter 11: Cognitive Behavioral Treatment for Problem Gamblers

In chapter 11, the authors discuss the cognitive and behavioral treatment methods used in the management of problem gambling at the Flinders Medical Centre in Australia. Their approach involves a variety of techniques, and the chapter is full of helpful suggestions on implementing a cognitive behavioral approach. In addition, the chapter provides both case studies and a formal evaluation of the efficacy of the service. It is a useful resource for clinicians and counselors.

Chapter 12: Psychopharmacological Management of Pathological Gambling

In chapter 12, the authors provide a very thorough and comprehensive summary of the research on the psychopharmacology of gambling addiction. While the data are promising, the results must be tempered with the knowledge that many studies contain methodological limitations and are based on very small sample sizes. The evidence is encouraging but continues to require further replication before becoming a standard component of any treatment package. This chapter is an excellent resource for anyone interested in conducting replication studies evaluating the efficacy of these medications.

Chapter 13: A Transpersonal Developmental Approach to Gambling Treatment

In chapter 13, the authors examine the application of Jungian psychology and ideas related to spiritual development to the treatment of problem gambling. According to the authors, Jung viewed addiction as a misguided spiritual thirst for a wholeness and union with God. The approach integrates psychological theories of development such as those of Piaget and Kohlberg with Eastern and Western philosophical notions of contemplative development. According to the authors, the approach is unique in that not only is it a developmental spectrum of pre-personal, personal, and transpersonal consciousness, but it also considers the possible pathologies as developmental barriers that can arise at each stage. The authors then discuss each of the ten stages of transpersonal development and include examples illustrative of the different approaches taken at each stage. The idea of the counterfeit hero archetype is rather interesting. The authors state that "the compulsion towards winning . . . is not fused with the mature Hero's understanding that he or she is not God." It is a really interesting way to describe the distorted mindset of the pathological gambler.

Chapter 14: How Science Can "Think" About Gamblers Anonymous

Gambler's Anonymous (GA) is a mutual aid fellowship modeled on the philosophy and principles of Alcoholics Anonymous (AA). It is probably one of the "interventions" that is utilized most by problem gamblers and one that maintains a culture of recovery distinct from AA. The authors argue that rigid conceptions of rationality and subjectivity can lead to a neglect of the important process of "thinking"; the neglect of "thinking" has created a gap between science and these types of mutual aid group. The authors of chapter 14 discuss two major topics: first, drawing from the work of several scholars, the authors discuss AA and how the organization is inconsistent with modern notions of individuality, rationality, and professional authority, among others; and second, the current literature as it pertains to GA and AA.

Chapter 15: Problem Gambling and Anger: Integrated Assessment and Treatment

In chapter 15, the authors discuss the issue of the treatment of anger for problem gamblers. As they point out, problematic gambling often includes a set of dysregulated emotions. Problems of anger and domestic violence appear to be particularly prevalent among gamblers, and accordingly, the authors set out to describe an effective treatment method for anger among problem gamblers. The chapter includes a discussion of how they set up their treatment, techniques used, and goals of the treatment, and then concludes by discussing in detail a case study.

Chapter 16: A Treatment Approach for Adolescents with Gambling Problems

In chapter 16, the authors provide an overview of their approach to treating youth with gambling problems. Given the consistent finding that attitudes and exposure to gambling are shaped in the early formative years of adolescent development, this chapter contains valuable advice on the treatment of youth derived from the knowledge base of highly experienced therapists and researchers.

Chapter 17: The Evolution of Problem Gambling Helplines

In chapter 17, the author discusses the evolution of problem gambling helplines. New Zealand's Helpline is an example of an effective model that is designed to enhance motivation for change and the provision of telephone/online counseling, referrals, and information services. The author notes that often, many problem gamblers appear to seek help in much the same way as they approach gambling: the quest for a "quick fix." Those who do desire help most often do not want to come in for in lengthy session of counseling. The New Zealand approach takes advantage of the window of opportunity, that is, an easy and rapid access to assistance via the telephone when the motivation to seek treatment is maximal. The author briefly examines the history of the helpline from its inception in the 1980s in New Jersey, and discusses the various functions that a helpline can serve. The author then examines three case studies in more detail including Ontario Problem Gambling Helpline, Britain's Gamcare, and New Zealand's Hotline and finally discusses the limitations of helpline services, future directions for each of these services, and where he would like to see such helplines develop in the future.

The collection of material in this book provides the reader with a wealth of diverse perspectives on the nature of gambling, problem gambling, and approaches to intervention. The primary goal of this book is to present a comprehensive and critical analysis of the conceptual and empirical literature surrounding gambling and problem gambling. Our aim is to provide the reader, from undergraduate students to clinician and active research investigator, a guide to the major issues. A comprehensive understanding of the psychology of gambling and problem gambling is fundamental if we are to maximize the benefits and minimize the negative aspects of this commercial product.

This book is targeted toward undergraduate and graduate students in psychology, sociology, public health, medicine, nursing, bioethics, mental health, addiction and political science. It is also intended for anyone interested in participating in the ongoing debate on gambling and problem gambling.

Acknowledgments We owe an enormous debt of gratitude to the pioneers in the field of gambling research. We are also indebted to the many colleagues whose guidance and insights we have benefited from during the completion of this book. This book would not have been possible without generous feedback and support from our consultants: James Westphal, Ruth Herd, Christine McKay, Amina Jabbar, and Jennifer Borrell.

Part I

Chapter 2
Explaining Why People Gamble

Michael Walker, Tony Schellink, and Fadi Anjoul

Human gambling is an enigma. It is difficult to understand why people are willing to stake money on the outcome of an unpredictable event when the expected return is less than the initial stake. Explaining the popularity of lotteries, electronic gaming machines, and totalizator betting is a challenge to currently accepted theories of human behavior. If psychology is the scientific approach to explaining human behavior, then we might ask how well a clearly self-defeating behavior such as gambling can be understood.

For the purposes of exploring this extraordinary behavior, it is necessary to limit its definition. Without great loss in generality, "gambling" can be defined as a monetary transaction between two parties based on the outcome of an uncertain event. One party wagers that the event will turn out one way while the other party wagers that it will turn out the other way. Depending on who is right, one party will be wealthier by the amount staked (the winner) and the other party will be out of pocket by the same amount. Since the winner receives from the loser the amount wagered, the contest can be conceptualized as a zero-sum game and the activity can be labeled "zero-sum gambling.". No wealth is created by zero-sum gambling; rather it is redistributed. Thus, winning games is associated with increasing wealth and losing games is associated with decreasing wealth.

The expected effect on wealth by playing a game can be calculated by the product of the probability of winning (p) and the amount of money that will be won (w) compared to the amount staked (s). The quantity ($pw - s$) is the expected effect on wealth. It is sometimes referred to as the value of the game to the player. A fair game is one in which $pw = s$, and taking part in a fair game is a fair gamble. The individual is able to anticipate increasing wealth by ensuring that $pw > s$. The prospect of wealth depends on the individual accepting a gamble in which either p is such that $pw > s$, or w is such that $pw > s$, or both. Thus, it is quite understandable why an individual will accept gambles in which the stake is sufficiently low, the payoff sufficiently large, or the prospect of winning sufficiently attractive. Presumably, gambling will thrive where both parties believe that the parameters of the game favor them.

Michael Walker
University of Sydney, Australia

M. Zangeneh, A. Blaszczynski, N. Turner (eds.), *In the Pursuit of Winning.*
© Springer 2008

Consider the bet on D'Oyley's marriage, made in 1815. Cartwright bet Berens ten pounds to one pound that some Jurist Fellow now of the College will marry before D'Oyley does. In the 19th century, bets such as this were made by Fellows of All Souls College, Oxford, and written down in *The Old Betting Book* (Oman, 1912). Although we do not know the winner, it is reasonable to speculate that both Cartwright and Berens believed that they had made a favorable wager. Cartwright was clearly confident that D'Oyley's marriage was highly unlikely; Berens thought otherwise. In a sense, the outcome of the bet indicates who had the more accurate understanding of the situation. If all gambling conformed to this example, then there would be little left for psychologists to explain. Remarkably, the bets recorded in *The Old Betting Book* have little in common with contemporary gambling.

In all legalized contemporary gambling, one of the parties can be labeled "the house" and the other party, the gambler. The house may be a casino, club, bar, or other venue for gambling. The rules for the gambling at a venue are controlled by law and, in most jurisdictions, the law is carefully patrolled and the gambling closely regulated. The interesting aspect of contemporary gambling, which differentiates it from that recorded in *The Old Betting Book*, is the "edge" to the house. All contemporary legalized gambling is controlled so that $s > pw$ for the gambler: the house expects to win. The extent of this edge varies from one form of gambling to another. In many casino games, the edge is small whereas in large lotteries the edge is large. There is a broad principle that governs the size of the edge and, at the same time, provides an insight into the attractiveness of gambling: the larger the prize for which the gambler plays, the larger the edge to the house. Thus, the edge in games where s and w are of similar size is usually only a few percentage points. In casino blackjack, for example, the edge to the house for skilled play by the gambler is less than 1 % (Walker, Sturevska, & Turpie, 2000). Where w is large compared to s, as in horse racing and slot machines, the edge is correspondingly larger and typically about 20 %. Where w is extremely large compared to s, as in lotteries, the edge to the house is large and frequently approaches 40 %. In economic terms, the price that can be obtained for the gambling product is determined to a large degree by the size of the largest prize.

If individuals were motivated to seek out and accept bets in which $pw > s$, then contemporary gambling would be most unattractive to the vast majority of people. Whereas the wager between Cartwright and Berens is understandable, that between the player and the slot machine is not. In explaining the attractiveness of contemporary gambling forms, some of the major assumptions of psychological theory must be questioned. We must ask whether the modern gambler fully understands the odds. If ignorance is not part of the explanation, and gambling is rational behavior, then what do gamblers receive for their expected losses? Alternatively, if gambling behavior is irrational, then what situational factors or unconscious drives motivate it? Of all the alternatives available, the only one that we can exclude immediately is that gambling is unattractive and therefore avoided by the vast majority of individuals.

Gambling and Human Nature

One of the common claims about gambling is that it has been part of the human scene since recorded history. It has been argued that certain archaeological discoveries point to an extensive history of gambling (Halliday & Fuller, 1974). For example, six-sided animal bones, called "astragali," that resemble modern dice have been found in ancient Egyptian tombs dated to c. 3500 B.C. Ancient Egyptian murals dating to the same period depict the playing of board games (David, 1962). Board games and astragali that date back to c. 2600 B.C. have also been found in the royal tombs at Ur in Mesopotamia (Woolley & Moorey, 1982). It has been assumed that these remains are evidence that gambling existed in early human society. This claim is then extrapolated to infer that the propensity to gamble is part of human nature (Thomas, 1901). Gambling, along with prostitution and alcohol consumption, are assumed to be vices grounded in human instinctual drives. According to this view, rather like the sexual and aggressive instincts, the urge to gamble is inherent in humans. Prostitution, for example, has occurred since civil societies were first established in Sumer, Egypt, and the Indus Valley. Thus, if prostitution is "the world's oldest profession," then gambling is the world's second oldest diversion (Thompson, 1997). Freud observed that one of the roles of society is to socialize the instinctual drives. The task of explaining individual differences in the attractiveness of gambling then becomes one of explaining why some people gamble so much and others are not attracted to gambling in the least. The Freudian metaphor here is that society, primarily through the parents, trains the child to inhibit the gratification of gambling impulses; variations in gambling behavior are, at least in part, explained by variations in appetite and self-control (Orford, 1985).

The claim that gambling has always been part of human culture is important because it implies a biological basis for the notion of "gambling urge" and places the activity in the "learn to control" sphere of human endeavor. These claims form a straightforward theoretical base for understanding excessive gambling in terms of addiction and impaired control (O'Connor & Dickerson, 2003). However, the historical account, on which the assumption of a biologically based urge is grounded, has recently been disputed (Anjoul, 2003). Gambling of the kind defined at the beginning of this chapter, unlike the widely promulgated view that it has always been part of human society, is likely to have been a relatively recent occurrence historically. It is likely that the necessary preconditions for gambling were not met before the 5th century B.C.

What are the preconditions for gambling in society? There appear to be three. First of all humans must be motivated to acquire wealth. Second, play must exist as a sphere of human activity. Finally, wealth must be easily transferable. Play behavior is common across primate species. The games that humans play can be traced in part to the inherent nature of humans. Similarly, the acquisition of wealth has been linked to principles of evolution and is evident from prehistorical finds. The conjunction of these two claims may well have led to wealth being transferred to the winners of sporting and gaming events. Early references to gambling-like behavior are likely to have involved gaming of this kind. The reason for this is that the third precondition for gambling as a popular activity and a part of culture was absent. Wealth could not be transferred or distributed with ease. Gambling as a popular activity did not arise until the invention of coins and their denominations in Greece in the 5th century B.C. Without coins in different denominations, gambling in the modern sense could not exist. If gambling became an accepted part of society as late as the 5th century B.C., then it is unlikely that gambling is an appetite inherent in human nature. What sense then can be made of the relics that predate the 5th century B.C.? There is no certainty that either board games or astragali were used specifically for gambling. The historical remains clearly indicate forms of game-playing. Evidence of game-playing can be found across all civilized societies and across all time periods. However, evidence of game-playing does not necessarily indicate gambling. The central difference between gambling and game-playing is that the former involves an exchange of wealth based on an uncertain outcome. Thus, the evidence for game-playing has been confused with evidence for gambling.

Gambling is unnecessary for survival or perpetuation of the human race. Gambling is essentially a mechanism for redistributing wealth. Monetary economies do not feature in hunter-gatherer modes of living. Indeed, the human species have spent more than 99 % of their existence to the present time living in tribal, noneconomic conditions. Hominoids or human-like creatures have been in existence for more than a million years. Human beings (*Homo sapiens*) have roamed Earth for tens of thousands of years. By comparison, the modern age is only hundreds of years old. It is very easy to lose sight of this fact, making it difficult to appreciate that modern economic institutions have not always dominated societies as they do today. From this perspective, there does not seem to be any good reason for expecting gambling to have been present among our early ancestors. They did not need to invent ways to distribute wealth because subsistence, the struggle to stay alive, was the basic order of their era.

Gambling and Culture

Culture may be defined as a set of shared ideas, values, beliefs, and moral codes that are transmitted across generations through socialization and form the basis of social behavior. This definition suggests that cultural differences in orientation to gambling will be related to differences between cultures in the basic nature of shared ideas, values, beliefs, and moral codes that form the basis of gambling.

There are at least two fundamentally different ideological frameworks for living: traditionalism and individualism. Traditionalists are characterized as theistic, heaven-oriented, and submissive (Riesman, 1954). An afterlife is assumed and given priority over the transience of life on Earth. Piety is of utmost concern because pious behavior is antecedent to a desirable afterlife. Social standing in this life is discounted, and virtue is preferred as the mark of an individual. Moreover, traditionalism encourages the acceptance of inequity and cooperation, not competition and covetousness. It is clear that such ideas and values do not facilitate a positive attitude to gambling. Within the traditionalist framework, gambling is regarded as a means to exploit others and, therefore is inconsistent with cooperative values.

A society in which most of its members adopt a secular, earthly, and progressive approach to universal problems is said to be one that is characterized by individualism. Most Western societies embrace individualism. Western societies are highly secularized, appealing to science and determinism to explain reality. Evolutionary theory is generally regarded as a matter of fact, and all events are seen to have material causes that are consistent with the laws of physics and chemistry. Religion and magic are removed from governing institutions, and designated to the private sphere. This means that life on Earth is given priority over the prospect of eternal life because life on Earth is deemed certain, whereas eternal life may ultimately prove to be a myth. Thus, the general approach to the future is one that encourages the individual to exploit his or her life on Earth. Also featuring in the earthly approach is the notion that destiny is in the hands of the individual. Such a belief forms the foundation for working diligently to achieve goals. Given the inclination toward the belief that there may not be anything beyond life to look forward to, individualism further advances a perpetual striving to better one's station in life, and hope is expressed in political and economic terms. The individual is assured that resisting social inequity and striving to compete will allow for an improved quality of living. Those who have made it to the top triumphantly display the indicators of their accomplishments. This is the essence of individualism and, in the cultural context, the basis of shared ideas, values, and beliefs that are conducive to gambling. The more that a society is based on individualism, rather than traditionalism, the more the spread and popularity of gambling would be expected. Certainly, modern Western industrialized countries are those in which a wide range of gambling has been legalized and in which a variety of forms of gambling are easily accessible (McMillen, 1996).

One of the major problems in researching cultural differences in attitudes and behavior is in finding samples of individuals who are equivalent. In an important study of values, Hofstede (1980) solved this problem. Hofstede developed a questionnaire to measure work-related values, which he distributed to IBM employees in 63 countries. The IBM employees represented "almost perfectly matched samples" in all respects except nationality (Hofstede, 1991). An analysis of the data suggested that four factors accounted for problems common to all employees: Individualism–Collectivism, Power Distance, Uncertainty Avoidance, and Masculinity–Femininity. These factors respectively describe the relationship between the individual and the group, social inequity, dealing with uncertainty, and concepts of masculinity and femininity.

Although Hofstede reported pronounced cultural differences in each of these factors, much of the contemporary research on the structure of culture has focused almost exclusively on the individualism and collectivism dimension (Kagitcibasi & Berry, 1989), suggesting researchers regard it as one of the most important tools for studying cultural differences in social behavior. The current cross-cultural literature defines individualism as the tendency to be more concerned with one's own needs, interests, and goals, whereas collectivism refers to the tendency to favor group cohesion and groups interests. Further, a person (or nation) with strong individualistic values necessarily has weak collectivist attitudes (Freeman & Bordia, 2001). Within individualism, factor analytic work by Triandis and Gelfand (1998) has identified the importance of winning as one of five dimensions.

Hofstede reported individualism factor scores for fifty countries and three multicountry regions. The results suggest that Westernized countries generally adopt an individualistic approach, whereas Arab countries and Eastern nations are more collectivist. This trend has been replicated in other recent studies (Briley &Wyer, 2001; Buda & Elsayed-Elkhouly, 1998).

McQueen (1995) has provided a comprehensive comparison of worldwide levels of gambling in a report of annual lottery sales across 87 countries. Anjoul (2003) cross-referenced the gambling levels of 38 countries from this report with individualism scores from Hofstede's research. The 1994 population of each selected country was estimated using a United States census bureau population estimator located at http://www.census.gov. The 1994 lottery sales for each selected country were divided by the estimated 1994 population, to yield a standardized per capita measure of gambling for that year. Anjoul found that there is a significant positive linear relationship between per capita lotto gambling expenditure and levels of individualism, $r_{(38)} = 0.336$, $p = .02$. Further, if Singapore is omitted from analysis, the correlation between lottery gambling expenditure and individualism is $+0.57$ ($p < .001$). This result suggests that gambling in Singapore is a special case. Anjoul's analysis represents the first empirical investigation of the relationship between levels of individualism and gambling in a society. The results suggest that increased levels of individualism generally correspond with increased levels of lotto (gambling) expenditure in a society.

Thus, both the historical evidence and the cultural evidence are consistent with the argument that gambling is a learned phenomenon that is heavily influenced by the values inherent in different cultures. This same evidence does not support the notion of an inherent, biologically based, drive to gamble, or of individuals who experience powerful urges to gamble that are wholly or partly outside their ability to control. Far from being a side issue in understanding why people gamble, the historical and cultural evidence points in the direction of society norms and values, socialization practices, personal goals, and motivations. That same evidence points away from biological, physiological, and brain-centered mechanisms that create urges in the way that such mechanisms create the urge to eat, drink, and copulate.

Gambling Skill

Eisler (1990) made a distinction between gambling games that are "fertile" and those that are "sterile." Fertile gambling games are those in which the skill of the individual in playing the game can affect the probability of winning and thereby the long-term outcomes. By contrast, sterile games offer no such opportunity. Among the fertile games are card games such as poker, blackjack, and bridge, sports betting and racing, and the large majority of private bets. Numbers games such as lotteries, bingo, and electronic gaming machines are sterile. The distinction is essentially the same as that made between games of skill and games of chance.

If individuals are motivated to maximize the monetary profit from gambling, then fertile games should be especially attractive. Given that all legally available gambling games are constructed so that there is an edge to the house, sterile games should be relatively unattractive. At the same time, games involving a great deal of skill may become too predictable to be widely attractive. Those with sufficient knowledge may wish to bet on the outcome but the majority without sufficient knowledge would want to avoid such bets. If both games of chance and high-skill games are likely to be less popular, then there remains a group of games, involving little skill, that would be expected to be the most popular forms of gambling. It is therefore surprising to learn that the most popular forms of gambling throughout the world are sterile gambling games such as lotteries and electronic gaming machines. The widespread popularity of simple games of pure chance requires further investigation. Again, both common sense and psychological theory are put to the test. What is it about lotteries that makes them the most popular form of gambling worldwide, or about electronic gaming machines that makes them the primary cause of problem gambling?

There are at least two explanations for why fertile gambling games are less popular than sterile games. The first explanation focuses on effort and reward. The simplicity of the modern electronic gaming machine is at the core of its attractiveness. Anyone can play. Anyone can win. Intelligence, status, and skill mean nothing. No group is disadvantaged. No special venue is required. According to this view, electronic gaming machines are attractive because they can provide a major win for minimum effort. All that remains to be resolved when individuals play gaming machines is who will be lucky and who will not. The alternative explanation focuses on the electronic gaming machine as close to the ideal in stamping in a simple set of behaviors through positive reinforcement. Modern electronic gaming machines provide a return on average once in five to six games and the games can be played repetitively at a rate of ten or more per minute. These "wins" provide partial reinforcement on a random schedule. However, from the player's perspective, a random reinforcement schedule may not be discriminable from a variable ratio reinforcement schedule. Variable reinforcement schedules are among the most powerful processes that maintain behavior (Walker, 1975).

Nevertheless, one would expect the opportunity to use a little skill to increase the payoff would certainly be attractive to the individual who seeks to win. However, the question of whether the opportunity to improve expected payouts by use of skill actually increases the risk of excessive gambling is not easy to answer. The prevalence and popularity of electronic gaming machines where outcomes are based on chance alone does not by itself resolve this issue. In many jurisdictions, the laws regulating electronic gaming machines preclude the inclusion of any element of skill. Nevertheless, electronic gaming machines, in which blackjack or draw poker are the games played ("card machines"), do permit an element of skill. For example, in draw poker, a pair of aces should be held in preference to the other three unrelated cards. Strategies for blackjack and draw poker exist and can be used by players to reduce the expected loss on these games. Interestingly, this element of skill does not make the games more popular than those that are purely chance events (Wagenaar, 1988). In New South Wales, since 1994, hotels have been permitted both card machines and machines based on games of pure chance. The pure chance games proved so popular that in many hotels the card machines were phased out. Nevertheless, preference alone does not answer the question of which machines are more likely to induce excessive levels of gambling. Card machines may have been less popular for any of a number of reasons: inferior prize structure, inferior graphics, or an inferior average payoff. The question is better approached by asking what happens when games of pure chance are modified so that an edge can be obtained through practice and skilled play. Machines in Britain give an insight into the answer.

Griffiths and his co-workers (Parke, Griffiths, & Parke, 2003; Parke, Griffiths & Turner, 2003) have described the structural differences between gaming machines in the United Kingdom and gaming machines in the United States. Whereas electronic gaming machines in the United States can be characterized as having highly valuable top prizes (sometimes running to millions of dollars), and game outcomes that occur according to fixed probabilities and random number generation that ensure that outcomes are fully independent from one game to the next, British machines are different. The American style machines have a high payout variability such that over the short term the average payout can deviate markedly from the long-term expectation of, say, 90 % of cash in. Since British machines often stand alone in small venues, it is desirable that the cash take remains relatively constant from one week to the next. For this reason, a compensator is built into the machines to adjust the payout probabilities so that, even in the short term, the 90 % return rate is maintained. In addition, British machines incorporate more complex game features. For example, players might strive to reach specific machine states (such as the letters ROULETTE on the screen) that are entry points to a range of games on a game board. These games have different payout options and may require eye–hand coordination skills. Players in Britain may thus acquire and exhibit real skill differences that are not possible on American machines. These skills may involve machine choice (knowing how to choose a machine that is likely to pay out) and machine play (eye–hand coordination). Despite the fact that British machines frequently have relatively small top prizes, such as £25, Griffiths reports that high levels of excessive play are generated.

An interesting point emerges from the comparison of electronic gaming in the United States and Great Britain. Habituation to machines can be facilitated either by large prizes or by opportunities for the use of skill. Independently of the machine, players exhibit similar illusions of control (Parke et al., 2003). It seems likely, then, that the basis of excessive gambling involvement is not the actual level of skill involved in trying to beat the machine, but the perceived skill. It is likely that, over the short term, players are actually unable to distinguish between results that can be attributed to actual skill and those which are attributed to mythical "skill" (Wagenaar, 1988). For example, blackjack is a gambling game that admits actual skill: "basic" strategy maximizes the monetary expectation of the player (card counting excluded). However, the majority of players deviate from basic strategy and prefer personal rules such as never hit a third time after two small cards (Wagenaar, 1988;

Walker et al., 2000). The rule "never hit a third time" is actually inferior to basic strategy, but the player is unable to perceive the small effect involved. Selective attention to confirming results can maintain an inferior strategy. Similarly, electronic gaming machine players may elect to play machines that have not recently had a large payout in the belief that the machines are now ready to pay ("hot"). Although there is no difference in the expected performance of "hot" and "cold" machines, players may be convinced that there is an actual difference in performance.

Accessibility of Gambling Games

The ready availability of gambling outlets can easily go unnoticed, yet accessibility is a major factor associated with use. Before the move to legalize casinos throughout many parts of the world, illegal casinos often thrived. Yet the percentage of adults who visited illegal casinos was low, partly because the locations of such casinos were generally kept secret. Regular play at casinos increases dramatically when legal casinos are introduced. Similar changes in the level of problem gambling can be observed when some types of gambling are legalized in a community. In Australia, states with electronic gaming machines legally available in clubs and hotels have much higher levels of problem gambling than states where such machines are not easily accessible (Productivity Commission, 1999).

Easy accessibility constitutes one among several factors that contribute to the popularity of any particular form of gambling. Lotteries, gaming machines, and betting on horses are all easily accessible, yet betting on horses is a male-dominated activity whereas lotteries and gaming machines are generally attractive to members of both genders (Schellinck & Schrans, 1998; Walker, 1992). Gender differences in gambling have been attributed to the presence of absence of a skill factor. However, it is unlikely that the claim that men prefer games of skill and women games of chance is the full explanation of gender differences. The game of craps, for example, involves little skill but attracts men rather than women, whereas gambling on bridge (a game of skill) attracts members of both genders. It would seem more likely that the factors that are important in making gambling attractive to both men and women are the perceived personal safety of the activity and gender role stereotypes associated with involvement in different forms of gambling.

Discrete and Continuous Gambling Games

An important distinction has been made between games in which bets can be made repetitively and those in which there is a significant gap in time between one bet and the next (Dickerson, 1984). Thus, casino games, betting on horses and dogs, gambling on cards, and playing electronic gaming machines are all classified as continuous because the betting is ongoing with many games or bets made consecutively in a session. Discrete games include lotteries, football pools, and many forms of sports betting. In addition, betting on specific horse races such as the Kentucky Derby, Grand National, or Melbourne Cup constitutes discrete gambling rather than the continuous wagering observed in betting shops. Discrete gambling games are not necessarily less popular than the continuous variety. In Australia, for example, the most popular form of regular gambling is Lotto, a form of lottery drawn several times each week (MacMillan, 1985). However, the importance of the distinction between discrete and continuous forms of gambling lies not in popularity but in the potential for continuous forms to condition the behavior of the individuals involved. Electronic gaming machines are frequently cited as clear examples of human behavior under the control of powerful partial reinforcement schedules (Dickerson, Hinchy, Legg-England, and Cunningham, 1992; Shewan & Brown, 1993). Thus, one explanation for excessive involvement in gambling involves the conditioning of gambling behavior and the prediction that continuous forms of gambling will be more dangerous from the perspective of consequent gambling problems.

The Genesis of Gambling-Related Problems

Different types of gambling vary in the potential to be linked with excessive gambling behavior and the associated problems. Lotteries, for example, are rarely linked with excessive gambling. By contrast, electronic gaming machines are a major cause of problem gambling wherever they are legalized. In New South Wales, Australia, 85 % of individuals seeking help in overcoming excessive gambling cite machine gambling as the primary cause of their problems (Walker, Blaszczynski, Sharpe, & Enersen, 2003). Why machine gambling should be so closely associated with excessive gambling behavior requires further explanation. Electronic gaming machines involve no skill, except perhaps in Britain. Thus, there is no rational basis for believing that one gambler may succeed through practice where another, perhaps a novice, is more likely to fail. All electronic gaming machine players should expect to lose and should be more confident in this expectation the more games that are played. Electronic gaming machines are usually easily accessed by the general public. This quality, on its own, however, does not explain the attractiveness of the machines. In casinos, the popularity of machines remains high despite the presence of attractive table games (McMillen, 1996).

In seeking to understand why electronic gaming machines, more than other forms of gambling, are associated with persistent play to the detriment of the life of the individual, various explanations have been put forward. One kind of explanation focuses on the fact that machines offer easy money. No great skill is required and anyone can be a winner. Assuming that large numbers of people are motivated by the chance of obtaining money in this way raises the question of why they persist when the evidence becomes clear that machines take money more often than they give it away. One possibility is that humans are far from objective in assessing risks and rather biased in their valuing of money (Wagenaar, 1988). Despite mounting losses, large wins remain attractive and may be perceived as relatively more likely than is in fact the case. Another possibility is that players do not appreciate that machine outcomes are independent from one game to the next (Ladouceur & Dube, 1997). Erroneous beliefs concerning machines and payouts have been recorded in many studies and may account for persistence in the face of loss (Delfabbro & Winefield, 2000; Toneatto, Blitz-Miller, Calderwood, Dragonetti, & Tsanos, 1997; Walker, 1990). For example, no matter how great the amount of money lost, it is always possible for a significant win to decrease the debt. The debt itself may be regarded as a sufficient investment to make a large payout seem likely (Walker, 1992).

The similarities between heavy consumption of alcohol and heavy involvement in gambling have led to another kind of explanation for excessive gambling. According to this view, gambling can become an addiction (Blaszczynski & Nower, 2002; Brown, 1987a; Orford, 1985). For some individuals the rewards of gambling create an urge that is difficult to resist. The nature of the rewarding mechanism is not fully agreed but may involve partial positive reinforcement by the occasional machine payouts or may involve conditioned arousal based around the excitement of playing. One other perspective is sometimes mentioned as an explanation for machine play. The gambler is assumed to be using gambling as an escape from other more negative aspects of his or her life (Carrig, Cheney, Philip-Harbutt, and Picone, 1996; Jacobs, 1987). As a means of coping with problems elsewhere in life, gambling is an avoidance coping method achieved by the narrowed focus on the electronic gaming machine.

There is little doubt that all of the explanations for gambling have some merit for some people some of the time. Further, individuals may gamble as a way of spending time with friends or of spending time outside the home. In searching for the best explanation of excessive play, it is important to note that the gambler does not necessarily have insight into the causes. The gambler cannot be expected to know that the value of the top prize has been overweighted or to grasp the slight probability of its occurrence. Similarly, the player is unlikely to know that cherished beliefs about beating the machine or being lucky are in fact invalid. Even the nature of the gambling addiction may not be fully understood. Under such circumstances, individuals are likely to rely on culturally available explanations such as "an uncontrollable urge to gamble" or being "weak willed." The reasons that individuals give for gambling may not be sufficient to explain either recreational or excessive involvement. Nevertheless, it is important to explore further the reasons individuals give for gambling and to examine whether the behavioral evidence is consistent with the self-reported evidence. It is important to examine whether the explanation of recreational gambling can also provide an explanation of excessive gambling.

Perspectives on the genesis of excessive gambling are divided on whether or not extreme levels of gambling involvement can be explained by reference to ordinary nonproblematic gambling behavior. Claims that pathological gambling is a clinical entity with a separate genesis, including physiological vulnerability, run counter to claims that pathological gambling is an outcome of learned skills such as self-control, or biased thinking such as belief in the gambler's fallacy. For a variety of reasons, these claims and counterclaims are best examined with respect to excessive involvement in playing electronic gaming machines. Gambling on such machines is not complicated by effects of skilled versus unskilled play. Involvement does not appear to be related to gender role stereotypes. Since one side in the gambling activity is a machine, which behaves according to known rules and constraints, the explanation of the other player is thereby simplified. Most importantly, the fact that machine gambling is strongly linked to pathological gambling is a good reason for focusing on the psychological processes of electronic gaming machine players.

Reasons Given for Machine Gambling

A wide variety of reasons are given by individuals for why they play electronic gaming machines. The most frequent explanation is that the activity is fun and a form of entertainment (Caldwell, 1974; Downes, Davies, David, and Stone, 1976; Schellinck & Schrans, 1998). Almost as many gamblers say that it is something to do, a way of passing time, perhaps to avoid responsibilities elsewhere in their lives. Making money is listed by about one-third of players as a motivation for playing. Other reasons given include socializing with friends and family, and giving in to the impulse to gamble, particularly when exposed to the machines. A small number of individuals say that they are addicted to the machines, that they are compulsive gamblers, and that they cannot overcome their urges to play the machines.

There is a question of whether people can report accurately the motivations for their actions (Nisbett & Wilson, 1977). This may apply to the reasons people give for playing electronic gaming machines. Consider, for example, the most common explanation that playing machines is fun. Hidden behind the response is a range of possible interpretations. What is it that is fun? The player may mean that the game itself is fun: that pressing a button and watching the reels spin is fun. Alternatively, the player may mean that the unfolding of chance events is fun: the resolution of uncertainty is rewarding in itself (Lovibond, 1968). Or the player may mean that the games where money is won are fun. If the game itself was the main cause of fun, then electronic gaming machines played without cash would have been marketed to exploit this interest of the public. Although computer simulations of slot machine games exist, there is no product sold to the public as a game without money. Again, if it was the unfolding of chance events that was entertaining, then games could be played quite inexpensively at one cent per line ("minimin" play). However, this strategy of play is rare (Haw, 2000; Williamson & Walker, 2000). It is difficult to avoid the conclusion that the fun of playing electronic gaming machines lies in the expectation and actuality of winning. Studies of rates of play support such an interpretation. Big wins disrupt play (Delfabbro & Winefield, 1999; Dickerson et al., 1992). Clearly, the fun and the winning are inextricably linked.

A similar analysis can be made of the idea that playing is a way of passing time. There is no reason to believe that this claim is false, but reason to question whether it is the complete explanation. If passing the time was the prime motivation, then minimin play is the least expensive way of achieving this goal. Since players do not use minimin strategies, it is unlikely that passing the time is the sole goal. "Passing the time" may be reasonably interpreted as "passing the time while having fun." Since having fun is inextricably linked with winning money, it can be seen that this reason too implies winning money as a motivation. Similar logic may show that the only motivation common to most players is the hope of winning money.

Among problem gamblers, almost half say that they are addicted to the machines and that they cannot control their impulse to gamble on them (Schellinck & Schrans, 1998). At the same time, a large number of problem gamblers still claim play the machines for fun and entertainment. About half of all machine gamblers, regardless of whether they are problem gamblers or not, say they really enjoy playing on the machines. This raises the question of why the remaining 50 % of players are gambling on the machines if they do not really enjoy playing. One of the common reasons given is to fill in time and to relieve boredom. However, such reasons are also not independent of winning money. Otherwise, the individual could attain the same ends less expensively by watching others gamble.

The Demography of Machine Gambling

The extent of gambling on electronic gaming machines depends to some extent on the accessibility of the machines. In general, the more accessible the machines the more similar the distribution of the players to the general population; the less accessible the machines the more likely those playing them will have distinctive demographic characteristics. In Australia, where machines are widely available in hotels, clubs, and casinos, those using the machines tend to be similar to the general population. In places where the machines are more restricted, such as in Canada, the demographic profile of regular gamblers is more skewed. In Canada, regular machine gamblers are more likely to be young (18 to 29 years of age), male, single blue-collar workers (Schellinck & Schrans, 1998).

The demography of gambling in a society has important implications for theory. Theoretical explanations that assume that the same processes of engagement and perseverance apply to all people equally lead to the expectation that the characteristics of those who gamble will be similar to those who do not. Theoretical explanations that assume that the motivation to gamble and the pathway into gambling vary across individuals may produce patterns of involvement that distort the demographic profile. Thus, explanations in terms of wealth creation are likely to be associated with socioeconomically biased profiles, whereas those that stress biologically based factors are less likely to produce the same bias. If problem gambling was associated excitement and risk-taking, an age-related skew to youth might be expected. If erroneous thinking about gambling was a cause of problems, then an educational skew to less education would be expected. In reality, problem gamblers do not differ greatly from regular gamblers in terms of demographics. In Australia, problem gamblers (primarily machine gamblers) have a mean age of 39 years, are more likely to be male (60 %), and more likely to live in cities (Jackson et al., 1998; Walker et al., 2003). Regular machine gamblers who are less likely to become problem gamblers are married or living with a partner and have children. The problem gamblers' profile in terms of gender, income, work status, and education is basically the same as for regular gamblers (Productivity Commission, 1999). The profile of problem machine gamblers in Canada is similar, with a few distinctive differences. Similar to the profile in Australia, those who are problem gamblers, compared to regular gamblers, are more likely to be separated or divorced and live in households with two adults and no children. However, in Canada, problem gamblers are more likely to have lower education, levels, less likely to speak English as a mother tongue, and are more likely to be 50 to 59 years old. Regular machine gamblers who have children, are homemakers or students, or have completed university are less likely to be problem gamblers.

Impaired Control Over Gambling Behavior

The core idea behind problem gambling is that the individual may continue to gamble far too long at a staking level that will cause problem levels of financial loss. Excessive gambling refers to that fact that such a gambler does not stop when it is prudent to do so. It follows that excessive gambling necessarily involves aspects of impaired control because the individual should stop but does not do so. The causes of impaired control are not as clear-cut. For example, impaired control may refer to the inability to cope with powerful urges to begin and continue gambling, or it may refer to the failure to set limits or accept limits on expenditure. The concept of uncontrollable urges suggests an addiction to gambling whereas the notion of excessive expenditure suggests poor money management.

One commonly cited cause of impaired control over gambling is that problem gamblers are often motivated to gamble as a means of emotional escape (Blaszczynski & Nower, 2002). There is strong evidence for an association between negative mood states and impaired control of gambling, although the direction of causation is less clear. Since excessive gambling is a cause of substantial monetary loss, depression following large losses would be expected (Walker, 1992). However, there is evidence for the view that gambling is an escape from depression. Dickerson, Baron, Hong and Cottrell (1996) found that 73 % of problem gamblers stated that they frequently gambled as a way of escaping depression.

Why should negative mood states be associated with the impulse to gamble? Several major explanatory ideas have been proposed by various authors. According to the relief of the negative mood state by gambling acts as a negative reinforcement. Negative reinforcement schedules have been demonstrated to be powerful activators of behavior (Rescorla, 1968). Thus, according to Hand (1986), the impulse to gamble as an escape from depression is an example of behavioral conditioning and does not depend on the cognitions of the individual. By contrast, Sharpe and Tarrier (1993) suggested that the mediator between mood state and gambling is coping strategy. Individuals with adaptive coping skills are able to use problem-focused strategies so that money is managed appropriately, and irrational thinking is challenged. In this way, the individual is better able to cope with the urges to gamble. Individuals with more emotion-focused coping strategies would be expected to be more vulnerable to the urge to gamble. This would be especially so for individuals who use avoidance-focused coping strategies where the existence or importance of negative feeling states is denied (Shepherd & Dickerson, 2001). A related explanation has been provided by Blaszczynski and Nower (2002) in their pathways theory of problem gambling. According to Blaszczynski and Nower (2002), there is an emotionally vulnerable subgroup of gamblers who gamble in order to regulate mood states. Thus, the gambling itself is viewed as a coping strategy.

How would gambling enable an individual to cope with negative mood states? There are at least two major views about the way in which gambling can regulate mood. First, the gambling can move an individual from one state of consciousness to another. Thus, for some individuals, gambling can be a relaxation following stress (movement from the "telic" state to the "paratelic" state), whereas for others it is a movement from boredom and loneliness to excitement (Brown, 1987b). Thus, the core idea here is that gambling modifies arousal in a way that is positively reinforcing (Anderson & Brown, 1984). An alternative view has been proposed by Jacobs (1987). According to Jacobs (1987), gambling enables individuals to gain an altered state of consciousness involving dissociation in which wishes are fulfilled. The primary motivation of pathological gamblers is to reach the refuge of the dissociated state of mind. Individuals who are gambling while in this dissociated state report being in a trance, losing a sense of reality, feeling numb, and having no memory of the events that occurred.

While there is little doubt that some individuals report aspects of dissociation while gambling, this account would appear to be more relevant to some forms of gambling than to others. In particular, becoming absorbed in play to the exclusion of all else and entering into imagined experiences has been reported primarily for electronic gaming machines. There does not appear to be comparable evidence involving dissociation as a major mechanism in problem levels of betting on horses, casino blackjack, or scratch lotteries.

Erroneous Beliefs About Gambling on Machines

Electronic gaming machines have a set return to the player. The random nature of the outcome of a game ensures that the return is an expected return in the long run. Thus, in Canada the expected return is 90 % to 95 % (depending on the Province) and, in Australia, 90 %. The expected return generates a number of erroneous beliefs. Players may believe that a given machine will return the set percentage of the money that they invest. Players may also believe that in the long run, the game return percentage also holds true across sessions and days. In fact, the average return to the player from any given machine is 60 % to 70 % and the average return for sessions of play may be as low as 40 %. The reason for these lower return rates is the reinvestment of winnings by the player. In the extreme case, provided that the individual plays for a sufficiently long time on a machine, the return to the player will be zero. However, players frequently cash out before all of their money is lost. Most commonly, players proceed to another machine, which explains why session returns (across multiple machines) are lower than single machine returns, in general.

Despite the random nature of machine payouts, players typically believe that various factors influence the likelihood that the machine will pay out (Toneatto et al., 1997). The cognitive error that is common to a range of erroneous beliefs is the failure to understand properly the meaning of randomness across independent events (Ladouceur, 1996; Ladouceur & Walker, 1996). A second major source of false beliefs is the failure to understand the meaning and implications of personal luck (Wagenaar, 1988). More than half of all machine gamblers will tell you that everyone has the same chance of winning on electronic gaming machines, yet they will also say that their chances of winning on a particular machine depend on how recently someone else won on that machine. This is known as the gambler's fallacy and believing that the chances of winning in the future are dependent on how many have won on that machine in the recent past is the most common misconception held by machine gamblers. Other commonly held misconceptions are that the chances of winning are influenced by the size of the bet, the type of machine or game they are playing, the time of day or day of week, and skill of the gambler in pressing the buttons (Schellink & Schrans, 1998).

Problem gamblers are more likely to hold these beliefs than other regular gamblers. In particular, they are much more likely to believe that machines in certain locations within the venue or their favorite/lucky machines are likely to win, that the specific make/manufacturer of the machine influences the chances of winning, and that the time of day and the size of the bet influence winning (Schellink & Schrans, 1998). They are also more likely than regular gamblers to believe that after a string of losses they are more likely to win. This conviction that a win is imminent grows stronger for problem gamblers as the string of losses lengthens, whereas for regular, nonproblematic gamblers it weakens (Ladouceur, 2004). Problem gamblers are not only more optimistic about winning despite cumulative losses, but they also begin each session with the belief that they are likely to win.

Relatively few of the erroneous beliefs of players have observable manifestations. Nevertheless, some players hold coins and lucky talismans while they play. Others play only certain machines, under special conditions (such as having the reserve light on), and in stylized ways that are believed to influence the outcome. Some players speak to their machines, sometimes encouragingly, sometimes pleadingly, and sometimes angrily. The false beliefs that certain actions will predispose fate toward good luck are called superstitions (Windross, 2003). Their superstitions appear to influence play very strongly. When individuals are prevented from using their superstitious practices while they play, session length and number of games played are decreased by 50 % (Walker, 1992).

Explaining Erroneous Thinking by Reference to Machine Characteristics

It is interesting and relevant to understand why and how erroneous beliefs form and persist in gamblers. Rosecrance (1985) pointed out that superstitious beliefs develop as a means of coping with uncertainty. To the extent that magical thinking and practices enable people to believe that they have some control over fate, so they reduce anxiety and facilitate an optimistic view. Lotto numbers in the range 1 to 30 are more popular than other numbers, presumably because of the good luck associated with birthdays. In Australia, horses with names containing an "r" as the third letter are commonly believed to be more likely to win races than horses with other names (Windross, 2003). The reason for this belief may be related to the fact that several of the earliest Melbourne Cups were won by horses with appropriate "r" names such as "Carbine." In the case of erroneous beliefs about electronic gaming machines, the false beliefs may be based on how the machines actually work, for although each spin may in fact be independent and random, how they are designed can often lead the gambler to believe this is not true.

One of the most common erroneous beliefs of gaming machine players is the efficacy of machine testing (Walker, 2001). Players commonly believe that machines have playing states. Some machines are seen as being in a winning state, and are more likely to make a big payout. Other machines are seen as "cold" or "hungry." The erroneous belief is that a small number of plays will provide a reading of the playing state of the machine. Thus, an advantage can be gained by playing a large number of machines for a small number of games on each, and then persevering with a machine that is in a winning state (as evidenced by a payout). Since machines are engineered so that the notion of playing states is untenable, it is interesting to examine what factors of machine structure facilitate such a belief. At least two machine characteristics have been investigated: prize structure and near misses.

Prize Structure

Most plays result in gamblers wagering their money and winning nothing. How often they win and how much they win depends on the odds and payout structure of the games. There can be anywhere from ten to thirty possible payout levels, each with its own probability of occurring during a play. The chances of winning the small prizes are much greater than of winning big prizes. Machines that have a very large top prize in comparison to the amount wagered must have a correspondingly low probability of that prize being won so that the total payout remains at some preset rate (often about 90%). For example, the probability of winning the top prize in many Australian machines is one in a million plays. The frequent small wins constantly strengthen the belief of the gambler that a big win is imminent. At the beginning of a session, the amount that can be lost is restricted by how much is bet on each game played. For example, if betting $0.50 a spin, 12 spins a minute, the most that can be lost in an hour is 720 spins * $.50 = $360.00. However, the amount that could have been won in that hour is much higher as each of those 720 spins could have won a big prize. This means that early in sessions, given the highly variable nature of the wins and losses, gamblers will quite often find themselves ahead in their games at some point. Thus, even though the trend is toward loss, there is a good chance of being in a "winning" situation near the beginning of a session. It is estimated that the player is winning more than invested at some point in the first hour in approximately 70% of sessions (Walker & Schellink, 2003). This is simply a fact that follows from the skewed payout structure of games. However, the experience of being ahead in the game at some near the beginning of the session has the potential to create the impression among players that they can choose a machine that will pay well and that they can thereby beat the machine. Players frequently lament not having quit while they were ahead.

Near Misses

The symbols that bring big wins (pyramids, swinging bells, etc.) are made to be much more easily recognizable to gamblers than the other symbols, and gamblers watch for them to appear on the screen. One of the most popular games in Australia provides a bonus of 15 free games when three or more pyramids appear on the screen. The pyramid symbol is distinctive in shape and color and pulses, unlike other symbols. Two scattered pyramids constitutes a "near miss" and is regarded as such. The ability of players to recognize near misses has been associated with perseverance in play (Reid, 1985; Strickland & Grote, 1967). These near misses heighten gamblers' beliefs they can win and their feeling that a win will occur soon. The fact that players are frequently ahead early in a game, and that near misses are frequent and easily identified, would be expected to contribute to the erroneous belief that playing states are real and that they can be detected.

The Gambling Life Cycle of Machine Players

From the literature, it may sometimes seem that playing electronic gaming machines is a monotonic descent into excessive gambling: the more you play, the more you lose, and the greater the consequent problems. Certainly, the extreme levels of pathological and compulsive gambling have been characterized this way (Custer & Milt, 1985; Lesieur, 1979). This emphasis on the development of gambling problems distracts attention from the fact that many regular and problem gamblers not only reach levels of excessive involvement but also return from those levels. The fact that pathological gamblers recover from the problem presents problems for assessment and measurement of the prevalence of the phenomenon (Walker & Dickerson, 1996). Research in the area of drug addiction has shown that natural recovery occurs for both alcoholism (Cunningham, Sobell, & Sobell, 1998) and for smoking (DiClemente, Prochaska et al., 1991). DiClemente and Prochaska (1998) point out that for most addictive populations, only approximately 25 % of those exhibiting the problem behaviors (DSM-IV disorders) enter professional therapy programs. Similar results have been found for problem gambling (Schellinck & Schrans, 2002), where only 19 % of electronic gaming machine problem gamblers (both those who had ceased gambling and those who continue) had ever contacted or used formal services in helping them overcome their problem gambling. Of those who claimed to have resolved their problem, 75 % had never contacted a formal service to seek assistance in overcoming their problem.

All individuals begin their lives as non-gamblers, but only a minority (approximately 10 %) in modern Western countries of any population do not gamble in any way throughout their lives (Productivity Commission, 1999). Most people gamble at one stage or another. The form of gambling that is tried depends on a range of factors, social and economic, of which one of the more important is accessibility. Electronic gaming machines are readily available to the adult population in most Western countries (Dickerson, 1996). The majority of those who try the machines do not develop an interest in playing the games. These players may play occasionally but do adopt a regular or frequent pattern of gambling on the machines (Walker, 1992).

Of people who try out the machines, only one in four goes on to become a frequent player (several times a month or more) (Schellink & Schrans, 1998). About half of those who become frequent players adopt regular play immediately, while a further 20 % do so within the next 2 months, and 30 % adopt regular play over a longer term. In Australia, about 15 % of adults gamble on the machines at least once a month while in Canada the figure is lower, at approximately 6 %. Some gamblers gamble regularly for a year or so, while others gamble regularly or sporadically on and off for up to 20 years. The average number of years that a machine gambler plays regularly, excluding those who develop problem gambling, is approximately 2 1/2 years (Schellink & Schrans, 2002). Those who develop into problem gamblers continue to gamble regularly for approximately 4 1/2 years. During this time, their gambling is more continuous and frequent in nature.

Since those who gamble regularly on average do so only from 2 1/2 to 5 years on average, there are many machine gamblers who are now past regular gamblers. When non-problem gamblers are asked why they stopped gambling, roughly half say they made a conscious decision to stop, usually because they felt they were wasting too much money on the games. For others, it is a combination of new interests and finding the games boring, the machines becoming less accessible to them, some personal event happening in their lives, or lifestyle changes such that it became less convenient to gamble regularly (for example, they stopped frequenting bars or pubs and so they stopped gambling on the machines). The majority of regular players are introduced to the games, play them frequently, either on a continuous or sporadic basis, over several years, and then, whether they decide to stop or something changes in their lives, they spend their time doing something else. Many of these regular gamblers realize the potential for problem gambling, or just spending too much, and adapt their gambling behavior to control their spending. If they decide they are spending too much they cut back or stop before it becomes a problem.

The transition from regular play to excessive play typically happens quickly (Schellink & Schrans, 2002). On average, those who gamble excessively on gaming machines begin to do so in slightly more than a year. Over the next 4 to 5 years, and up to 15 years in some cases, the individual becomes increasingly aware of the problems being caused by the time and money being spent on gambling. Approximately 70 % of these gamblers decide to stop at some stage each year but fail to do so. About 25 % of problem gamblers may seek some kind of assistance from sources such as gambling counselors or Gamblers Anonymous during the time they are problem gamblers. Importantly, approximately 75 % of individuals who are gambling excessively, and suffering serious problems as a consequence, decide to cut back or stop their gambling without seeking professional assistance (Schellink & Schrans, 2002).

The importance of these results is that they enable problem gambling to be seen as related to and continuous with regular gambling. Further, the evidence is consistent with the proposition that "pathological" and "compulsive" gambling are simply extreme examples of excessive gambling behavior. Nevertheless, the available evidence is not sufficient to rule out the possibility that within the segment of the population that gambles excessively on gaming machines, there are subgroups that for psychological or biological reasons are more vulnerable to the attractions of machine gambling, to the point where medical intervention is necessary (Blaszczynski & Nower, 2002).

Explaining Why People Gamble

The evidence available suggests that the desire to win money (or item of value) is the core motivation of the gambler. Although such a claim may seem to be a tautology, it is not. This becomes clear when it is realized that competing claims for the role of core motivation include excitement and diversion. According to such views, the monetary aspect of gambling is secondary. However, the evidence that winning money is central to understanding the gambling phenomenon is compelling. Popular gambling did not arise until monetary denominations were invented. Gambling is more popular in societies that stress materialism and individualism. The larger the prize, the more attractive is the gamble as judged by the amount individuals are willing to pay to take part. Gambling is heavier within sectors of society that are less wealthy. Thus, while people may gamble for amusement, for excitement, for escape, for company, or for induced states of altered consciousness, the common denominator is the desire and hope of winning money.

Given that the desire to win money is the central motivation, there remains the question of why a majority of people in many Western countries attempt to win money in an endeavor that is set up so that they will lose money. Gambling is a bad investment, so why is it so popular? Part of the answer lies in the ability of some gambling prizes to transform the life of the winner. A lottery ticket may be a very poor investment, but from where else can the average person in the street hope to obtain such a sum of money? However, not all forms of gambling offer such an attraction. Much lower prizes may be attractive because the games offer an element of skill. Every regular punter may believe that he or she can pick winning horses better than the average punter. Blackjack players may believe that their skills are sufficient to beat the bank. Most of all, every person who makes a bet may think that he or she will be lucky.

Despite these arguments, the most important aspect of gambling that remains to be explained is why some people become regular gamblers, persisting with gambling even to the point where the loss of money begins to cause problems elsewhere in their lives. Since all legal gambling is constructed to take money from the public, persevering with the activity increases the likelihood of loss until it approaches certainty. If it is assumed that the individuals who gamble are rational human beings, why do they not they stop once it becomes clear that the venture is failing? There are three important answers to this question. First, many individuals hold mistaken impressions about the likelihood that they will win. Second, the short-term losses of gamblers are often offset by large wins. Finally, problem gamblers do stop gambling; even pathological gambling has a life cycle. There is considerable evidence that gamblers hold a range of mistaken beliefs about their preferred form of gambling. Perhaps the most important of these is a form of the gambler's fallacy: that the worse the run of luck, the more certain you can be that a change in luck is near. Further, often luck does change, as the random or unpredictable nature of outcomes should lead us to expect. Thus, persistent gambling is incorrectly perceived as a descent into debt. Rather, it is a trend into debt interspersed with relatively large wins. It is likely that these occasional wins strengthen the erroneous beliefs that the gambler already holds about the activity. Nevertheless, gambling may continue to a point at which the monetary loss is beyond recovery and the accumulated debts decrease the well-being of the individual. At any point, one might ask why such an individual does not stop. The answer lies in the fact that no matter how large the debt, a large win will improve matters. A large win will mean that the most insistent creditors can be paid. Such optimism will be destroyed eventually. Approximately 75 % of problem gamblers cease gambling at excessive levels without professional help. Among those who seek help, perhaps the most difficult step has already been taken. In seeking help, the individual confesses to knowing that the game is up.

Is there a group of gamblers for whom this kind explanation fails? The consensus view is that this kind of cognitive explanation does not account for all pathological gamblers. Alternative views stress that there is a minority of individuals for whom upbringing and biology conspire to create a vulnerability to gambling that is impossible for the individual to manage. Whether or not this is true is essentially an empirical question.

Chapter 3
Games, Gambling, and Gambling Problems

Nigel E. Turner

> *It is said that the Goddess of Fortune, once sporting near the shady pool of Olympus, was met by the gay and captivating God of War, who soon allured her to his arms ... the result of the union was a misfeatured child named Gaming. From the moment of her birth this wayward thing could only be pleased by cards, dice, or counters ... As she grew up she was courted by all the gay and extravagant of both sexes, for she was of neither sex, and yet combining the attractions of each. At length ... she ... gave birth to twins—one called DUELLING, and the other a grim and hideous monster named SUICIDE.*
>
> *The Goddess Fortune ever had an eye on her promising daughter— Gaming; and endowed her with splendid residences, in the most conspicuous streets, near the palaces of kings. They were magnificently designed and elegantly furnished. Lamps, always burning at the portals, were a sign and a perpetual invitation unto all to enter.*
>
> *Steinmetz, 1870*

In this chapter I summarize my own insights into the nature of gambling and random chance, taking into account my research, simulations of games, interviews with gamblers, and my own experience in each of these games. I begin by placing gambling in its social, economic, mathematical and intellectual context and then focus on the major types of gambling games that people play. I end with a detailed examination of random chance and the house edge.

Gambling is a very exciting waste of money. I am a recreational gambler, but occasionally ask myself why I enjoy this utter waste of money. Oddly enough, I was a non-gambler until 1997 and therefore have a very good memory of my first adult gambling experience— winning $80 playing roulette. I have some ambivalence about the hobby. I know too much about most of the games to really enjoy them. I love the sound of a roulette ball rolling around the wheel and enjoy the anticipation of the potential win, but my mind too easily works out the expected loss on each spin and I end up questioning the wisdom of another bet. I prefer games that involve an element of skill because I can fool myself into believing that I can win in the long run. I use the phrase "fool myself" because in truth I have not acquired the necessary skills to do so. I know enough about card games, cards skills, and the mathematical

Nigel E. Turner
Centre for Addiction and Mental Health, Canada

M. Zangeneh, A. Blaszczynski, N. Turner (eds.), *In the Pursuit of Winning.*
© Springer 2008

theories behind strategies such that I could beat the house edge. However, I lack the motivation to perfect these skills. In short, I am too lazy to win consistently at the poker or blackjack table.

Gambling serves no truly useful function in society other than giving people something to do together. However, the same could be said about music, parties, the arts, sports, drinking alcohol, or anything else we do to momentarily forget our mortality. I do believe there are psychologically healthy aspects of gambling. Studies have shown that elderly adults who play bingo are mentally and physically healthier than elderly adults who do not (Desai, Maciejewski, Dausey, Caldarone, & Potenza, 2004). But this must be weighed against the incredible harm that results when a person becomes addicted to gambling. Even in the context of the article by Desai et al. (2004), it is unknown if gambling *caused* people to be healthier or being healthy merely *allowed* people to get out to the bingo hall or casino. I believe that bingo in particular involves considerable cognitive exercise that would likely be beneficial to the mental health of non-problem players. Card games may also provide some benefit, but I doubt that slot machines and other electronic games of chance would provide much cognitive exercise. Nonetheless, getting out and enjoying oneself may in itself be healthy. However, it is very likely that people could get those same health benefits via activities other than bingo (e.g., playing bridge, lawn bowling, shuffle board, or other non-gambling games). Non-problem gamblers are in general psychologically healthy people, and this group can tell us much about the nature of problem gambling and about healthy living in general.

Why do people gamble? This is a complex question. For many people, gambling is fun, exciting, or thrilling. It can provide a person with a dream of untold wealth. Anyone can dream, but the dream you buy when gambling is strong because it is actually possible (though very unlikely). In addition, gambling can provide people with a way of proving their worth compared to other people (e.g., bragging rights of winning a poker game or pool contest).For men this effect of gambling touches upon very basic instinctual desires to out-compete other men.

Gambling provides us with a delimited form of risk taking in which the possible consequences are known and relatively safe: win, lose, or break even. In contrast, the possible consequences of climbing a mountain are much more open-ended. One could succeed and successfully reach the top of the mountain. However, other possibilities include falling off the mountain, losing one's climbing buddies in a crevasse, freezing to death, or making the cover of next month's *National Geographic* magazine. Ignoring the risk of addiction, gambling itself is a relatively harmless activity. However, there is always the potential that an individual may develop a severe dependence on gambling. Gambling addition can lead to financial loss, problems with relationships, lost job opportunities, depression, and even suicide. For people who do develop a severe gambling problem, mountain climbing would probably have been a safer activity.

Most often gambling makes sense only if it is viewed as a hobby or entertainment. This is not to say that gambling is just harmless entertainment, but it is entertainment nonetheless. I suspect that part of the thrill of gambling is the potential for loss. Just as standing on the precipice of a mountain cliff is more exciting than seeing it from a safe distance, risking everything at the gaming table is part of the thrill of gambling. With the exception of a small number of professional gamblers (e.g., some poker players, computer-based horse or sports bettors, card counters) gambling for money is a poor financial choice. According to the annual report highlight listed on Ontario Lottery Gaming (2006) Web site, in 2004–2005 18 million customers spent $1.6 billion at Ontario's four resort casinos. That translates into an average spending of $89 per visit. This is more expensive than renting a movie, or going bowling, but cheaper than a night at the opera or a weekend trip to Trinidad. Unique to gambling is the ever-present (though extremely unlikely) possibility that the player could come home rich. This is something that is not likely to happen at the movie theatre, bowling alley, opera house, or Trinidadian beach. An integral part of the thrill of gambling is the dream of the big win. The problem with gambling as entertainment, however, is that much of the entertainment inherent in gambling comes from ignoring the odds against winning. What is more interesting is that the gambling industry goes out of its way to ensure that everyone knows that they are making a great deal of money. Figures 3.1 and 3.2 illustrate the incredible show of wealth that has been a part of the gambling industry for at least 200 years (see Asbury, 1938 for a discussion of the splendid hells of previous generations). Far from discouraging play, this display of wealth attracts more customers to the glamour and bright lights.

Without the potential for a win, gambling just would not be fun. Take away the money and most games of chance are really very boring games, for example, pressing the spin button on a slot with no chance of a prize. Even poker, arguably the most skill oriented of the commercially available forms of gambling, depends to a great extent on money to generate excitement. It is simply not possible to bluff someone out of a poker hand unless there is money at stake. In contrast, video games (e.g., *Age of Empires* and *Tomb Raiders*) and other non-gambling games

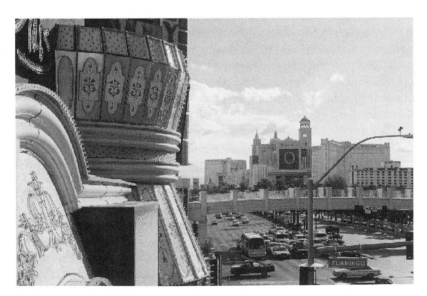

Fig. 3.1 Hotels crowding the skyline of Las Vegas

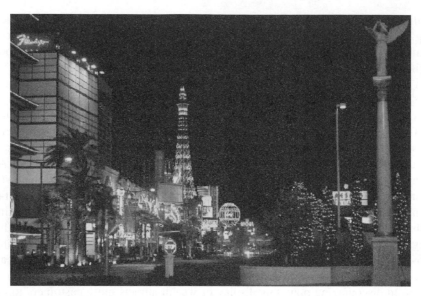

Fig. 3.2 Las Vegas at night

(e.g., chess, checkers, and lawn bowling) are designed to be inherently fun to play without the prospect of winning money. Certainly people can and do sometimes bet on games that involve skill (e.g., chess, bowling, golf, and video games), but games of skill are in general fun even without money riding on the outcome. In contrast, commercial gambling games are typically very simple games in which each bet is completed after only a few seconds. Contrast this with non-gambling games such as Monopoly, chess, and video games, which can take several hours to complete. There are exceptions, however; people do make private bets on games such as gin, backgammon, pool, and bowling, and such bets may take several minutes to be resolved. However; most commercial gambling is based on extremely simple games. Even commercial sports bets are reduced to a simple numbers game such as Team X will win by 6 points over Team Y or Team X will win and the total score will be under 40.

Gambling venues as entertainment are predicated on their ability to draw in people for the fun and excitement of winning, even though at the end of the day, the player is more likely to be the loser than to be the winner. Casinos could not exist without a house advantage of some sort. Therefore, the entertainment value is intrinsically tied to players' erroneous beliefs about their ability to win. Erroneous beliefs are more common among people who suffer from a gambling disorder; however, most people (including myself) will display some flaws in their reasoning when it comes to random chance. Over the past few years, I have conducted numerous studies on gambling in various populations. One of the main topics that interest me is the extent to which a misunderstanding of random chance can explain problematic and pathological gambling. To measure this concept, I developed a test called the Random Events Knowledge Test. In every study that I have conducted, I have found a small negative correlation between erroneous beliefs and the severity of problematic gambling. Non-problem gamblers typically answer between 70 % and 75 % of the questions correctly, while pathological gamblers typically answer between 60 % and 65 % of the questions correctly (Turner & Liu, 1999; Turner et al., 2006b). I view the lower scores of the pathological gamblers as an issue of knowledge, rather than as a measure of intelligence or distorted thinking. People are not really taught about the true nature of random events. Non-problem gamblers score higher than pathological gamblers, but still answer a substantial portion of the questions incorrectly.

Why Society Encourages Gambling

Although faulty reasoning in the mind of the individual gambler may explain some aspects of problematic gambling, gambling is not just an individual activity. In the past 20 years, broad sweeping changes have occurred in the legal status of gambling in countries around the world. In Canada, most forms of gambling were illegal until recently. Over the past 10 years in Canada, provincial governments have played an active role in promoting the construction of new gambling venues. Similarly, in the United States new casino ventures are often the result of a negotiation between the gaming industry and politicians or among the gaming industry, politicians, and a native band. Governments around the world are becoming dependent on gambling revenue.

Throughout history, governments have alternated between encouraging gambling and prohibiting gambling (see Asbury, 1938; Rose, 2003; Skolnick, 2003). Some citics tried to stamp out gambling (New York, 1902), but others cities used gambling to raise money to build public institutions (e.g., Yale University). Several cities, including Macau, Monte-Carlo, Las Vegas, Baden Baden, and Atlantic City, have relied on gambling proceeds for a substantial portion of their economic wealth. In countries where gambling is illegal, organized criminals will step in and satisfy the citizens' apparent need to gamble (Asbury, 1938; de Champlain, 2004). Interestingly, 120 years ago, card games such as faro were available in local bars across much of North America. These gambling dens generated a very strong anti-gambling sentiment in the general public that led to riots in the 1830s (Asbury, 1938; Turner, Howard, & Spence, 2006a) and in the 1890s to the election of politicians who promised to get rid of the gambling. A good case study is New York City from 1890 to 1902. In the 19th century, gambling was officially illegal; however, for years casinos operated openly with payoffs to the local police and the "gambling commission" (e.g., $1000 per month for a large casino; Asbury, 1938). In the mid-1890s a reform-minded mayor was elected and the corruption was gradually cleaned up. William Travers Jerome became District Attorney from 1901 to 1909 for New York County and systematically harassed the gaming clubs until he was able to close them down. Jerome chased the rich casino barons such as Canfield out of New York City, but left a void that was later filled by the likes of Lucky Luciano and his cohorts (see de Champlain, 2004). It is apparent in these historical facts that a segment of

the general population wants to gamble and another segment of the population wants
to outlaw gambling. The relative power of these two segments of the population has
seesawed over the past 200 years.

In recent years, governments have found that the general public does not like
tax increases. To balance the books, they have turned to gambling to raise money.
Given a choice between legalizing gambling and a tax increase, people who want to
gamble will vote for gambling, and people who do not want to gamble will vote yes
so that other people will pay the (tax) bills. As evidence for this, a survey of attitudes toward gambling in Niagara Falls just before the opening of a casino (Turner,
Ialomiteanu, & Room, 1999) found approval of the casino was predicted by high
scores on positive attitude toward gambling, low scores on anticipated problems,
and perceived economic benefits.

In this context, gambling is often portrayed as a booster to jump-start the local
economy. There is no question that the Las Vegas economy has benefited from
gambling. Figures 3.1 and 3.2 indicate a city that is overflowing with wealth. Other
cities, jealous of the bright lights, want a piece of that action for their own communities. At least in some cases gambling casinos do provide economic benefits to
communities that permit their construction (see Eadington, 2003; Stitt, Nichols &
Giacopassi, 2003; see Grinols, 2003 for a contrasting view).

In 1993, the Ontario government permitted the opening of a casino in Windsor.
In 1996, the government permitted the opening of a casino in Orillia and another
in Niagara Falls. Surveys conducted before and after the casino opened indicated
that the majority of the residents were in support of the casino (Room et al., 1999;
Turner, Ialomiteanu, & Room, 1999). I examined the Statistic Canada records of
cross border travel near Windsor and Niagara Falls between 1993 and 2002. In both
communities, there was a remarkable increase in the number of people crossing the
border into Canada after the opening of the casinos (see Figure 3.3). It is unknown to
what extent this increase was due to the casinos themselves, the improved economies
of both countries, and the lower Canadian dollar. However, it seems reasonable to
attribute at least some of the cross-border traffic to the opening of the casino. Ontario
Lottery and Gaming is proud of its achievements in stimulating the economies of
these two cities. For example, they report at the Ontario Lottery and Gaming (2006)
Web site that they have created 29,500 direct and indirect jobs and have generated $23 billion in gaming proceeds since 1975 for worthwhile causes throughout
Ontario.

The city of Niagara Falls once attracted tourists from around the world, and was
one of the most popular destinations in the world for a honeymoon vacation. By
the 1980s it had degenerated into the status of a cheap honeymoon, and by 1993,
its economy was in ruins and the unemployment rate was around 16 %. Politicians
scrambling for a quick fix to the city's problems held a referendum to determine
support for opening a casino. The casino was supported by a 1995 referendum and
Casino Niagara was opened in late 1996. Today the economy of Niagara is doing
very well. Some of this success is very likely a direct result of the casino. When
one compares the unemployment rate in 1993 with the rate in 1997 (see Figure 3.4),
there is a huge improvement. However, the improvement actually occurred before
the casino was even opened, perhaps in anticipation of the casino. Further, the

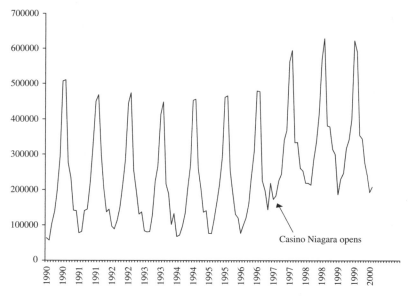

Fig. 3.3 Number of US residents entering Canada by the Rainbow Bridge before and after the casino opened

unemployment rate actually increased slightly immediately after the opening of the casino (perhaps because of the end of construction work associated with building the casino). Figure 3.4 also includes the unemployment rate from a number of other cities in Ontario to show how the unemployment rate in Niagara Falls was quite similar to the unemployment rate[1] in other communities around Ontario during the same time period. However, it is impossible to determine if the unemployment rate in Niagara Falls would have fallen if the casino had not been opened. Another factor is the value of the Canadian dollar. Niagara falls is on the border with the United States, and as such, a fall in the value of the Canadian dollar would result in a boost to the economy of Niagara as products such as gasoline, clothing, and furniture became less expensive relative to similar products available in the United States. The relationship between the value of the Canadian dollar and the unemployment rate is shown in Figure 3.5. As the dollar fell, after a lag of 4 or 5 months, the unemployment rate in Niagara also fell. Part of the reason for this association is that the lower Canadian dollar provided an opportunity for Americans to save money by shopping in Canada and increasing the market for exports from Canada. However, more recently there was also a remarkable construction boom in Niagara Falls, Ontario, much of which was due to the construction of an even larger permanent casino. To the residents of Niagara, the essential facts are that before the casino was built, the economy of Niagara Falls was very depressed. Today, the economy is doing very well. Thus on balance the casino appears to be good for the city.

---

[1] Tables showing the unemployment rate, construction permits, and cross border travel can be downloaded from the Statistics Canada Web site for a small fee.

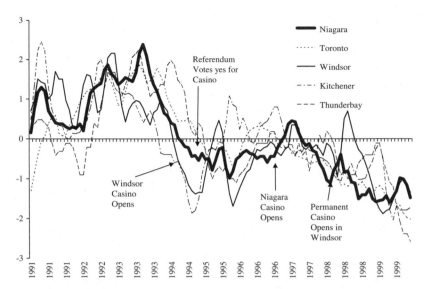

Fig. 3.4 Unemployment rates relatively to average for each community (in z-scores) from 1991 to 1999

However, according to Grinols (2003), all this is irrelevant. He argues that the only economic benefit of gambling is the value of gambling to the people who live in a community: jobs, revenue from gambling, tourist spending, and so on are irrelevant. The only real benefit in opening a casino is that gambling becomes more

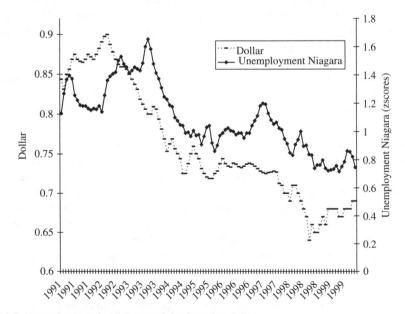

Fig. 3.5 Unemployment in Niagara and the Canadian dollar

convenient to non-problem gamblers in that community. When this convenience is weighed against the increases in crime and problem gambling, gambling turns out to be a bad choice economically (Grinols, 2003). Interestingly, Eadington (2003) makes the opposite case, that destination casinos marketed to tourists are the most beneficial to a community (e.g., Niagara Falls, Las Vegas), whereas convenience gambling marketed to local residents (e.g., electronic gambling machines in bars or convenience stores) tends to be associated with the highest rates of problematic gambling.

Room, Turner, and Ialomiteanu (1999) found a statistically significant increase in problematic gambling behavior after the introduction of the Niagara casino. Similarly, Shaffer, Hall, and Vander Bilt (1999) have shown that as the availability of gambling opportunities have increased across North America, the rates of problematic gambling have also increased. Further, employment might improve locally, but this provides local jobs; it does not provide any overall benefit to the country. According to Grinols (2003), when gambling is viewed from a national or international perspective the net economic impact of gambling is negative.

A Brief History of Gambling

Gambling has been around for thousands of years. Steinmetz (1870) argued that gambling is a universal characteristic of people all over the world. Random events are unpredictable and mysterious. Historically, games of chance were often associated with religious rituals to divine the will of the gods (Gabriel, 2003). Dice are perhaps the oldest know gambling device (Grunfeld, Zangeneh, & Diakoloukas; see chapter 9, this volume). Originally people used sheep knucklebones as dice to make bets; today dice are still often called "bones." Later during the Roman era, betting on chariot races or lotteries became popular (Steinmetz, 1870). Gaming houses of some form have appeared in numerous countries around the world. According to the *Oxford English Dictionary*,[2] our current word casino is derived from the Italian word *casini,* which means little house. In the early 1700s, casini were popular places in Italy for rich merchants to meet, trade, and gamble. By the mid-1800s, casinos could be found in numerous cities around Europe. Crucial to the development of casino gambling was the invention of gambling games with a house edge that would provide the house with a steady profit. Roulette, faro, blackjack, baccarat, and craps all date from this time period.

The game of faro is a particularly interesting case, in part owing to its extraordinary success for about 300 years and because of its subsequent extinction (Turner et al., 2006a). In faro, one of the oldest known games, the players are pitted against a bank run by the casino rather than against each other. According to Asbury (1938), the roots of faro can be traced back to the Middle Ages. It attained its modern form at the court of King Louis XIV of France (Asbury, 1938); however, additional rules

---

[2] Downloaded February 21, 2007 from http://www.askoxford.com/concise_oed/casino?view=uk.

continued to evolve throughout the 19th century. According to Arnold (2000), it was the most popular game in America in the last half of the 19th century. Faro dealers often traveled with their gaming equipment from town to town, setting up their faro banks and often risking their personal fortunes in a private home, saloon, or on a riverboat. Despite its long history, in modern times even references to the game of faro have all but disappeared. For example, books, Western films, and popular Western TV shows of the 1970s all disregarded faro in favor of poker (Turner et al., 2006a). Today, it is essentially an extinct game of chance. The game died in the United States during the early part of the 20th century as the temperance movements achieved increasing political power that eventually culminated in the National Prohibition Act of 1919 banning the possession of alcohol. However, unlike blackjack, lotteries, poker, craps, slot machines, and roulette, which gradually all re-emerged from the underground, faro died.

The death of faro is rather interesting from a number of perspectives. Exactly why it died is not clear. Epstein (1976) attributes the game's demise to the small house edge if the game is played optimally. Turner et al. (2006a) determined that the game yields a house profit of from 1.0% to 2.9 % depending on the type of bet the player makes and 13.9% for a call of the turn. However, a unique feature of faro is that it can be played with no house edge at all. Today, blackjack could also be unprofitable if most players played in an optimal manner (e.g., basic strategy plus card counting), but very few people play blackjack in an optimal manner (Wagenaar, 1988). Beating blackjack is a complicated process of counting the relative number of high and low cards and increasing one bet when the remaining deck has more high cards than low cards. With faro, optimal players merely need to be selective about their bets and bet only on "case cards" (when only one card of a particular rank is left in the deck). If we accept the idea that faro died because of optimal play, then we are faced with a puzzle: why did so many casinos and other gambling venues offer the game for such a long period of time (see Asbury, 1938)? In addition, in the 1890s, Canfield's was famous for claiming to run honest casinos, and yet his casinos were apparently very profitable (see Asbury, 1938). Perhaps, like in blackjack, today few players played in an optimal manner so that the game was still profitable. It should also be noted that there were rule variations such as Hockelty that would guarantee a profit for the house. With Hockelty, from which we get the phrase "in hoc," all bets were required to remain on the board until resolved and any bet on the very last card (known as hoc) was claimed by the dealer (see Turner et al., 2006a). Turner et al. (2006a) determined that with hockelty and optimal play, the player would face a house edge of 1.75% per resolved bet. This existence of rules that guarantee a house edge means that the extinction of the game cannot be attributed simply to optimal play.

Another possibility is the reputation of the game as a cheater game. Because the cards never left the hands of the dealer, the dealer most often did the cheating. According to Asbury (1938) and every other source we have looked at, faro games were most often run dishonestly. In support of the cheater game hypothesis another game also died at the same time—bunco. Bunco was a game played with cards or dice. It was so often used as a cheater's game that is it became synonymous with fraud, and today the police unit assigned to investigate fraud is sometimes known as the bunco squad. The idea that gamblers are cheats was one of the negative stereotypes of gambling, used by 19th century reformers to garner popular support for the prohibition of gambling (Asbury, 1938; Flavin, 2003). However, cheating in itself is not sufficient to explain the demise of faro. Poker was also a cheater's game (see Twain, 2004 for a vivid description of the 19th century poker scene); however, today poker is more popular than ever. It is likely that a combination of factors led to the death of faro including the reputation of the game, the problem of keeping the game profitable when players played it optimally, and the suppression of gambling during prohibition.

Games People Play

One does not need to know how to play a gambling game in order to understand disordered gambling; however, having some knowledge of the games the clients are playing may provide some insight into the gambler's motives for gambling. Most gambling games fall into one of four categories based on the role probability plays in the outcome: games of pure chance, games of both skill and luck, games of true skill, and games of subjective probability.

The author's knowledge of these games comes from reading books (see Turner, Fritz, & Mackenzie, 2003), attending conference presentations about game strategies (e.g., 13th International Conference on Gambling and Risk-Taking), conducting simulations (see Turner & Fritz, 2001), and playing the games himself. For more information about specific games, I recommend Ortiz's *On Casino Gambling* (1986), Wong and Spector's *The Complete Idiot's Guide to Gambling Like a Pro* (1996), Reber's *The New Gambler's Bible* (1996), and Harroch, Krieger, and Reber's *Gambling for Dummies* (2001). They each give detailed accounts of the rules and attempt to correct some of the common errors that people make regarding gambling.

Games of Pure Chance

In games of pure chance, the underlying events on which gamblers bet are both random and independent, and the player has no real opportunity to make a profit in the long term. The outcome of the game depends entirely on the results of a random number generator such as dice, bingo balls, or a slot machine. Examples of games of pure chance include lotteries, keno, bingo, slot machines, roulette, craps, and baccarat.

Lotteries and other similar numbers games are the most popular form of gambling (Room et al., 1997; Turner et al., 2006b). Lotteries appear to be less problematic than some other forms of gambling. However, they often represent the first type of commercial gambling that people have access too. The basic premise is straightforward: the player buys a ticket and wins if the numbers on the ticket match the numbers that are drawn. In most lotteries, players can win smaller prizes by matching only some of the numbers drawn. The chances of winning a lottery can usually be determined precisely by computing the number of unique combination of the numbers that are possible. The math for this computation is often beyond the skill of the individual player; however, many lotteries are required by law to publish the player's chance of winning.

In some lotteries, the top prize changes with each draw. If no one wins, the prize money is rolled over so that the prize on the next draw is larger. With the Lotto 6/49 prize offered in Ontario, for example, if the potential prize for a $2 ticket is greater than $28 million, the expected return is positive and long-term profit is theoretically possible. However, because these lotteries usually allow more than one person to buy the same ticket number, there is a chance that the prize will have to be split between multiple winners. The larger the prize, the more tickets are sold and the greater the chance that the prize will be split. As a result, even when the prize exceeds the odds against winning it, the players may still be playing against a negative expected return.

Keno is a type of lottery in which a player buys tickets made up of between 1 and 15 numbers chosen from a total of 80 numbers. That is, a player's ticket might consist of 3, 4, or even 15 numbers. Twenty numbers are drawn randomly from either ball cages or a computer generator. The player wins if some of his or her numbers are drawn. The more of a player's numbers that are drawn, the higher the prize. The more numbers the player bets on, the more numbers he or she must match in order to win a prize. A player who bets on only one number triples his or her money if it is drawn. But if a player selects 6 numbers, matching 1 number pays nothing. Matching 15 numbers pays a very large prize.

A wide variety of games are now sold as instant lotteries. In general, the player matches three symbols or prize values by scratching off a removable plastic coating. Nevada tickets, pull tabs, and break-open tickets are essentially the same as instant lottery tickets, but the symbols are hidden by a cardboard flap and the symbols are similar to slot machine symbols (e.g., lemons and cherries). Other instant lotteries are based on bingo, keno, or crossword puzzles. With instant lotteries, the win is determined when the ticket is made. Computers in the factory where the tickets are printed determine if the ticket will be a winner or not.

Bingo is a numbers game; however, winning is related to numbers and their location on the card. The game involves matching randomly drawn numbers to numbers printed on a card in a 5 × 5 grid. Typically, prizes are awarded for the first person to complete a line (five numbers in a row horizontally, vertically, or diagonally), two lines, or the entire card. Players stamp or cover the matching numbers on their card(s) until the matched numbers form the required pattern. The player who completes the pattern yells "Bingo!" to claim the prize. A "runner" verifies the bingo win by calling out the serial code of the card to ensure that the win is legitimate. If two people win at the same time, the prize is split. A typical bingo session might consist of 10 games. Bingo is a social game, but the socialization takes place between games. Winning at bingo is purely a matter of luck, but playing multiple cards simultaneously requires well-developed memory and attention skills, which likely generates a strong illusion of skill. Keeping up with the caller is quite challenging, and the cognitive exercise of playing multiple cards may even be beneficial to some players. The sight of elderly ladies successfully playing 16 or more cards while I had difficulty monitoring 6 cards was quite a humbling experience. However, multiple cards do not enable a person to overcome the house edge; the chance of winning is increased, but cost is also increased. Games with progressive (growing) jackpots and networked games with super jackpots are now available; however, the players' odds of winning in these games are lower. Another recent innovation is the introduction of electronic bingo that automatically fills in the numbers that are called, thus eliminating any cognitive benefit of playing the game.

Slot Machines, Video Lottery Terminals, and Electronic Gambling Machines

The following is a brief introduction to the nature of slot machines. For a more comprehensive discussion of slots, see Turner and Horbay (2004). The basic game of a slot machine involves setting three or more reels into motion by pressing a "spin" button, a spin icon on a computer screen or, on older machines, pulling a lever. When the reels stop spinning, if matching symbols from all three line up on a payline, the player wins. Some machines have five reels or multiple paylines. Common symbols include lemons, cherries, lucky sevens, and diamonds. The amount of the win varies depending on the rarity of the symbol. A slot machine can have either actual physical reels or a video display. The game play is essentially the same on either reel or video slots; however, the video display allows the programmer to incorporate a much greater variety of gambling experiences (e.g., bonus features) into the game than is possible with physical reels.

A video lottery terminal (VLT) technically is a gambling machine that is run as a remote terminal by a lottery corporation, and is located outside a casino (typically in a bar, restaurant, or other venue). It is called a terminal because the random numbers are often generated by a central system, rather than within the machine itself. The central determination system allows such machines to be legally classed as lotteries rather than slots, but from the players' perspective this distinction is irrelevant. VLTs typically provide a variety of games, including simulated slot machine games, video poker, and blackjack; however, some casino video gambling machines now are also multigame platforms.

There are no real differences between a lineup slot game played on a traditional slot machine, a video slot machine, a VLT (North America), a pokie (Australia), or a fruit machine (Great Britain). What is important is the nature of the game (e.g., no skill vs. some skill) and the location of the game (e.g., casino vs. bar). There is no skill in slot play, but some electronic gambling machines also offer blackjack and video-poker games that do involve some degree of skill. It is important not to lump all electronic games into a single category because the game play of a slot game is quite different from the game play of a semiskilled game such as video poker. Both no skill (slots) and some skill (video poker) games are potentially addictive, but they appeal to different people. Semiskilled games are more action oriented because the player has to make choices that affect the outcome. Slot games may appeal more to the escape gambler. Semiskilled and nonskilled games may be associated with different erroneous beliefs. A slot player cannot influence the outcome of his or her game whatsoever. A video poker player can influence the outcome of the game, but the prizes are generally set so low that even with optimal play the player would still lose.

Because of bonuses and progressive jackpots, the payback percentage will vary and in some cases may even reach a positive expected return. In addition, apparently there are some video poker games in which a positive return can be obtained with expert play; however, these are restricted to the highly competitive Nevada market. Older fruit machines in England were required to meet their long-term payback targets within a short time frame. As such, these fruit machines were random without replacement and it was possible to make a profit by waiting until the machine was "due" to pay out. As a general rule, electronic gambling machine cannot be beaten.

When slot machines were first invented more than 100 years ago, they consisted of three flywheels that were set in motion by the pull of the lever. The force of the spin would, to some extent, determine how far the reels would turn. It was possible to manipulate the outcome by carefully controlling (or tampering with) the lever. Some players still believe that it is possible to win by controlling the lever. Modern slot machines are computers. The reels themselves only serve to tell the player if he or she has won or not; they do not determine if the play wins. A random number generator (RNG) determines the wins and losses on a slot (see Turner & Horbay, 2004 for details on the implementation of the RNG in slot games). Computerized RNGs produce an erratic sequence of number but they are not truly random; they are pseudorandom. To overcome this limitation of the technology, slots run their RNG all the time and poll the current values when the spin button is pressed. This added uncertainty ensures that the RNG code of the slot machine cannot be broken.

A typical slot machine reel might have 11 pictures on it (e.g., oranges, cherries, diamonds), and blanks between each picture. The odds of a symbol landing on the payline have little relationship to the number of images on the reel. Instead, the computer generates a number between 1 and 64, and maps this number on to one of the stops on the physical reel; this mapping is called the virtual reel. Perhaps only 1 out of the 64 virtual stops points to the diamond symbol, but 10 of the 64 virtual stops point to a bar symbol. This mapping process allows the slot to offer large prizes, but also makes the game seem to have better odds than it actually has. The pictures that land on the payline itself are determined randomly; however, the pictures above and below the payline and the spinning reel itself offer a distorted impression of the player's chance of winning.

There are numerous myths about slot machines. For example, many people believe they have to stay at a particular machine because it is due to win. Each spin is an independent random event. The history of the machine's play is irrelevant. A machine is never due to win. In addition, because a computer, not the actual reels, determines the outcomes of a slot, there is no such thing as a near miss. A near miss is simply a loss (see Turner & Horbay, 2004, for a discussion of other myths about slots).

Roulette

Roulette is one of the oldest banked games (i.e., a game in which the house runs a bank and the players play against the bank rather than against each other). It consists of a fixed outer rim and a rotating inner wheel. Roulette is not very popular in North America, but is quite popular in Europe. Although in North America roulette takes up a only a small portion of a casino's floor space, the game appears in a large number of gambling-related advertisements, suggesting that it is a very potent symbol of the elegance and excitement of casino gambling. Roulette can be played in a variety of ways. People who play for large wins can place bets on single numbers. People who prefer frequent small wins can place bets on all 18 red or all of the 18 black slots for an even money payoff (bet $10, get paid $10 for a win). Column bets cover 12 numbers and are paid a profit of $2 for every $1 bet. Streets (three numbers), double streets (six numbers), and corner bets (four numbers) are also available. The math behind roulette is quite clever in that there are many different types of bets available, but nearly all have the same house edge of 5.3%.

Craps

Craps is a table game that gives the player a wide range of betting options and a very slim house edge. Craps is one of the fastest, most exciting, and noisy casino games. There is no skill involved in winning, but because of the complexity of the game and the fact that the player gets to hold the dice, there is a strong illusion of skill. A unique aspect of craps is that a single bet, of say $10, can last for several rolls of the dice.

There are several types of bets, but the main ones are called passline, don't-pass, come, and don't-come bets. The payback percentage in craps varies from 98.6% for passline, don't-pass, come, and don't-come bets to as low as 83.3% for a bet on the numbers 2 or 12. Players take turns rolling the dice. Any player can bet on the shooter's throw by placing money on the passline. On the first roll the shooter wins if he rolls a 7 or 11, he or she wins or loses if he or she rolls a 2, 3, or 12 (craps). However, all others numbers (4, 5, 6, 8, 9, and 10) are neither winners nor losers, but become the player "point." To win, the shooter has to roll his or her point again before rolling a 7. If the player rolls a 7, he or she loses the bet. A don't pass bet is the opposite of pass bet. Adding to the complexity of the game, after a point number has been established, the player can increase the size of his or her bet with a free-odds bet. Free-odds bets are paid out according to the true odds against winning, so there is no house edge on them (payback is 100% on the free-odds bet). The average expected loss for a $100 passline bet is $1.40. If a player has a $100 bet on the passline and then backs it with a $100 free-odds bet, the expected loss is still $1.40. The complexity of craps and the availability of free-odds bets give the player a strong illusion of skill. Free-odds bets increase the volatility of the game, and which enhances its roller-coaster feel.

There are numerous other betting options in craps, including placing a bet that 6 or 8 will come up before a 7, betting that the next roll will be a 7, betting that a 6 will come up as a double 3 ("hardways"), or betting that a specific number (e.g., 12) will come up on the next roll. The players, including the shooter, can place several different types of bets at the same time.

Games of Both Skill and Luck

Although a random number generator plays an important role in these games (e.g., a shuffled deck of cards), the player's success also depends on his or her knowledge, strategies, and decisions while playing. A good player can minimize losses with poor hands and maximize wins with good hands. Examples of games of both luck and skill include blackjack, poker, and dominoes. Video poker and other forms of poker played against a casino (e.g., Caribbean stud poker) involve some skill, but the skill is insufficient to overcome the house edge. Turner et al. (2003) labeled these games semiskilled games. To make the issue more complicated, there are special circumstances such as large progressive prizes under which slot machine, lotteries, and even bingo can be played with a positive expected return.

Blackjack

The object of the card game blackjack is to get a hand that scores as close to 21 as possible without going over. The players play against the casino. If a player's hand is closer to 21 than the dealer's, then the player wins; if the dealer's hand is closer, the dealer wins. If both the player and the dealer have the same number, they tie, or "push," and the player neither wins nor loses. If the dealer and the player exceed 21, or "bust," the dealer wins. The house edge in blackjack comes from the fact that if both dealer and player bust, the dealer wins. Face cards and tens are worth 10, aces are worth either 1 or 11, and all other cards are worth their face value. A "blackjack" or "natural" occurs when a player gets any combination of an ace with a ten, jack, queen, or king.

The dealer deals two cards to each player and to him- or herself. The dealer presents one card face up and one face down. If the dealer has a blackjack, then all players automatically lose unless a player also has a blackjack, in which case the game is a push (the player neither wins nor loses). If the dealer does not have a blackjack, the dealer then proceeds clockwise around the table, asking the players if they wish to "hit" (take another card) or "stand" (not take another card). If a player has a blackjack (and the dealer does not), it is an automatic win. Otherwise, the player indicates a hit either verbally or by scratching the table toward him- or herself. The player can continue to draw cards until his or her total exceeds 21. If a player's total exceeds 21, the player loses.

If a player is happy with the total points of his or her hand, then he or she can stand. The player also has the option of doubling down (doubling the bet, but only drawing one more card), or splitting a pair (e.g., turning two 8s into two separate hands). Some variations of the game, such as Spanish 21, allow the player to surrender (giving up two units of his or her bet and quitting the hand). Once the dealer has dealt additional cards to all the players, the dealer draws cards for his or her hand. The dealer must stand on 17 or higher and hit below 17. A win generally pays even money; however, if the player wins with a natural, the natural pays 3 to 2, or 1.5 times the bet.

The main skill involved in blackjack involves knowing when to stand, draw, double-down (increase the bet), or split (divide a pair into two hands) based on the cards one has and the dealers up card. The Basic Strategy is a set of rules for how to play every given combination of player and dealer cards. However, even the most skilled basic player will still lose money in the long run. However, if a player keeps track of the cards that have already been dealt (card counting), he or she can use this information to vary his or her bets and take advantage of situations when the dealer is more likely to bust (more high cards left in the deck). With careful play, the player can achieve a positive expected return. In practice, however, card counting is very difficult and few people can master the mathematical and emotional skill (e.g., suppression of excitement) needed to succeed.

Poker

Poker appears to have been derived in the United States during the 19th century from a variety of different games, which may have included *brag, as nas (dsands), post and pair, primero, gilet, brelan, bousilotte, ambigu, and poque* (Asbury, 1938). Today, poker is played around the world by millions of people. In recent years there has been a rapid growth in the popularity of poker tournaments, much of which is related to the highly publicized huge prizes awarded at the World Series of Poker held in Las Vegas. These poker games are now televised as if they were sporting events. Poker is important in a discussion of gambling problems because it is often the first real gambling that a lot of young people engage in. Teenagers may not legally be allowed to engage in commercial gambling at casinos, racetracks, or lottery stores, but there is no law that can stop them from making private bets with each other.

There are probably several hundred different ways of playing poker. Casino poker games can be divided into "house" games played against the casino and true poker played against other players. House games such as Caribbean stud, pai gow, let-it-ride, and joker poker are banked games in which the player plays against the dealer. Althoughsome skill is involved in these games, they are all designed to ensure a payback of around 95%. Video poker also belongs in this category and may be one of the more skill-oriented house games.

True Poker

Playing Against Other Players

True poker is played between players. Poker games can be found in kitchens, bars, the backrooms of restaurants, card casinos, poker rooms in large casinos, and on the Internet. Most players learn to play recreationally at home games, sometimes called "kitchen table" poker. In Ontario, home games of poker are legal as long as the entire pot goes to the winner of each hand. That is, no third party takes a percentage of the pot as profit. When poker is dealt in a casino, the house charges a "rake" as a percentage of each pot or an hourly rate. With tournaments, the casino charges an entrance fee. People knocked out of the tournament can often "rebuy" into the game by paying an additional fee. Typically, 90% of the players lose their entrance fee, and 10% of the players win back more than their entrance fee. The last few people in the tournament win large prizes. In recent years, the world series of poker tournaments held at Binions Horse in Las Vegas have paid prizes in the millions. The casino makes money by keeping a percentage of the total entry fees.

Kitchen poker includes a wide variety of games; usually the choice of the game is up to the dealer. The most common games dealt in a casino are seven-card stud, Texas hold'em, and Omaha hold 'em.

In seven-card stud poker, a player is dealt seven cards and makes the best poker hand using five of his or her cards. The player is initially dealt three cards, two down and one up. This is followed by three additional cards, dealt face up one at a time. The last card is dealt face down. There is a round of betting after the third, fourth, fifth, sixth, and seventh cards.

Texas hold 'em, is played at a table that seats up to 10 players. Each player gets two cards face down. These are the player's pocket or hole cards. After players bet on their pocket cards, three cards are placed face-up in the middle of the table. These cards are called the "flop." They are community cards that all players can use to make a hand. A second round of betting occurs. The fourth and fifth community cards are also dealt face up, each followed by a round of betting. Players make their hands by selecting the best five-card combination of their pocket cards and the table cards. The winner is the player who can make the best five-card hand. If two players have an equal combination of cards, the pot is split between them. Omaha hold'em is very similar to Texas hold'em, but each player receives four pocket cards, and five community cards are placed in the middle of the table. In Omaha, players must use two pocket cards and three table cards to make their hands.

In most forms of poker the ace is the highest card, while 2 is the lowest, and the players try to obtain the highest hand possible. The rules of each game vary, but the status of the various hands is inversely related to their probability of occurrence and is the same for most poker variations. The hands, ranked from lowest to highest, are (1) no pair with highest card, (2) two pair, (3) three of a kind, (4) a straight (sequential cards with no gaps, e.g., 4, 5, 6, 7, 8), (5) a flush (five cards in the same suit), (6) a full house (three of one kind, two of another), (7) four of a kind, (8) a straight flush (sequential cards in the same suit), and (9) a royal flush (10 to ace in the same suit). Two pair weak hand in a game with wild cards or several draws, but can be a fairly strong hand in a game such as Texas hold 'em.

In low-ball poker games, the players try to obtain the lowest possible hand. A winning hand would have no pairs, and be made up of low cards (e.g., 2, 3, 5, 7, 8). In some low-ball games, ace is a high card, while in other low-ball games ace is a low card. In Omaha high-low split, players can try to win with either a high card or a low card hand. The high hand and low hand split the pot. However, to win the low, a player cannot have any pair or any card higher than an 8.

To a large extent, poker is a game of skill, but if the players are well matched it becomes more like a game of chance. Mathematical and psychological skills are involved in the game. A skilled poker player has to judge the relative chance of winning with his or her starting cards and be able to take into account the size of the pot, the players' betting positions, the number of players still in the game, the number of players that have yet to act (e.g., bet, fold, or call), and his or her knowledge of the habits of the other players. A skilled poker player must be able to bluff convincingly (bet with a weak hand), or slow play (not bet a strong hand) in such a way that the other players do not know what he or she is holding. In addition, the player has to have enough emotional control to avoid letting excitement, anger, or frustration influence his or her play. Some players also possess the ability to put other players off their game by provoking their anger, intimidating them, or charming them.

Kitchen poker with friends is self-limiting in that excessive gambling is not likely to be encouraged or tolerated. Even in a casino, poker players will sometimes criticize foolish actions made by other players or offer advice or playing tips. However, poker can be very predatory, with skilled players intentionally trying to put the other players off their game so that they can take advantage of them. For example, McManus (2003) described how Amarillo Slim is able to sweet-talk other players into folding or calling depending on what he has in his hand. Basil Browne (1989) found that many players go in and out of tilt, ranging from nonproblematic to problematic at different times. However, poker can be very predatory, and some players will purposely try to put other players on tilt in order to take their money.

The advent of online poker may have changed poker into a much more problematic game. With online games, there is no longer a social barrier to excessive play because online players do not know each other and are unlikely to offer advice. In addition, online games are much more widely available and the stakes that are available range from bets with pennies up to hundreds of dollars. The low stakes make it easier to initiate a habit; the higher stakes make chasing losses possible. Another distinct feature of poker today is the game that most people are playing: no-limit Texas hold 'em. The very name "no-limit" reveals the main problem with this game. At any point in the game any player may push all of his or her chips into the middle of the table. This particular version of poker may be more dangerous than other forms because the players can either suffer substantial losses very quickly or, potentially worse, substantial wins.

Another recent phenomenon is the broadcasting of poker tournaments on television. One troubling aspect of these shows is the incredibly loose play of the players shown on television. A skilled poker player is very selective about the hands he or she pursues (Warren, 1996). He bides his time waiting for good cards. In tournaments the blinds (a forced bet that the first one or two players after the dealer have to make) increases as the tournament progresses. As the blind become very large, the players are under pressure to either make their move with mediocre cards or be forced to play out their remaining chips with the random cards dealt when it is their turn to make the blind bet. A starting hand of pair of 5s may be a weak hand, but it is more likely to win than a randomly selected pair of cards. As a result, the players in the televised games often make bets (e.g., going all in with a pair of 5s) that would be a poor choice if the player were not under the pressure of increasingly large blind bets. In addition, the players often start to act as if the game were a matter of pure random chance. By the time players reach the final table of a world series or other tournament, all the players are highly skilled. Turner and Fritz (2001) showed through simulations that if all the players in a game are equally skilled, a poker game becomes a game of pure random chance. As such, the very poor plays made during the final tables of these tournaments and that in other circumstances would be considered bad choices are a logical response to the circumstances. The problem is that these final tables are aired disproportionately often on television, which might result in amateur players being encouraged to make similarly bad choices in ordinary cash games.

Games of Subjective Probability

In all the games discussed so far, repeatable events (e.g., dealing cards or rolling dice) play a large role. When we move to betting on sports games, horse races, or stock trading, we are talking about events that are not repeatable under identical conditions. Some investments can be thought of as a type of gambling. Long-term investments are generally viewed as being a relatively safe way to build wealth. Typically, the value of a stock increases over time and if the company earns a profit, it pays out dividends. However, there are numerous other types of investments that are more like gambling. For example, buying commodity futures, speculating on new companies, day trading (e.g., buying and selling stocks in a very short time frame), or shorting a stock (e.g., arranging to sell stocks that you currently do not actually own) are three forms of speculative investment that can be called gambling.

The complex nature of the games and the inclusion of uncertain events (e.g., pitching, batting, catching, running, rumors) add some degree of random chance to the outcomes of the games. However, these games are not random, and the outcome of one event (a game this week) is not independent of other games played with the same players. In addition, because the players in the teams or the horses being run actually do differ in terms of ability, it is often possible to predict the outcome of a particular game with a level of accuracy well above a random guess. If all the players had to do was to pick the winner, there would not be much profit in the field of sports betting. To overcome this problem, in these games a bettor is pitted, not against the actual outcomes of the games, but against the subjective guesses of the gambling industry about the outcomes (e.g., the odds, point spread, or money line set by a bookie) and against the mass habits of other bettors (e.g., pari-mutuel odds or the fluctuating prices of the stock market). In this context, skill involves not merely guessing the winner, but also in outthinking the rest of the betting public. For example, suppose a bookie determines that one team is more likely to win an American football game by 6 points over the other team. This number is then used to determine the point at which a bet wins. A bet on the favorite (the team expected to win) has to win by 6 points of more before the gambler wins the bet. This line maximizes the uncertainty of the gamble by removing the difference in skill between the two teams. In other games such as horse racing and stock market purchases, this process is accomplished by the mass betting behavior of the betting public in competition with each other. A gambler who has special information about a team, horse or stock can theoretically beat the rest of the betting public.

However, if the market is efficient (Heakal, 2002) in that all information is equally distributed to all players, these games become essentially random. With stock market investments, a strong potential for future earnings or growth will drive up the cost of a stock. Therefore, the future prospects of a stock are quickly factored into its price. Similarly a sports team that is going well will attract a large number of action (bets), pushing up the line (increasing the amount the team has to win by in order for the bet to win), and making it harder for the bettor to make a profit. However; because information is never evenly distributed, some good betting opportunities will always be available. In addition, people are not particularly rational when making decisions, and as such may overreact to good news or bad news or ignore the information altogether. Because of this inefficiency, it is possible to make money on these forms of gambling.

Games of True Skill

Sometimes people place bets on skilled games that they are engaged in. These are private bets between individuals and are dealt with only briefly in this chapter. Examples of common games of skill that people bet on include golf, chess, hoops and one-on-one (forms of basketball), pool, bowling, and darts. Unlike games of both skill and luck, such as cards and dominoes, which include a random number generator, in games of true skill, no random number generator is used. A dart or bowling ball will not always go where the player aims, but as the player's level of skill increases, uncertainty is reduced. Many players will offer a handicap to their opponent to make the bet more even. Typically these games can be thought of a zero-sum games because the total amount bet is paid to the winner. However, if one includes the cost of equipment, greens fees or other game related costs, and transportation to and from the game, the average player is in fact playing against a negative expected return.

On Random Chance

In the Cydonia Mensae region of Mars there is an enormous face that stares out into space. Some people have speculated that it is evidence of a past civilization on Mars. Similarly at the entrance to Thunder Bay Ontario lies a mountain of a man guarding his treasure of silver—the sleeping giant. These are examples of how good the human mind is at finding meaningful patterns in random chance. Some people take such humanlike images very seriously, interpreting the face on Mars as proof of an ancient Martian civilization. More generally, deviations from expected results, such as winning or losing streaks, are perceived as too unlikely to be a coincidence. Anyone who has worked with gamblers comes to realize that they often have a number of erroneous beliefs and attitudes about control, luck, prediction, and chance. In this section I examine the nature of random chance to help the reader understand what random chance is and how it fools us into believing that we can beat the odds.

Some people believe that "random" events have no cause and are thus mysterious. As a result, they may believe there is a greater opportunity to influence the random outcome through prayer or similar means. In the past, some religions have used dice games to divine the will of the gods (Grunfeld, Zangeneh, & Diakoloukas, see chapter 9, this volume). Related to this is the notion that everything happens for a reason and thus random outcomes must contain a message. Other gamblers believe that there is no such thing as a random event and that they can therefore figure out how to win.

Randomness is difficult to define. Random events are unpredictable, erratic, unplanned, and independent of each other. However, random events sometimes appear to form a pattern or serve a purpose. For example, there are areas in the night sky, such as Orion's "belt," where stars appear to form a straight line. Given enough opportunity, any pattern could form by chance alone. An infinite number of monkeys on typewriters could eventually type out the complete works of Shakespeare. Although random events appear to happen without a rule or cause, they are in fact the result of material causes (e.g., gravity and friction), but an exact list of forces acting on a random number generator (e.g., dice) may be unknown or impossible to specify precisely.

How does a mechanistic universe create an unpredictable event? A random event occurs when a difficult problem such as controlling the exact speed, movement, and height of a pair of dice is combined with a complex process such as rolling the dice across a table and bouncing them against a bumper on its far side. This combination leads to complete uncertainty as to what will actually occur. During the past 30 years, physicists and mathematicians have come to realize that "tiny differences in input can quickly become overwhelming differences in output" (Gleick, 1987, p. 8). *Chaos* describes the unpredictable effects associated with small changes in a complex system (Gleick, 1987). For example, given the exact same weather conditions, the flapping of a butterfly's wings might make the difference a week later between a thunderstorm and a sunny day. This "butterfly effect" is actually a rather romantic exaggeration of the phenomenon. It is very unlikely that a butterfly would have any effect. However, it illustrates the idea that the outcome of a complex process is dependent on the exact initial conditions of that process. The notion of sensitive dependence on initial conditions is an important property in understanding the behavior of complex systems. A more topical example is the behavior of a dice that after rolling across a table lands for a millisecond on its edge between the 1 and the 4. Extremely tiny differences in the manner in which the dice was held (e.g., height, position) before it was thrown or the speed with which it was thrown might determine if the dice were to land on the 1, the 4, or some other side.

All physical events are determined or caused by something. Mechanical randomizers such as bingo balls, roulette wheels, and dice use the laws of physics to maximize uncertainty. The basis of all random-like events is a combination of initial uncertainty and complex or nonlinear relationships.

Uncertainty simply means that we do not know the exact values of all the variables with absolute precision. Uncertainty is an inherent part of measurement; nothing is ever 100% certain. A car driving at 70 kilometers per hour in cruise control will vary in speed by 1 or 2 kilometers per hour. Thus there is some uncertainty as to the exact speed at any given moment. Orkin (2000) illustrates this problem with the question "How many fish are exactly 12 inches long?" Suppose a type of fish is usually 12 inches long. In all cases, 12 inches is only an approximation. If a fish is 12.000001 inches long, it is not exactly 12 inches long. It is not possible to measure something so precisely as to completely eliminate uncertainty.

A complex or nonlinear relationship is one in which a small change in the input causes an unpredictable change in the outcome: sometimes a large change, at other times a small one. For example, there is a nonlinear relationship between caffeine and performance. Too little caffeine and a person might have trouble staying awake; too much and the person might become agitated and unable to concentrate on what he or she is doing. Suppose a researcher wanted to know how caffeine affected performance on a task. Initial uncertainties in this example would be factors such as how much sleep the research participants had the night before, how many cups of coffee they had that morning, and how much coffee they usually drink per day (i.e., their level of tolerance). If the researcher did not control for these factors, the uncertainties combined with the nonlinear effect of caffeine could produce chaotic test results. A person who came in after downing five cups may be agitated by a single dose of caffeine, whereas another person who had missed his or her morning coffee might still be sleepy after two doses.

All true random events are the result of chaos. Roulette wheels, dice, cards, and slot machines are essentially designed to maximize uncertainty. Slot machines use a mathematical formula called a congruential iteration to produce "random" events (see Turner & Horbay, 2004). This algorithm produces a complex sequence of numbers, but this sequence is not random because the entire cycle will eventually repeat itself. To attain a closer approximation to random chance, the RNG in slot machines runs continuously. Most of the numbers are not used. When a player presses a spin button, the current value of the RNG is polled. A split second later, a different outcome would occur. In this way, the outcome is completely unpredictable.

Sports games are also random number generators. Many aspects of games involve a chance outcome (e.g., a skilled baseball player may hit a ball only 30% of the time). Games are complex systems that produce a great deal of chaotic uncertainty. Similarly, prices on stock markets fluctuate in a chaotic manner as the competing forces of demand, supply, and rumor drive the price up or down. However, if all that gamblers needed to do to win money was to pick the better team or better stock, they could win most of the time by simply betting on the favorites. Unfortunately for the punter, most of the difference between team is removed though the use of differential payouts (e.g., odds), differential prices (e.g., stocks), or some other equalization methods (e.g., the line). If the information about a particular game, stock, or race was equally distributed (as would occur in an efficient market), then no punter would able to win on these types of games. However, information is often not equally distributed, giving people who know how to utilize the information a potential advantage.

In Turner (1998), I argued that one of the reasons people develop problems with gambling is that they have an incorrect mental model of the nature of random chance. The naive gambler has the notion that random chance has to be consistently erratic. That is, the outcomes are erratic and are always erratic. Strong deviations from the norm are not possible. In taking this position, the gambler discounts unusual events such as winning streaks or losing streaks. When a winning streak occurs, as they occasionally do, the gambler is faced with a problem. The player might think, "How can 7 come up 3 times in a row by random chance? It's just not possible!" Ideally, the gambler at this point would alter his or her mental model of random chance and develop a more complete understanding that might include the idea that unusual outcomes are possible. Gamblers typically do not alter their mental model. Rather when faced with this outcome the gambler would either (1) assume the game is biased or that 7 was lucky and bet on 7, or (2) assume that 7 will not come up again and bet against 7. Why do people not learn form this situation? I believe the reason is that in all circumstances one of these two possibilities will occur. The gambler does not know which, but 100% of the time one of these two naïve beliefs will be supported. The same people often hold both theories and apply them when needed. If they back 7, and 23 comes up, instead of thinking that their theory about the 7 bias is wrong, they might think, "darn, I should have known that 23 was due to come up."

House Edge

The house edge is the basis by which the casino makes money from games of chance. I am often asked how a random game can have a house edge. The truth is that the house edge has nothing to do with the randomness of the game. The house edge is simply the fact that a win is too small to make up for the times when the player loses. This is accomplished in a number of different ways and is often subtly hidden by the nature of the game. Roulette is unique in that the house edge is clearly marked so it is particularly useful to illustrate how the house edge works. The American roulette wheel contains 36 numbered slots that are colored black or red (1–36) and two slots that are colored green (0 and 00), for a total of 38 slots. European roulette has only 1 green slot, but otherwise the game is very similar. If a player bet on one number on the America wheel, the probability of winning is 1/38, but the payout for a win is only 36 chips. If the player bets a one-dollar chip on 17 and the ball comes to rest in slot 17, the player is paid $36. (Note that this consists of a win of $35 plus the player's original $1 bet for a total return of $36). Roulette is in fact that only commercial game that I know of in which the house edge is clearly marked; the 2 green slots conveniently represent the house's profit per bet (2 chips for every 38 chips bet). However, it is not the green slots per se that determine the house edge, but the fact that the player is paid only 36 chips for a win (not 38). If a player was given an additional 2 chips, the game would be fair (no house edge), but unprofitable for the casino. In summary, the payback for playing the American roulette wheel is 36/38 (94.7%). The difference between the payout and the number of slots on the wheel —2 chips—goes to the house as profit. The European version of the game has only one green space and consequently has a much smaller house edge, 2.6%. The greater popularity of roulette in Europe may be related to the smaller house edge.

Lotteries, slots, bingo, blackjack, and other games essentially operate in the same manner—the money paid for a win does not make up for the chances of not winning. In most games the house's portion is not easily to identify (not painted green). For example, in European roulette an even-money bet (e.g., red, green, even, odd, low, or high) might appear to have no house edge at all. If the ball lands on the one green slot on the wheel (0) the player loses only half of his or her bet. On the surface this would seem to make the game fair (i.e., no house edge) because you get half of your money back for a 0. However, when the long-term results are computed, the house edge is 1.3%. The extinct game of faro used a similar strategy to hide the house edge. A player bet that a card would come up on a pile of winner cards, rather than on a pile of loser cards. If it came up as a winner and loser on the same turn, the player would lose half of his or bet. In blackjack there are three asymmetries that hide the house edge: (1) players are paid more (1.5 to 1) for a blackjack, giving the player an advantage; (2) the player can choose to hit, stand, or surrender, whereas the dealer has to follow very strict rules, giving the player an advantage; and (3) when the both dealer and the player both bust (exceed 21), the house still wins, giving the house an advantage. Working out the net edge for the player is actually fairly complicated. In games such as slots or bingo, the probability of a win is unknown to the player, but the mechanics of how the house makes its money are the same. However, even in games where the probability of a win is precisely known and publicly available (e.g., lotteries), people still place their bets.

In horse racing, the true odds are unknown but can be estimated based on a horse's previous performance. The racetrack guarantees a profit by taking a cut off the top of the total pool of money bet, and then distributes the rest to the winners. However, this profit is hidden in the odds that are posted. Mathematically odds are a ratio of two events. Odds of 3 to 1 mean that the first event is three times more likely to occur than the other event (e.g., a horse has three chances of losing for every one chance of winning). Odds of 3 to 1 actually translate into a $\frac{1}{4}$ (25%) chance of a win (i.e., win/(win + lose) = 1/(1 + 3) = $\frac{1}{4}$). However, when the track posts the "odds" of a horse winning it is actually posting the payout for that horse if it wins. A horse might be posted as 2 to 1, meaning that a gambler will win a profit of $2 for every $1 wagered. Mathematically, 2 to 1 should mean that the horse has a 1/3 (33%) chance of winning. In reality, the quoted odds are in fact an exaggeration of the horse's ability. The horse might only have a $\frac{1}{4}$ (25%) chance of winning. In exaggerating the odds, the race track guarantees a profit by paying out less for a win ($2 for every $1 bet) than would be needed to make up for its chance of losing ($3 for every $1 bet). The profit, however, is hidden because the track quotes the payout odds, rather than the true mathematical odds.

In the game of poker, the players are either charged an hourly fee to play at the table or the house retains a portion of the total amount bet (e.g., the rake) on each hand of the game (e.g., for each $10 in the pot they might keep a $1 chip, up to a maximum of $5). With a rake, only winners pay the house edge. This is quite clever because the winner is too happy raking in his or her chips to complain about the small amount the casino is keeping. In fact, most winners will also give away an additional chip or two to the dealer as a tip, increasing the size of the house edge substantially.

Other games might use a commission (e.g., stock market, baccarat, some sports bets) to ensure a profit. One of the most well hidden house edges is found in sports bets. With sports betting, the house edge is usually ensured by charging a commission to the winners called the vig or vigorish (e.g., $1 for every 10 bet). If a player places a $10 bet on a team, he or she would have to pay an additional $1 commission or vig. If the player wins, he or she gets back $21. This $21 consists of the amount won ($10), the amount bet ($10), and the commission paid ($1). Given these numbers, it would seem that the winner is in fact getting the entire commission or vig back. The player might be under the impression that there was no house edge. The house edge comes from the fact that the bettor is not getting paid any winnings on the extra $1 vig that was risked. The $1 extra that is bet results in a house edge of 4.5%. Thus it's not the vig that is paid that leads to the house edge, but the absence of a win paid on the vig.

For slot machines, the house edge is impossible to determine because the odds of the events are unknown. Slot games are extremely volatile in that the outcome of a bet can vary from $0 back to $2000 or more back. The occasional wins result in huge swings of fortune. This volatility makes it impossible to determine the house edge for any short sequence of bets. In addition, through virtual reels mapping the reels in fact give a distorted impression of the player's chances (Turner & Horbay, 2004). A reel of 22 pictures might include a jackpot winning symbol, suggesting that the jackpot had a 1 in 22 chance of landing on the payline and that the jackpot would therefore occur 1 in 10,648 spins. In reality, through the use of virtual reel mapping, the chance of getting a big win symbol of the payline might be 1 in 32, so that the chance of a jackpot might be 1 in 32,768. Even worse odds of 1 in 64, or even 1 in 256 are possible using virtual reel mapping. The payline itself accurately displays the outcome of the game, but the reel as it rolls by, and the lines above and below the payline, will display the large winning.

The experience of gambling is also related to the volatility of gambling. A very volatile game is one in which there are large swings in the player's outcome from play to play. Volatile games have a mixture of frequent small prizes and less common large prizes. Slot machines, lotteries, and bingo are relatively volatile games, with prizes that can be anywhere from one times the bet to several million times the bet. In contrast, blackjack, roulette, baccarat, and craps are not volatile and typically have prizes that are equal to the bet. Figure 3.6 shows the difference between the outcomes of a game with high volatility and one with low volatility. Based on simulations, we estimate that there is a strong positive relationship ($r = .63$, $p < .05$) between the volatility of a game of the size of the house edge. Slot games, for example, have a house edge that averages around 10%. Baccarat, on the other hand, has a house edge of only 1.2%. This relationship between volatility and house edge is even true in the game of craps. A passline bet has a house edge of 1.4% but only

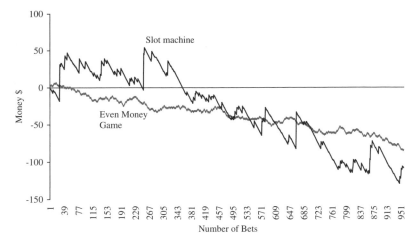

Fig. 3.6 A comparison of a volatile slot game with an even money game (red and black on roulette)

pays even money (1 to 1), whereas a bet that the next roll will be a 12 pays 30 times the bet with a house edge of 16.6%. There are two reasons for the relationship between the volatility and the size of the house edge. First, a volatile game is more of a risk for the operator. A player could win the jackpot on a slot machine on the very first spin. A large house edge is necessary to protect the casino or lottery from unexpected large wins. Second, it is possible to charge a larger house edge on a volatile game because the game's volatility hides the house edge. On the other hand, with games that pay out only small prizes (e.g., blackjack, craps), a large house edge would be too obvious and the players might be discouraged from playing. In summary, volatility is another means by which the house edge is hidden.

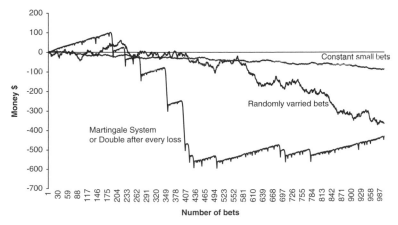

Fig. 3.7 The Martingale system of doubling after each loss compared to the random walk of a constant bets or variable random betting

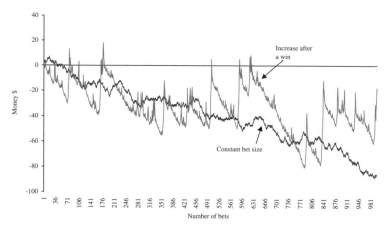

Fig. 3.8 Increasing ones bet after each win on roulette

However, the volatility of the game also depends on how people play the game. In craps, for example, most players place their bets on the passline or comeline for even money payoffs (bet $1, win $1). However, after the first (come out) roll, players can also add a "free odds" bet to their initial bet. The additional bet can greatly increase the volatility of the game. In addition, variations in bet size also increases volatility. Problematic gamblers often increase their bets over the course of a gambling session. Turner and Horbay (2003) have argued that players who vary their bets systematically push around the random outcomes of the game in such a way that they increase the volatility of the outcome. Figure 3.7 depicts the outcome from two different betting strategies: a constant even-money bet and a double up strategy. As can been seen in the figure, the variability of the outcome for the constant bet condition is rather small. The constant bets produce a random walk that meanders up or down very gradually. In contrast, when the player is using a doubling strategy it augments the bet-to-bet variance in the player's outcome. The player's experience is very different from the random walk. Another strategy of play is to increase the bet after a win. As shown in Figure 3.8, this betting strategy produces a pattern very different from the other two figures.

Action and Escape

I have heard of several attempts to group different types of games into categories. One common distinction is the idea of Action and Escape games. The stereotype is that men tend to play action games and women tend to play escape-oriented games. There are a few women who also play action-oriented games, and there are a number of men who play escape games. I believe this distinction between the two types of games is actually quite important, but it is by no means a clear-cut distinction in terms of games, but more a distinction in terms of the player's approach to the game. At the 13th International Conference on Gambling and Risk-Taking, Rachel Volberg (2006) examined some empirical evidence for this split, focusing on early- and late-onset gamblers. She found that here data supported the split to some extent but there were a number of puzzles. One problem was that the so-called action players also reported playing electronic games of chance. I pointed out that some types of electronic games of chance involve skill (e.g., video poker) and therefore may appeal to action gamblers.

Another problem with this distinction is that it depends on how the game is played. Skill may be a crucial factor in defining an action game; however, many people believe they can play games of pure chance (e.g., lotteries, slot machines) as if they were playing a game of skill. A while back, I interviewed a problem lottery player who believed that he had a system that gave him an edge. His system involved tracking past wins and looking for patterns from one draw to the next that predict which numbers will come up next. The system was actually quite logical and if he was searching through information that was not random (e.g., weather forecasts) it might work. To make matters worse, he kept finding patterns after the fact that convinced him that the game could be beat. Unfortunately for this individual, he was searching through random numbers for patterns that just simply were not there. There are numerous Web sites and books that cater to people who have similar beliefs by providing information about past lottery draws or strategies on how to profit from games of chance (see Turner et al., 2003 for several examples).

Both action and escape players are escaping from some aspect of their lives, but they are escaping in a different manner. Escape gamblers want to lose themselves in the dream of a better world. Action gamblers want to dream about being big shots, high rollers. Escape gamblers are more likely to be by themselves; an action gambler wants to be the center of attention. Escape games tend to be games requiring no skill that anyone can play (e.g., bingo, slots, lotteries). The advantages of these games are that every player has an equal chance of winning and that the player does not have to think about the game. One essential feature is that an escape game has a mixture of small prizes and large prizes. Small prizes provide frequent positive feedback, but the large prizes are essential in order to facilitate the escape into a dream world.

Most action games, in contrast, involve some element of skill, but skill in not essential. For example, craps, roulette, and baccarat are also often seen as action games. I think the most important features of action games are that they tend to often frequent small prizes, but usually do not have any large prizes. Many action games are in fact even money games (e.g., baccarat, craps, blackjack, many sports bets) where the win matches the size of the bet (bet $10, win $10). As such the only way to win a large amount of money is to make a very large bet (bet $1000, win $1000), This is especially true for action games that do not involve any skill (e.g., craps). An action game is one that either provides the player with frequent small prizes with no large prizes available (e.g., craps, roulette, blackjack) or one that provides the player with a strong sense of control over the outcome (e.g., poker, horse racing, sports betting).

Concluding Remarks

Gambling has been around for thousand of years. It is a form of entertainment that can become very problematic. There will always be a segment of people in society who want to gamble. Historically, governments have varied from the extremes of promoting gambling and exploiting gamblers to prohibiting gambling and arresting gamblers (Skolnick, 2003). Currently we are in a promotion wave (Rose, 2003).

It is important to understand the games people play. Games are not equally likely to cause problems. The games that appear to be the most problematic (e.g., electronic gaming machines, blackjack) are those that are fast, continuous, have relatively small minimum bets, and are widely available. If gambling is inherently addictive, one of the great puzzles of gambling is why so many people in society (estimates range from 63% to more than 80%) gamble nonproblematically. More research, however, is needed with non-problem gamblers to determine how they manage to avoid problematic play. What do they do right?

Problem gambling is a complex process that likely requires a complex explanation. There are probably a number of reasons that some people develop a gambling problem. Most likely gambling is a cyclical process involving an interaction between a person's mood, his or her experience playing, and the game itself (e.g., machine). In the present chapter, I have examined the games, how they are played, and the peculiar nature of random chance in the hope of promoting a better understanding of this disorder. It is important that we understand the games themselves so that we can understand the experience of the player. According to Blaszczynski and Nower (2002), pathological gambling is the result of a number of different risk factors (e.g., wins, beliefs, mood, impulsivity). It is likely that a gambling addiction is the result of the experience of the game itself in combination with the player's mood, and expectations, and needs. I believe that to understand problem gambling we need to understand the games. We especially need to understand how random chance, skill, volatility, and market efficiency operate in each of the major types of games available. In addition, we need to develop an understanding of the nature of random chance itself, and how it affects the human mind. Finally, we need to understand the motivation of the non-problem gambler. Why is it that these people (e.g., myself) do not develop a problem?

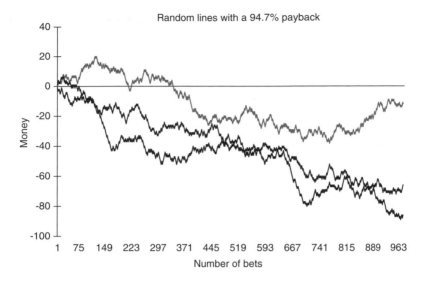

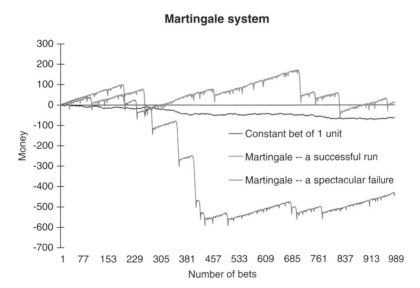

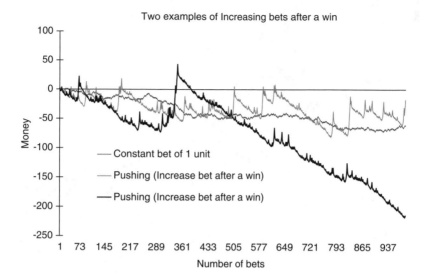

Two examples of Increasing bets after a win

Chapter 4
Exploring the Mind of the Gambler

Psychological Aspects of Gambling and Problem Gambling

Ewa Czerny, Stephanie Koenig, and Nigel E. Turner

The psychological factors that contribute to the development and maintenance of problem gambling are complex and interactive. A theory of gambling must touch upon many aspects of psychology. Which factors contribute to the acquisition of gambling behavior? What makes some individuals more vulnerable to developing problem gambling? How do other individuals influence a gambler's behavior? In this chapter we examine the psychological factors that have been studied in empirical research, which include associative learning such as classical conditioning, operant conditioning, social learning theory, and implicit learning. We then examine heuristics, biases, superstitions, and cognitive dissonance. Throughout this chapter, we investigate each of these factors in detail. It would be erroneous, however, to think that each factor can be isolated in its effect on gambling behavior. In fact, it will become clear that many of these concepts overlap.

Learning Theories

A number of different theories of behavior postulate that the environment plays a primary role in how humans behave. Taking little regard of internal motivations, these theories center on how stimuli in the environment impact, mostly on an unconscious level, the way in which humans behave in a particular situation. Despite not taking account internal motivations that may play another major role in how one behaves in a given situation, it is important to consider the different learning theories, and how each explains human behavior, especially in relation to problem gambling.

Ewa Czerny

Centre for Addiction and Mental Health, Canada Jeffrey Derevensky, McGill University, Canada

M. Zangeneh, A. Blaszczynski, N. Turner (eds.), *In the Pursuit of Winning*.
© Springer 2008

Classical Conditioning

Classical conditioning, a type of learning made famous in the late 1800s by Ivan Pavlov's experiments with dogs, has since been applied to many areas of psychology. Pavlov presented dogs with food, and then measured their salivary response. Pavlov then began to ring a bell just before presenting the food to the dogs. He noted that after numerous bell-food presentations the dogs began to salivate on hearing the bell, before the food was presented. He concluded that the dogs had learned to associate the sound of the bell with the presentation of the food. Classical conditioning occurs when any instinct drive response becomes associated with a novel stimulus. Stimuli that organisms react to without training are called primary or unconditioned stimuli (US); in Pavlov's experiment, food would be the US. Stimuli that organisms react to only after learning has occurred are called secondary or conditioned stimuli (CS); since Pavlov's dogs began to physiologically react to the bell in the same way as food, the bell would be the CS (Baron, 1995).

This type of learning has been applied to gamblers and problematic levels of gambling. In a gambling situation, wins, which are the US, produce arousal, a naturally occurring *reaction* to winning. A number of studies have demonstrated that gambling produces increased heart rate (Anderson & Brown, 1984; Brown, 1988; Griffiths, 1996; Leary & Dickerson, 1985), a state of subjective excitement (Dickerson, Hinchy, & Fabre, 1987), and dissociation (Jacobs, 1986). With repeated pairings of wins and arousal in a gambling environment, stimuli that are associated with the gambling environment also come to bring on this state of arousal (Dickerson, 1979; Sharpe & Tarrier, 1993). For example, the sound of slot machines may induce a feeling of excitement for an individual who has experienced many wins on the machines. This feeling of excitement may then motivate the individual to "try his or her luck" on the slot machines.

Second-order conditioning is also possible. Second-order conditioning occurs when the initial conditioned stimulus becomes associated with a different conditioned stimulus (Pearce, 1997); gambling cues come to elicit an urge to gamble that perpetuate the cycle of problematic gambling. Excitement can thus be experienced in anticipation of, during, or in response to exposure to gambling stimuli (Rosenthal & Lesieur, 1992). Blaszczynski (March, 2000) highlights how this process of conditioning can be used to support the theory that gambling is an addiction, produced by the effects of positive and negative conditioning, tolerance, and withdrawal.

Operant Conditioning

While classical conditioning occurs when two different stimuli are associated, operant conditioning (also known as instrumental conditioning) involves the association of a behavior and a consequence. There are four terms which are frequently used to describe either the occurrence or termination of behavior after exposure to either positive or negative stimuli. If something positive occurs or is presented after the behavior, the behavior may increase. This is called positive reinforcement. Conversely, if something good terminates or is taken away after the behavior, the behavior may decrease. This process is called negative punishment. Behavior may also occur in reaction to negative stimuli. If something negative occurs or is presented, a behavior may decrease; this is termed positive punishment. Conversely, if something negative is terminated or taken away, a behavior may increase, referred to as negative reinforcement. Thus, there are a number of behaviors that may occur as a reaction to either positive or negative stimuli (Baron, 1995).

Popularized by Skinner in the 1950s, operant conditioning is a very powerful explanation of human behavior, including problem gambling. Skinner developed his theories based mostly on animal research in which a hungry rat or pigeon would be placed in a box (a Skinner box) and rewarded for particular behaviors (usually with food pellets). A rat would be trained to press a lever; a pigeon would be trained to peck a target. Skinner found that different reinforcement schedules would produce differences in the rate of learning, the rate of response, and resistance to extinction. All animals would first be trained with continuous reinforcement; however, Skinner found that once a behavior was established, the behavior could be maintained with noncontinuous or intermittent reinforcement. Skinner described four basic intermittent reinforcement schedules: (1) fixed-interval schedule—reinforcement is delivered after a specific interval of time has elapsed, (2) variable-interval schedule—reinforcement is delivered after a variable amount of time has elapsed, (3) fixed-ratio schedule—reinforcement is delivered after a fixed number of responses has occurred, and (4) variable-interval schedule—reinforcement is delivered after a variable number of responses has been performed. While continuous reinforcement schedules arc good for establishing new behaviors, variable schedules are more effective at maintaining behavior (Baron, 1995). Gambling behavior is reinforced with a variable-interval schedule: after a variable number of responses, behavior is reinforced by a win. Gambling behavior is maintained because the individual does not know exactly when the next win will occur, but understands that he or she needs to continue to gamble if he or she is to win again.

According to Skinner (1953; Weiten & McCann, 2007) learning can take two forms: positive and negative reinforcement. When a rat is given a food pellet for pressing a lever, it is called positive reinforcement. Negative reinforcement is the removable of an aversive stimulus as a reinforcement for the behavior. For example, a rat might experience a mild electric shock through the floor of its cage until it presses a lever to stop the shock. The animal learns to press the level or run to the other side of the cage in order to escape the aversive stimulus (e.g., electric shock). Escape learning is considered to be a model for phobia. According to Weiten and McCann (2007), phobics are internally rewarded for avoiding their feared object. Phobics reinforces their own avoidance behavior by removing an internal aversive stimulus (anxiety) by avoiding their feared object. The idea of internal aversive stimulus has important implications for pathological gambling.

Negative reinforcement is often confused with punishment. Punishment is an attempt to decrease the behavior, whereas reinforcement is an attempt to increase the behavior (Weiten & McCann, 2007, p. 247). An example of punishment would be a shock given after a lever was pressed that would discourage the behavior (decrease lever pressing).

Both negative and positive reinforcement play a role in gambling. Wins are obvious examples of positive reinforcement. Many gamblers find that gambling provides them with an effective way of relieving their sense of stress, anxiety, depression, or other negative moods. Relief of these negative moods leads to negative reinforcement of the gambling behavior. Similar models have been proposed to explain drug and alcohol abuse (Marlatt & Gordon, 1985). I believe that the prospect of a big win facilitates this escape through gambling. The possible big win allows players to dream about escaping from their lives. The games that are most often associated with escape gambling tend to be games that offer a mixture of small and large prizes (e.g., lotteries, bingo, slot machines). Data provided by (Turner et al. 2006a; Turner, 2006b) suggest that the negative reinforcement may be more important than positive reinforcement. This might be because positive reinforcement from gambling is intermittent, and because of the house edge in the long run is usually insufficient to make up for the times that the player loses. Conversely, negative reinforcement occurs all the time with every gamble. One of our interview subjects told us that no matter what the outcome of a bet is, as long as the player has enough money to make another bet, he "could still dream about the big win."

There are several limitations to operant conditioning as an explanation for problem gambling. First, operant conditioning does not incorporate internal factors such as beliefs and expectations into the explanation of problem gambling. In addition, many individuals who are exposed to the irregular schedules of reinforcement inherent in the gambling context do not develop a gambling problem. It may be that those individuals who do not develop a problem gave up before winning. However, it is important to point out that gambling outcomes are random, not intermittent. A random sequence of outcomes is actually more erratic than a typical intermittent schedule used in a laboratory. In addition, a rat placed in a Skinner box does not start out with variable reinforcement. Instead, the rat is first rewarded for being near the lever, then for touching the lever, then for pressing the lever. Rewarding of successively close approximations to the desired behavior is called shaping (see Skinner, 1953). Casino gambling, however, does not involve any overt shaping process. As stated in the preceding text, casino gambling is completely random in nature. A player might experience several wins in a row, or could lose for hours without winning. Anything is possible. Perhaps the lack of shaping explains why most people who gamble do not become addicted to gambling. Turner et al. (2006a) found that early winning experiences, and the size of first wins, were associated with the severity of problematic gambling. Interviews with problem gamblers confirm that early gambling experiences are often remembered fondly. Perhaps problem gambling is established by randomly occurring shaping experiences that occur during the gambler's early exposure to a game, and later maintained through intermittent reinforcement. If this explanation is correct then the reason that most people who gamble do not become hooked is that most people have not had their behavior shaped in a way that would lead to problematic gambling.

Social Learning

Also called differential association, social learning theory states that individuals model, learn, and maintain behaviors that are observed, appealing, and reinforcing (Gupta & Derevensky, 1997). A very important factor in the development of any behavior is human interaction. Humans are very social creatures, and consequently reactions to an individual's behaviors impact his or her future behavior.

It is believed that within the gambling context social facilitation may maintain gambling behavior. When discussing problem gambling, it is very important to analyze how other individuals influence an individual's gambling behavior. How does the presence of others affect how an individual gambles? The answer seems to depend on whether the other individuals are gamblers themselves. Hayano (1982) found that both professional and regular poker players form a subcultural core that fosters social interaction. In addition, gambling venues are places where venue-specific group norms constrain and shape the gamblers' behaviors (Ocean & Smith, 1993). Studies on inveterate horse players suggest that some gamblers may persist in the act of gambling if the social rewards outweigh the costs (Rosecrance, 1988, 1989). Thus, it appears that within a gambling institution powerful social influences exist and significantly shape a gambler's behavior.

Group solidarity is often evident since players perceive that they are on the same side; playing against the enemy, the house (Ocean & Smith, 1993). According to Ocean and Smith (1993), emotional and moral support are social rewards that are also available to casino regulars. Gambling friends provide comfort and help reduce anxiety, especially to those that have sustained large monetary losses. Being a casino regular can also help an individual develop a salient identity, and increase social status and self-esteem. Outside relationships may suffer if a gambler desires to spend more time with other gamblers who make him or her feel better about him- or herself (Ocean & Smith, 1993). Ocean and Smith (1993) state, "Casino regulars who are marginalized from society face a dilemma when they start gambling; their commitment to the casino makes it harder to thrive in the outside society, which drives them even more urgently to the gambling institution to meet their needs for esteem, achievement, and status" (p. 331). A "double reinforcement" process thus occurs as social rewards positively reinforce commitment to the gambling institute, whereas conflicts with outside society are negative reinforcers that are removed as a gambler spends time within the gambling institution (Ocean & Smith, 1993). Thus, social rewards within a gambling institution reinforce gambling behavior and consequently promote future casino gambling commitments.

An important question, however, is how the presence of others specifically affects a gambler's behavior. Several researchers have demonstrated that individuals tend to be riskier in the presence of others than when gambling alone (e.g., Blascovich, Ginsburg, & Howe, 1976; Blascovich, Ginsburg, & Veach, 1975). Holtgraves (1988) and Goffman (1967, as cited in Holtgraves, 1988) both discuss how the amount of money an individual wagers has character implications. First, betting a large amount of money allows a person to be viewed in a particular way; individuals who are aware that other individuals are wagering large amounts of money may increase their wagers in order to avoid being seen in a negative context. Second, the style or pattern of a person's wagers can express his or her character in a positive way; an individual may be seen as being a competent gambler if he or she manages to increase wagers during a succession of positive outcomes. Finally, the outcome of a person's bet is evaluated by others, with winning resulting in the more positive outcome (Holtgraves, 1988). Individuals, as a result, may take more risks in group settings as a way of displaying "character" and thus enhancing their self-image.

Some interesting research has been conducted on the relationship between social facilitation and gambling success. Researchers have found that the public at a race-track is more accurate at estimating probabilities of winning than any individual expert or combination of expert selectors (Fabricand, 1965 as cited in Metzger, 1985; Figlewski, 1979 as cited in Metzger, 1985). In addition, it seems that the public tends to underestimate high probabilities and overestimate low probabilities (e.g., Ali, 1977 as cited in Metzger, 1985; Fabricand, 1965 as cited in Metzger, 1985). Thus, it appears that individuals in large groups tend to estimate probabilities differently than individual bettors.

It is important to highlight that even if the initial reasons for gambling revolve around social rewards, the continuation of gambling behavior may result from an entirely different reason. Griffiths (1990b) suggests that gamblers who experience problems are more likely to be individuals who play on their own. Griffiths (1996) additionally found that most problem gamblers report that at the height of their problem gambling, it is a solitary activity. In other words, even if individuals travel to casinos in groups, the actual act of gambling may be solitary in nature (Griffiths & Minton, 1997). Moore and Ohtsuka (1999) suggest that once a gambler's behavior is out of control, the perceived attitudes of friends and family are no longer salient to him or her. Griffiths (1990b) proposes that although social rewards may play a role in the development and maintenance of social gambling, the development and continuation of problem gambling behavior may also be mediated by psychological and physiological variables. Thus, the impact that other individuals have on a gambler may diminish as gambling behavior escalates to a problematic level. Interestingly, Specker, Carlson, Edmonson, Johnson, and Marcotte (1996) found that women were more likely to gamble alone and choose activities, such as slot machines and video poker, that involve minimal levels of social interaction. Thus, gender differences may also exist in the degree to which individuals gamble with other individuals.

Griffiths (1999) suggests that technological advancement is contributing to a shift from gambling as a highly social activity to one that is solitary in nature. He states, "Many argue that gambling is a social activity, however, to reiterate what was argued earlier—technology is essentially turning gambling from a social pastime to an asocial one" (p. 279). The growing popularity of Internet gambling makes it possible for individuals to not be around one another when gambling. Technology, therefore, is altering the way in which gamblers interact with other gamblers and may ultimately change the way in which future gambling research is conducted.

Implicit Learning

Implicit learning involves the automatic absorption of regularities in the environment. The basic idea is that learning about patterns or regularizes in life does not require rewards; it merely requires consistency until the pattern is learnt. Implicit learning is a type of associative learning that may be very important for understanding the development of problem gambling. Most research conducted (e.g., Gaboury & Ladouceur, 1989; Toneatto, 1999; Walker, 1992a; Walker, 1992b) suggests that gamblers hold erroneous beliefs about the nature of random events and construct irrational thoughts about gambling. Researchers who examine the development and maintenance of problem gambling, however, have rarely studied the role of implicit learning. Implicit learning is a mechanism that might help us understand erroneous beliefs.

Every day, individuals are exposed to an infinite number of stimuli that are either actively attended to or are left out of conscious processing. Individuals are constantly extracting information from the stimuli that occur in our environment (e.g., color, speed, number, and frequency). These, and other properties, can be understood either explicitly or implicitly. A person who engages in actively trying to make sense out of his or her world is engaging in explicit learning. However, a second mechanism operates unconsciously all the time, absorbing regularities and expectations from experience. Reber (1993) described implicit learning as a process by which individuals acquire complex knowledge about their environment, independent of conscious attempts to do so, and in a way that the resulting knowledge is difficult to express. Implicit learning essentially enables individuals to automatically absorb patterns or regularities in everyday experiences. Until recently, the mechanisms for the operation of implicit learning were unknown. However, recent advances in neural net modeling of human learning and information processing (McClelland & Rumelhart, 1985) offer a means of understanding how the human mind is capable of absorbing patterns of regularities from the environment without reinforcement, conscious effort, or even awareness (see also Reber, 1996).

These patterns or regularities are then incorporated into rules that help people act appropriately in future, similar situations. Many studies of implicit learning have been conducted using an artificial grammar learning paradigm (see Berry & Dienes, 1993 for a review). In a typical study, subjects are asked to memorize grammatical strings of letters (e.g., MTTTV, VXTXRX, MTV) that are generated by a finite grammar. The subjects are informed about the existence of a complex set of rules that limits the letter order, and are asked to classify whether new strings are either grammatical or nongrammatical. Subjects are not reinforced for right or wrong answers. In this task, subjects perform significantly better than expected via chance (e.g., 69 % correct, where chance is 50 %; Berry & Dienes, 1993). Studies on the artificial grammar learning paradigm therefore demonstrate that people are capable of learning about events and extracting regularities without being reinforced to do so. The participants are often able to articulate some of the rules that were used to generate the items, but their performance in the task exceeds their awareness of the rules (Reber, 1993). As with real grammar, often people can determine that a sentence is grammatically incorrect, but may not be able to articulate exactly what rule has been violated. A sentence may just simply sound wrong.

It is normally adaptive to be able to learn implicitly about regularities because they enable individuals to interact appropriately with others (e.g., individuals are able to produce sentences that are grammatically correct and will be understood by others who use the same rules). Implicit learning mechanisms, however, were not "built" to deal with random occurrences. It is argued that the ability to accurately absorb regularities "breaks down" when individuals are exposed to events that are the result of chance. In the natural world, individuals rarely encounter purely random events. Many experiences in life are somewhat chaotic, but very few experiences are completely unpredictable. Traffic accidents, for example, may seem to occur randomly, and yet most accidents can be avoided by careful driving and good maintenance. Gambling games, however, are most often based on true random chance (e.g., dice, roulette reels, lottery balls, etc.). The problem is that by random chance, patterns of events do sometimes occur that appear to be predictable. Every researcher understands this principle because the validity of research findings is measured against statistical probability of occurrence by chance alone. Typically a result is evaluated at the .05 level of significance. At this level of significance an apparent difference between two groups when there was in fact no actual difference between the group would occur 1 out of every 20 times the study is replicated. No matter how large a difference is observed between two means, it is still possible that the results observed were merely random variation from a single distribution. We argue that in a similar manner, 1 out of 20 times (or perhaps even more often), a gambler will experience a pattern of results that could lead him or her to induce rules based on pure random chance. In summary, people have an instinctual tendency to induce rules about the world around them. According to Turner (2000), "our minds are designed to find order, not to appreciate chaos" (p. 6). As a result, individuals are susceptible to forming erroneous beliefs about the nature of random events. Problem gamblers may have experienced events (unusual winning streaks) that led them to induce mental rules that led to excessive gambling. Problem gamblers may also have set themselves up to induce incorrect rules by the manner in which they bet. As shown by Turner (chapter 3, this volume) in his Figures 3.5 and 3.6, certain betting strategies push around random events in such a way that a sequence of a random walk no longer looks random.

Heuristics, Biases, and Erroneous Beliefs

Numerous studies suggest that people exhibit many errors when reasoning about the probability of an event occurring (Gaboury & Ladouceur, 1989; Toneatto, 1999; Turner, Wiebe, Falkowski-Ham, Kelly, & Skinner,, 2005; Turner et al., 2006; Tversky & Kahneman, 1990a; Walker, 1992a, 1992b) suggest that gamblers hold erroneous beliefs about the nature of random events and construct irrational thoughts about gambling. Turner et al. (2006) found that problematic gambling was negatively associated with accuracy on a test of knowledge about random events

(REKT), $r = .34$, $p < .001$. The average score for non-problem gamblers on questions involving reasoning about randomness was 71% correct (SD = 16.5%), whereas for pathological gamblers the average score was 59.4% (SD = 16.4%). This difference was significant, $d = .72$, $p < .01$.

Individuals also have a stereotyped expectation of what a random event looks like. We expect random numbers to look random. For example, a lottery ticket with the numbers 5–6–7–8–9–10 will be perceived as less likely to win in comparison to a ticket with the numbers 1–3–14–27–37–41, though both tickets have the same chance of winning (Turner, 2000). Thus, people have distorted notions of randomness, leading to irrational understandings about the nature of gambling. Turner et al. (2005, 2006) found that only 51% of the general public correctly answered false to "A random series of numbers, such as 12–5–23–7 is more likely to win than a series of numbers in sequence, like 1–2–3–4," indicating a very poor level of understanding regarding random chance in the general public. However, Turner et al. (2006) found that pathological gamblers managed to perform worse on this question, with only 38% accurately responding false (Turner et al., 2006).

Tversky and Kahneman (1990) argued that human reasoning is based more on various heuristics ("mental" rules of thumb) than on strict logical analysis. Heuristics are not inherently irrational. Heuristics are often very efficient shortcuts that allow an individual to respond to a situation quickly. As with grammatical rules, heuristics and biases are rules that people do not realize they are using. In general, these rules are useful strategies because they reduce uncertainty, but they can also lead to severe and systematic errors. Tversky and Kahneman (1990) discussed the different heuristics and biases that individuals rely on when making judgments about uncertain events.

The two main heuristics described by Tversky and Kahneman (1990) are the availability heuristic and the representativeness heuristic. The availability heuristic involves evaluating the probability of an event by the ease with which instances or occurrences can be brought to mind (Tversky & Kahneman, 1990). Essentially people use the ease with which things come to mind as a measure of the event's actual occurrence in the world. This strategy works well for language concepts and the interpretation of ambiguous stimuli. Studies of probability learning (Reber, 1996) suggest that humans are remarkably good at learning real-world frequencies of events. Unfortunately, the distribution of information in our world often does not match its occurrence. Plane crashes are more widely reported, whereas car crashes are often not reported. People may therefore overestimate the chance of a plane crash and underestimate the chance of a car crash. Returning to the topic of gambling, the life stories of lottery winners are published in local newspapers or television; the names of the thousands of losers are not published. Another example is the asymmetry of wins and losses during a gambling session. On most electronic games of chance, an individual bet is quite small loss. Typical bets might range from 5 cents to 5 dollars. The wins, on the other hand, occur less frequently but are much larger. The asymmetry of wins and losses may be especially true for early gambling experiences because a novice gambler would most likely not risk a large sum of money the first time he or she played, but instead make small bets. After playing 25 cents per spin on a slot machine for 1 hour at a 90 % payback, a person would have perhaps a 75 % chance of losing around $30, a 24 % chance of having a small win (e.g., $10), and a 1 % chance of a large win (e.g., $500). It is likely that the 1 % of people who experience a large win will have a much stronger memory of the event than the 75 % who lost $30. Studies of the experiences of gamblers have found that problem gamblers often report experiencing a series of big wins early in their "gambling careers" (Custer & Milt, 1985, cited in Conventry & Norman, 1998; Dube, Freeston, & Ladouceur, 1996; Moran, 1970; Shubin, 1977; Turner, Ialomiteanu & Room, 1999; Turner et al., 2006;). The experiences of wins remain very accessible to the player, encouraging continued player despite subsequent losses. The effect might not just be an issue of memory; a win tells the player that it is actually possible to win. It may be particularly difficult to convince players that their beliefs about a particular game are wrong because they have had experiences of wins; they know that *it is* possible to win. The availability heuristic therefore contributes to the continuation of gambling.

The other heuristic described by Tversky and Kahneman (1990) is the representativeness heuristic, used to evaluate probabilities by the degree to which A resembles B. This heuristic is essentially the belief in small numbers, the belief that global properties will be reflected in local series, for example, tossing a coin 10 times must produce an even number of head and tails (i.e., 5 heads and 5 tails) and that long runs of one outcome (i.e., 10 heads) will not occur. The representativeness heuristic may be directly related to the gambler's fallacy; the belief that the probability of winning is increased after consecutive losses. Problem gamblers seem to make a logical inference that if random events are consistently erratic (unpredictable, but not favoring one side or the other), then a strong deviation from the expected pattern (e.g., a series of 5 heads in a row) must be followed by a few extra tails in order to balance the random distribution. The flaw with this reasoning is in the first premise; gambling is not consistently erratic; it just simply unpredictable. One cannot gain an edge by studying previous outcomes of a game.

The gambler's fallacy may also lead to the gambling behavior known as "chasing." Chasing occurs when players bet increasingly larger amounts to win back what they have lost. Gamblers, in other words, assume that a series of losses will be followed by a win; that if they increase their bet after each loss (i.e., chase), a win will recoup the amount they have lost (Stripe, 1994). Turner (1998) found that chasing is successful 99 % of the time; people may therefore come to believe that this strategy is infallible, and thus will gamble despite severe monetary losses.

According to Wagenaar (1988), the strongest effect of the representativeness heuristic is that it underlies the belief in luck. Since players do not expect long runs of wins and losses, they perceive good and bad luck respectively as the cause of these runs. Many gamblers describe luck as a wavelike roller coaster effect of wins and losses (Turner, 2000). The belief that good and bad luck last for certain lengths of time motivates the player to try to learn to detect times of good and bad luck. As a result, losses will be attributed to a lack of skill in the ability to detect luck patterns, rather than adverse odds (Wagenaar, 1988). Consequently, players will deceive themselves into believing that the next time they will be more alert to the signs of good luck/bad luck, and gambling behavior continues.

The representativeness heuristic stems from the belief that chance/randomness is self-correcting. Gamblers, however, fail to realize when using the representativeness heuristic (and the belief in small numbers) that each gambling event is independent of the others, and that knowing past event outcomes and about luck will not help individuals predict future successes more accurately (Wagenaar, 1988).

The availability heuristic and the representativeness heuristic, both implicitly acquired, are responsible for the development of cognitive distortions in gambling. Heuristics and biases have the effect of reducing uncertainty because they provide gamblers with insight and "specific knowledge" that will help them overcome the odds (Wagenaar, 1988). As a result, heuristic reasoning causes gamblers to underestimate the role of chance in gambling situations, and thus prolongs gambling behavior.

Attribution, Illusion of Control, and Other Biases

Numerous studies also report that gamblers elicit more irrational than rational verbalizations about their gambling skill while gambling (Gaboury & Ladouceur, 1989; Ladouceur & Gaboury, 1988; Ladouceur, Dube, Giroux, Legendre, & Gaudet, 1995). Ladouceur and Gaboury (1988) evaluated the perceptions of gamblers who played roulette and slot machines and found that 80 % of their subjects' perceptions were erroneous. Many subjects attributed their success to personal factors such as skill, meanwhile attributing their losses to external factors such as bad luck (Ladouceur & Gaboury, 1988). Gaboury and Ladouceur (1989) also suggest that gamblers who encounter a succession of wins tend to "automatically" believe that skill led to their success.

It is important to note that many games are actually designed to enhance the illusion of skill. In roulette, for example, the casino provides players with a list of the previous 20 winning numbers. In craps, players are provided with the opportunity to add an additional free odds bet after a point has been established. Craps is in fact a rather complicated game to play, but the complexity hides the fact that the game is one of pure chance. Some slot machines have stop buttons that appear to give the player a means of controlling the outcome of the game. The stop button merely fast forwards the game to the end, which has already been determined. In addition, there are numerous socially shared myths about the games such as the belief that a slot machine that has not paid out in a while is due to pay out. Many books on how to gamble also promote myths about gambling (Turner et al., 2003). In summary, when evaluating the illusion of skill one must consider the extent to which the game or socially shared myths may have caused those beliefs.

Walker (1992a) suggests that problem gambling is maintained by irrational thinking. He identifies two aspects of irrational thought: illusion of control and belief in luck. While the illusion of control is more prominent in games that have an element of choice, involvement, familiarity, and competition (Langer, 1975), a gambler's belief in luck is not conditional to such factors (Walker, 1992a). Toneatto (1999) states that gamblers see luck as being either controllable or uncontrollable. Gamblers who are superstitious tend to report that they have control over luck; other gamblers believe that luck is uncontrollable and that they will experience periods of both good and bad luck (Toneatto, 1999). Studies suggest that gamblers who believe that luck is an uncontrollable event wait for periods of good luck, and wager during those times (Gaboury & Ladouceur, 1989; Walker, 1992a).

Gamblers who win big early in their gambling career may develop a distorted concept about the role of their skills in their gambling. Researchers suggest that early wins can act as a precursor for the future development of problem gambling (Custer & Milt, 1985, cited in Conventry & Norman, 1998; Moran, 1970; Shubin, 1977). These early wins usually result in distorted expectations. For example, the "early win" phenomenon is demonstrated in a study by Langer and Roth (1975), who grouped subjects into one of three conditions: (1) subjects who won 50% of the time, predominately at the beginning of the game; (2) subjects who won 50% of the time, predominately near the end of the game; and (3) subjects who won randomly throughout the game. Langer and Roth (1975) found that subjects who won predominately early in the game believed they were more skillful than other players, remembered more wins, and believed they would be successful in the future. Langer (1975) defined such behavior and beliefs as the "illusion of control." Factors such as involvement in the game, competition, choice, and familiarity with the game caused subjects to feel inappropriately overconfident (Langer, 1975).

Interpretive biases also contribute to the maintenance of problem gambling (Toneatto, 1999). The two main interpretive biases discussed by Toneatto (1999) include the attribution bias and the hindsight bias. The attribution bias occurs when gamblers overestimate personal factors such as skill and/or knowledge to explain wins and underestimate situational factors such as chance. When a gambler is losing, however, he or she is more likely to attribute his or her losses to situational factors and thus underestimate the role of dispositional factors such as skill. This interpretive bias allows problem gamblers to explain away repeated losses and therefore maintain continued gambling (Toneatto, 1999).

Toneatto (1999) suggests that hindsight bias is another interpretative bias that can perpetuate problem gambling. After a win, gamblers tend to recall or evaluate their gambling choices as being correct (Toneatto, 1999). When gamblers evaluate their choices after a loss, they usually explain the loss away by stating that they should have anticipated or foreseen the outcome, and therefore avoided it. A gambler may say "I knew I should have played the other slot machine" or "I know better than to play 9 in the lottery" (Toneatto, 1999, p. 1599). Evaluating their behavior based on whether they won or lost enables gamblers to "delude" themselves into believing that they will experience a "big win" only after they have perfected their gambling strategies. Thus, players continue to gamble and gain experience that they think will bring them ever closer to a "big win."

In addition to magnifying their skills, having an illusion of control, and exhibiting interpretative biases, problem gamblers also tend to selectively remember events. Kahnemann and Tversky (1982) suggest that problem gamblers have an easier time recalling wins rather than losses because wins are rare events as compared to losses, which tend to be numerous and not as salient (Lord, Ross, & Lepper,

1975). Babad and Katz (1991) suggest that gamblers recall more wins than losses in order to comply with their wishes and expectations. In addition to remembering more wins, the monetary size of wins is overestimated and the size of the losses is underestimated (Toneatto, 1999). Since wins are more easily remembered, and since the amount won tends to be overestimated, gamblers believe that winning is to be expected.

Superstition

Griffiths (1996) suggests that problem gamblers are susceptible to perceiving illusory correlations and attributing causality to salient features in their environment that they believe are related to gambling outcomes. In gambling, "big wins" occur rarely and are therefore highly salient events compared to losses or small wins; the gambler may therefore remember the context in which the big win occurred even if such an association is noncontingent (Gaboury & Ladouceur, 1989). Thus, the gambler will try to reconstruct the exact context in order to repeat the big win, and will avoid events contiguous with heavy losses, even if noncontingently related (Toneatto, 1999).

Langer and Roth (1975) suggest that while problem gamblers understand that gambling outcomes are the result of randomness (especially in games of pure chance such as the slots and roulette) they may simultaneously believe in the existence of a reliable means of manipulating gambling outcomes in both games of skill (e.g., poker, blackjack) and in games of pure chance (e.g., roulette, slot machines, lottos).Thus, gamblers will use various methods in an attempt to directly influence gambling outcomes in their favor. According to Toneatto (1999), "such behavior is based on the gambler's (often implicit) assumption that specific objects, behaviors, or cognitions can causally influence gambling outcomes even though they occur at a physical and/or temporal distance from the gambling event and do not reflect easily verifiable mechanisms of action (e.g., magic)" (p. 1596). These assumptions are therefore superstitious in nature.

Superstitious beliefs can be classified into three main groups; talismanic, behavioral, and cognitive (Toneatto, 1999). "Talismanic superstitions include beliefs that the possession of certain objects will increase the probability of winning" (Toneatto, 1999, p. 1596). The possession of "lucky" objects (e.g., rabbit's foot, lucky pen), objects with personal significance (e.g., family heirloom; King, 1990), specific attributes (e.g., pink), and use of certain numbers (e.g., the birthdays of family members, past addresses; Wagenaar, 1988), all of which are associated with a previous win, are often reused to influence the outcome of the current game. For example, an individual who wins big at bingo may associate the win with the use of a specific colored inker (e.g., blue) and may use the same inker, or an inker of the same color, in future games in an attempt to influence the outcomes in his or her favor (King, 1990).

"Behavioral superstitions include beliefs that certain actions or rituals can increase the probability of winning" (Toneatto, 1999, p. 1596). Oldman (1974) found that games demanding behavioral involvement such as lotto and slot machines tend to evoke skill-like behaviors and lead to the belief that the outcome can be controlled even when it is evident that such behavior has no effect on the outcome (Griffiths, 1996). For example, individuals may purchase lottery tickets from a particular store, play bingo in a specific hall, play on certain slot machines, or gamble only on specific days of the week. Further, gamblers often engage in verbal (e.g., repeating a certain number they want to win on the roulette wheel, encouraging their favorite horse, uttering a specific word or phrase) and nonverbal behavior (e.g., kissing the dice, clapping, snapping fingers, throwing the dice softly for low numbers and hard for high numbers; Henslin, 1967) during the game in an attempt to increase the probability of winning.

Another behavioral superstition that has been described extensively is entrapment (Walker, 1992a). Entrapment is commitment to a goal that has not yet been reached. Walker (1992a) states that a main motivating factor that leads to the continuation of gambling behavior despite losses is the fact that the individual has expended many resources (e.g., money, time, energy) while gambling; if the individual should stop gambling, a winning event may occur, thus wasting the money, time, and energy he or she has expended. These individuals therefore believe that with perseverance they will eventually win. Entrapment is often observed in lotto and lottery players who bet on every draw, and slot machine players who do not leave a machine (Toneatto, 1999). Players who regularly buy the same lottery tickets might feel that they have to bet every week just in case their numbers come up.

Finally, "cognitive superstitions include beliefs that certain mental states can influence the probability of winning" (Toneatto, 1999, p. 1597). Superstitions of this type can include hope, prayer, positive expectations and attitudes, and a strong belief that winning is imminent (King, 1990; Toneatto, Blitz-Miller, Calderwood, Dragonetti, & Tsanos, 1997). For example, some gamblers believe that playing the game passionately will help to increase the possibility of winning, whereas other gamblers believe the opposite, that playing dispassionately will be more effective (Toneatto, 1999).

We have suggested that erroneous beliefs such as illusory correlations are the source of superstitious beliefs. In addition, we have discussed at some length the three main types of superstitions. The final point that needs to be addressed is the role of superstition in gambling behavior. What is the function of superstition, and how does it bring about an individual's future gambling? We will discuss one possible function, namely that superstition induces the illusion of control.

Past research (Wagenaar, 1988; Toneatto et al., 1997) suggests that one of the main cognitive distortions in heavy gambling is the illusion of control. Toneatto et al. (1997) claim that superstitious beliefs and behaviors are at the root of illusory control over gambling outcomes. The illusion of control is characterized by statements of overconfidence and excessive self-efficacy that might encourage excessive or persistent gambling (Toneatto et al., 1997). Langer (1975) defined the illusion of control as being "an expectancy of a personal success inappropriately higher than the objective probability would warrant" (p. 311). Langer's research verified her hypothesis; in certain situations, people will produce skill orientations toward chance events. Langer assumed that these "certain situations" involved factors of choice (e.g., whether to bet on red or black in the game of roulette), familiarity (especially after having previous exposure to the game), involvement, and/or competition (e.g., playing blackjack against the dealer) that may stimulate the illusion of control to produce skill orientations. Illusory control over gambling outcomes may induce players into believing that they are able to make a large number of decisions, enabling them to blame losses on their lack of skill instead of on the odds (Toneatto, 1999). As a result, gamblers will likely ignore the fact that the odds of winning (especially in games of chance) are very low, and they will assume that a big win will occur when they have understood the system (i.e., perfected their gambling strategy; Wagenaar, 1988). Once a small win or a near win has occurred, biased evaluation (e.g., biased attribution) of the outcome will maintain the illusion, as the gambler may conclude that with diligence and persistence a big win is imminent (Walker, 1992a). These biases will also be enhanced by advertising, socially shared myths, or features of the game designed to enhance the illusion of control. The player continues to gamble believing that he or she is on the right track to winning big.

Jahoda (1969) found that superstitions increase when individuals are not completely in control of the situation (i.e., during chance events). Walker (1992b) also suggests that utterances of superstitious beliefs occur more frequently in slot machine players than in poker players (in whom skill/control already plays a large factor in the game). He states that "if slot machine players believe that they can influence the machine to display winning combinations then it follows that they may be able to extract an edge where [they believe] other less fortunate or more ignorant players cannot" (Walker, 1992b, p. 259). It is not surprising, therefore, that some gamblers attempt to further increase their perception of control in a game of chance through the use of superstitious behavior (Ladouceur, Arsenault, Dube, Freeston, & Jacques, 1997). Tobacyk and Wilkinson (1991) found that individuals who are believers in superstition, psi, and precognition may be primed to develop illusory control beliefs in gambling situations. This research suggests that individuals who are already believers in superstition, psi, and magic are attracted to games of chance, and that through frequent gambling their erroneous beliefs about causality are promoted, leading to the illusion of control and to the maintenance of gambling behavior in this mutually reinforcing cycle.

Cognitive Dissonance

Thus far we have examined the roles that classical conditioning, operant conditioning, social learning, implicit learning, heuristics, and superstition play in problem gambling. Cognitive dissonance can also be used to explain the maintenance of gambling behavior and cognitive entrapment. The relationship between the results of a gambling action and a gambler's cognitive rules may result in either perceived consistency or dissonance (Abt, McGurrin, & Smith, 1985). Festinger (1962) describes cognitive dissonance as a feeling of uneasiness that occurs when an individual's actions are incongruent with his or her attitudes. As a result, the individual attempts to decrease the aversive feeling by justifying his or her behavior or by altering his or her attitudes, and/or by avoiding any situation that might further increase dissonance (Festinger, 1962). How does the gambler justify his or her continued gambling behavior when he or she experiences repeated losses? As mentioned previously, gamblers use many heuristics and interpretive biases (that arise out of conscious and implicit learning) such as the availability heuristic, representativeness heuristic, attributional biases, selective memory, hindsight bias, and learning from losses to justify their gambling habit (Toneatto, 1999).

In explaining wins, gamblers tend to overestimate dispositional factors (e.g., skills, abilities) and to underestimate situational factors (Gaboury & Ladouceur, 1989; Ross & Sicoly, 1979). To explain losses, however, gamblers may prefer using bad luck or idiosyncratic events instead of dispositional explanations (Lau & Russell, 1980). In addition, problem gamblers may selectively recall wins and have difficulty recalling losses (Lord, Ross, & Lepper, 1975); this effect may be due to saliency since larger wins are more rare and come to mind easier than losses (Kahnemann & Tversky, 1982). Babad and Katz (1991) have also suggested that gamblers may be motivated to recall wins and discount losses in order to sustain the hope or "wish" of winning. Toneatto (1999) states that the size of a win may be overestimated, while the size of a loss underestimated.

Gamblers may retrospectively evaluate gambling decisions as being correct or incorrect on the basis of whether they led to wins or losses (Toneatto, 1999; Wagenaar, 1988). Gamblers may believe that there is a skill to gambling and that an outcome can be controlled by the gambler. Gamblers may reframe repeated losses as learning experiences, which then provide feedback on the efficacy of a specific gambling system, gambling strategy, or the gambler's luck status (Bem, 1972). When close losses or near wins occur, gamblers may believe they are acquiring the skill to win larger amounts, that their gambling system is an effective one, or that their luck is shifting favorably (Griffiths, 1996; Reid, 1986).

These interpretive biases essentially enable gamblers to convince themselves that their only chance of regaining money lost is by perfecting their gambling techniques through further gambling (Toneatto, 1999). Gambling behavior is therefore sustained. Not all gamblers, however, may believe that their game involves skill; slot machine players typically report that their game is a matter of chance, not skill (Leary & Dickerson, 1985; Walker, 1988). In addition, when asked to state their thoughts aloud while gambling, gamblers who prefer slot machines emit more irrational statements regardless of the type of game being played (Walker, 1992b). There is thus a discrepancy between how often slot-machine gamblers emit irrational beliefs and their own beliefs regarding the amount of skill involved. Nonetheless, there may exist important differences in cognitive biases between individuals who do and do not prefer slot machines.

Abt et al. (1985) highlight how the very structure of a gambling institution provides a variety of mechanisms and conditions to assist a gambler in reducing dissonance. A gambler is offered separate opportunities to re-enter and to re-test a gambling situation, which then give the gambler new possibilities for more favorable outcomes than those that have already occurred. In addition, gamblers in casinos or race tracks are relatively cut off from the outside world, shielded from distractions, and exempt from outside demands. A supportive network of gamblers at the institution may reinforce a gambler's behavior by offering consonant explanations for temporary setbacks. Even the way the gambling situation is structured allows a gambler to ease cognitive dissonance, being able to maintain his or her gambling behavior.

Summary

We have examined how different psychological factors may play a role in the development and maintenance of problem gambling. First, we discussed different learning theories such as classical conditioning, operant conditioning, social learning, and implicit learning, and how each explains the way in which humans behave. It should be noted, however, that these theories do not take account of internal motivation, and focus only on how stimuli in the environment impact the way in which humans behave in a particular situation. The environmental stimuli that affect an individual can include other individuals. We examined how the presence of other individuals affects a player's gambling behavior. Research has documented how gamblers form a social core within a gambling institution, and how these groups shape gambling behavior. A "double reinforcement" process may occur as social rewards positively reinforce commitment to the gambling institute, whereas conflicts with outside society are negative reinforcers that are removed as a gambler spends time within the gambling institution. Thus, social rewards within a gambling institution reinforce gambling behavior, and consequently promote future casino gambling commitments.

We also discussed how humans have an ability to deal with regular patterns in the world. Implicit learning mechanisms, however, were not "built" to deal with random occurrences. Our ability to accurately absorb regularities "breaks down" when we are exposed to events that are the result of chance. Pathological gamblers may be prone to deceiving themselves into believing that random events are predictable. Problem gambling behavior is therefore maintained. Next, we examined how gamblers use various methods including superstitious behavior and thought in an attempt to directly influence gambling outcomes in their favor. Research suggests that through frequent gambling, erroneous beliefs about causality promote the development of an illusion of control, helping to maintain gambling behavior.

Finally, we discussed how gambling behavior may be viewed as a way of dealing with cognitive dissonance, which is a feeling of uneasiness that occurs when one's actions are incongruent with one's attitudes. As a result, individuals will attempt to decrease this aversive feeling by justifying their behavior or by altering their attitudes, and/or by avoiding any situation that might further increase dissonance. The very structure of a gambling institution may provide players with ways in which to ease cognitive dissonance, leading to the continuation of problem gambling behavior.

While a number of various factors in the development and maintenance of problem gambling have been discussed, it is important to keep in mind that these and other factors interact in order to affect behavior. Thus, biological/genetic, psychological, social, and environmental influences also need to be considered in relation to one another in order to get a more complete understanding of problem gambling behavior. As Lamberton and Oei (1997) state, "affective, cognitive, and behavioral variables may play different roles at different stages of problem gambling and may interact with each other in different ways during the causal sequence" (p. 91). Researchers usually seek the simplest explanation for a particular behavior. Such explanations, however, are hardly ever complete because complex behaviors result from an interplay of many factors.

Chapter 5
Individual Factors in the Development and Maintenance of Problem Gambling

Masood Zangeneh, Alex Grunfeld, and Stephanie Koenig

In chapter 4, the authors examined factors such as associative learning, consciousness, superstition, and cognitive dissonance, and their possible role in the development and maintenance of problem gambling. In this chapter, we explore individual factors, such as anxiety and arousal, temperament, attention-deficit/hyperactivity disorder, narcissism, and coping skills, as well as their potential relation to problem gambling.

Anxiety and Arousal

An individual difference factor that has received some empirical attention is anxiety and its relation to gambling. On the one hand, a body of research such as Orford's (1985), for example, has confirmed that problem gamblers do experience pronounced levels of social anxiety. On the other hand, not all studies have found similar high levels of anxiety in problem gamblers when compared to a control group or the general population. In an investigation of the differences in anxiety levels between problem gamblers and a control group by means of the SCL-90-R, a 90-item test that assesses psychological distress along nine symptom dimensions, Raviv (1993) could not discover any statistically significant difference in the mean responses of the two groups. A study by McCormick (1994) found that problem gamblers show deficits in coping repertoires, have limited strategies, and lack flexibility in choosing an appropriate skill in order to deal with stressful situations. Gambling behavior, therefore, is maintained in part because problem gamblers frequently lack the ability to cope with it.

As well, some convincing evidence has been uncovered of gender differences in the degree to which anxiety is correlated with gambling behavior. A comprehensive study by the Australian Addiction Research Institute (Coman, Burrows, & Evans, 1997) reports that two-thirds of problem gamblers are male, and that the two genders have markedly different gambling patterns. Women appear more prone to gamble as

Masood Zangeneh
Centre for Research on Inner City Health, St. Michael's Hospital, Canada

M. Zangeneh, A. Blaszczynski, N. Turner (eds.), *In the Pursuit of Winning.*
© Springer 2008

a way of dealing with stress, anxiety, boredom, and loneliness. Men, on the other hand, typically gamble for financial reasons, excitement, pleasure, and, to a lesser extent, for stress reduction.

Anxiety can be a risk factor for gambling, a consequence of gambling, or both. For an individual, gambling is frequently a way to escape from overwhelming personal or familial problems. According to Dickerson et al. (1996), gamblers begin to play as a way to escape depression or frustrating days. Suggest that the difficulty experienced by problem gamblers in ceasing to bet results in part from an increase in their emotional response to certain aspects of their previous gambling, such as the extreme excitement felt when listening to a race (McConaghy, Armstrong, Blaszczynski, & Allcock, 1983). As a gambler spends more time at casinos or race tracks, however, adverse consequences may result (e.g., loss of money or isolation from friends and family), which further increase his or her level of anxiety. It therefore appears likely that anxiety is both a risk factor and a consequence of gambling.

Learning theorists propose a further way in which anxiety leads to gambling behavior (e.g., Jenike, 1983; Salzman & Thaler, 1981). According to these theorists, neurotic/obsessive thoughts continually increase an individual's anxiety until the act of gambling reduces anxiety back to lower levels. Some empirical data (e.g., Raviv, 1993) indicate that the impulse to gamble is indirectly related to the presence of neurotic/obsessive thoughts. The correlation of anxiety and gambling may therefore be the result of a third factor, that is, neurotic and obsessive thoughts.

The *behavior completion mechanism model* (Blaszczynski, 1993; McConaghy, 1980; as cited in Coman et al., 1997) provides another practical means of conceptualizing the relationship between anxiety and gambling. According to this model, an individual feels tension when he or she is unable to engage in gambling behaviors. Further, attempting to control their own behavior leads gamblers to experience tension, irritability, and depression, which can be reduced only when the individual becomes engaged in gambling. The reduction of tension is thus a negative reinforcer, while the excitement produced by the act of gambling is a positive reinforcer. After these associations are made, any negative emotional state can act as a cue for further gambling.

Another important model focuses on the relationship between social influence and anxiety. A *social learning model* contends that gambling behavior may initially arise from social interactions, but that frequent gambling behavior causes gambling to take on an adaptational function. At this stage, anxiety precipitates gambling as an arousal escape or stimulation mechanism (Brown, 1987a). The influence of peers and family on gambling has been studied extensively, especially in the case of adolescents (Browne & Brown, 1994; Griffiths, 1990). Researchers have largely found support for the idea that adolescents who gamble are initially highly influenced by their peers and family. Browne and Brown (1994) studied the causes of gambling in a group of 208 college students. In line with the conjectures of the social learning theory, they found that having parents or friends who gamble was a significant predictor of student gambling. Following Griffiths (1990), Browne and Brown (1994) posited that, in gambling, students sought to emulate those whom they valued the most—their family and friends.

Jacobs (1988) has outlined a model that proposes that gambling behavior is maintained by both an abnormal arousal level (either hypo- or hyper-) and a childhood or adolescence marked by a sense of rejection by parents or other significant others. The feelings of rejection then stimulate behaviors and activities that produce relief from this psychological distress. The model thus combines physiological and social factors in explaining the maintenance of gambling behavior. Although Jacobs' (1988) model is interesting, it has yet to be widely accepted by researchers.

Regardless of which model we adopt, there appears to be a strong relationship between anxiety and gambling behavior. Raghunathan and Pham (1999) have investigated negative affect and decision-making, and offer three ways in which negative affect may influence an individual's decision-making: (1) by coloring the content of one's thoughts; (2) by altering the process through which people make decisions; and (3) by shaping the decision-makers' motives. The authors suggest that anxious (and therefore more aroused) individuals are likely to bring an implicit goal of uncertainty reduction and risk avoidance to a decision-making task, and thus prefer the lower risk-lower reward gamble. This finding, however, has not been completely supported by empirical research. In contrast to Raghunathan and Pham (1999), for instance, Mano (1994) found that arousal increases risk-seeking behaviors. In addition, situational anxiety has been found to increase risk-seeking in lotteries (Mano, 1992). Leith and Baumeister (1996) explain how arousal appears essential in triggering increased risk-taking when one experiences negative affect (e.g., anxiety); neither arousal alone nor anxiety alone is sufficient in triggering risk-taking. It therefore appears likely that it is not anxiety per se that increases risk-taking, but the combination of arousal and anxiety.

Zuckerman (1979) posited a link between gambling and a trait termed *sensation-seeking*. Sensation-seeking is a biologically based personality dimension that differentiates individuals who do and do not seek novel or complex experiences or situations. Individual differences for this trait could explain differences in risk-taking, and thereby differences in the continuation of gambling behavior. According to Zuckerman (1979), individuals who gamble excessively are trying to maintain their optimal level of arousal.

Anderson and Brown (1984) extend the idea of sensation-seeking, and suggest that gambling is very exciting; that some form of arousal or excitement is a major reinforcer of gambling behavior for regular gamblers; and that individual differences in sensation-seeking are involved with gambling behavior. By measuring changes in heart rate, the authors found that the presence of arousal resulted in different gambling behavior (Brown, 1986). There has been some empirical support (e.g., Dickerson & Adcock, 1987; Leary & Dickerson, 1985) for the idea that levels of arousal (as measured by heart rate and subjective ratings of arousal) are higher in regular players than in infrequent players. Griffiths (1990) also found that problem gamblers reported more excitement and arousal while gambling than did social gamblers. Leary and Dickerson (1985) argue that differences in arousal may occur because of an association between play and large sums of money won and lost. However, as this suggestion has not received empirical support (Dickerson & Adcock, 1987), the precise explanation for these observed differences in arousal remains largely unknown.

The view that problem gamblers are greater sensation seekers, however, has not been fully embraced by researchers. In a study by Blaszczynski, Wilson, and McConaghy (1986), for example, problem gamblers were compared to the general population on several anxiety and sensation-seeking measures. Blaszczynski et al. (1986) observed increased Psychoticism, Neuroticism, State, and Trait anxiety scores, and significantly lower Sensation-Seeking scores in problem gamblers. The authors argue that problem gamblers are not necessarily sensation seekers, but that avoidance or reduction of noxious physiological states or dysphoric moods, in conjunction with a behavior completion mechanism, is a major factor in explaining persistence in gambling.

While it is clear that stress may trigger gambling behavior, Coman et al.(1997) caution that it is not clear why some individuals become problem gamblers. Their research shows that gambling behavior increases stress, anxiety, and depression, since the gambler has to wager larger amounts of money in order to cover losses or receive the same amount of reinforcement from gambling. What types of individuals are prone to become problem gamblers, however, is as of yet not well established.

Temperament

Temperament refers to the usual mood or disposition of an individual. A large amount of the research conducted on temperament in the area of gambling has been concerned with the mood of individuals before, during, and after the act of gambling, as well as the rate of affective disorders seen in gamblers. In this section, we explore these topics, as well as the ways in which mood may contribute to the development and maintenance of gambling behavior.

As discussed in the previous section, the avoidance or reduction of noxious physiological states or dysphoric moods is seen as a major factor in the persistence of gambling (Blaszczynski et al., 1986). Dickerson et al. (1996) found that gamblers report commencing play as a way of escaping from depression or frustrating days. This relationship is recognized in the Diagnostic and Statistical Manual of Mental Disorder—Fourth Edition (DSM-IV, American Psychiatric Association [APA], 1994), where the fifth criterion for pathological gambling states that "the gambler gambles as a way of escaping problems or of relieving a dysphoric mood (e.g., feelings of helplessness, guilt, anxiety, depression)."

In this vein, a number of studies have focused on the relationship between depression and gambling behavior; these studies suggest that mood and gambling behavior may interact differently in different types of gamblers. Dickerson, Hinchy, Legg-England, and Cunningham (1992) found that greater average losses over time were associated with depressed mood immediately before the session of play; depression could even affect the degree to which gamblers will persist after gambling losses. Corless and Dickerson (1989) showed that negative moods (i.e., frustration, dysphoria) were associated with greater persistence when losing in high-frequency players, but were also associated with lower persistence in low-frequency players.

There have also been studies investigating the rate of occurrence of depression in various groups of gamblers. McCormick, Russo, Ramirez, and Taber (1984) diagnosed 76% of 50 gamblers seeking treatment as meeting the Research Diagnostic Criteria for major depressive disorder; of these individuals, 86% stated that gambling preceded their depression. Similarly, Black and Moyer (1998) found that 60% of their subjects had a lifetime mood disorder. Specker, Carlson, Edmonson, Johnson, and Marcotte (1996) found that gamblers in treatment, compared with untreated controls, were about three times more likely to meet the criteria for major depressive disorder. Ramirez, McCormick, Russo, and Taber (1983) reported that 50% of their sample was depressed. In Spain, Becona, Del-Carmen-Lorenzo, and Fuentes (1996) investigated depression rates for problem gamblers and found that 21.1% of their sample were depressive, providing further support for the relationship between gambling and mood disorders.

McCormick et al. (1984) noted that patients in a Virginia hospital who were gamblers and depressed stated that gambling was the only activity that seemed capable of energizing them and altering their depressed mood. Investigated problem gamblers attending a U.S. Veterans Administration treatment center and found they had more depression, lower self-esteem, lack of assertiveness, inability to handle stress, and inability to identify or express feelings. The authors hypothesize that the production of positive mood and cognitive states, and the reduction of negative affect, during the act of gambling reinforces further gambling behavior via operant conditioning (Blaszczynski & McConaghy, 1989).

Other studies, however, have found no relationship between gambling and depression. Thorson, Powell, and Hilt (1994) found no association between scores on a depression scale and reported gambling behaviors, but the prevalence of gambling in this sample was low, and the researchers did not evaluate the relationship between gambling frequency and depression, and so any conclusions drawn from this study are dubious. What is clear from the studies conducted thus far is that there does seem to exist at least some association between depression and gambling, but more sound research needs to be carried out to delineate the precise way in which depression and gambling behavior interact.

There has already been some speculation about the exact relationship between depression and gambling behavior. Murray (1993) states that "depression appears to coexist frequently with compulsive gambling, but the antecedent-consequent relationship is unclear and both conditions may form part of a larger personality disorder as yet uncategorized" (p. 798). Boyd and Bolen (1970) view gambling as a manic defense against helplessness and depression secondary to loss.

Another group of studies has investigated the relationship between gambling and bipolar disorder. McCormick (1993) found that 38% of Veterans Administration patients hospitalized for gambling were diagnosed with hypomania. A very early study in this field (Winokur, Clayton, & Reich, 1969) revealed a high prevalence of gambling among families of individuals with bipolar disorder. Specker et al. (1996), however, found no difference between problem gamblers and controls for bipolar and dysthymic disorders. It therefore remains unclear whether gamblers actually have a higher prevalence of bipolar disorders.

Some researchers, however, do not support the conclusion that gambling and mood disorders are highly comorbid. Crockford and el-Guebaly (1998), for example, suggest that the high prevalence of mood disorders frequently reported may result from a sampling bias, and not from comorbidity. What is clear is that more empirical research needs to be conducted in order to ascertain whether there is, in fact, a nonspurious relationship between gambling and mood disorders. If that indeed turns out to be the case, a further question of interest would be whether it is gambling behavior or a mood disorder that appears first. Perhaps both are the result of a third factor, such as financial need.

The correlation between mood disorders and problem gambling has very important clinical implications. Marlatt and Gordon (1985) argue that negative emotional states (e.g., boredom, loneliness, dysphoria) have been reported as common causes of relapse in substance and non–substance-addictive behaviors (which would include gambling). In a retrospective analysis of affective states in problem gamblers, Linden, Pope, and Jonas (1986) noted that 28% experienced recurrent episodes of major depression; about two-thirds of the subjects who had stopped gambling had since experienced at least one major depressive episode. The general conclusion to be drawn from studies in this vein is that if a problem gambler seeks treatment, the presence of depression or a negative emotional state may necessitate a different treatment strategy.

Attention-Deficit/Hyperactivity Disorder

Several researchers have noted that there appear to be elevated rates of childhood attention-deficit/hyperactivity disorder (ADHD; Carlton et al., 1987; Carlton & Manowitz, 1995) and adult ADHD (Castellani & Rugle, 1995) among problem gamblers. Specker, Carlson, Christenson, and Marcotte (1995) examined the occurrence of attention-deficit disorder (ADD) and impulse-control disorders in problem gamblers. The authors found a strong association among problem gambling, attention-deficit, and other impulse-control disorders; attention-deficit disorder was seen in 20% of the subjects.

As Carlton and Manowitz (1995) noted, ADD behavior, like excessive drinking or gambling, reflects a relative lack of behavioral restraint in that the impulsivity characteristic of ADD refers to an inability to "hold back"—to inhibit a range of behaviors. The attention deficit seen in ADD implies an inhibitory deficit, because focusing attention requires inattention to competing stimuli, the functional impact of which must be inhibited if they are not to disrupt the attentional process itself.

Substance abusers are also reported to exhibit a high rate of childhood histories of ADHD. A number of researchers have noted that substance abusers and ADHD patients exhibit a deficit on tests with complex visuospatial stimuli and those measuring abstracting ability (Ackerman, Dykman, & Peters, 1977; Brandt, Butters, Ryan, & Bayog, 1983; Douglas, 1984; Parsons & Farr, 1981). Posner and Presti (1987) suggest that this pattern of results is related to a deficit in higher-order attentional capacity.

According to Posner and Presti's (1987) model, attention consists of hierarchically ordered functions. The first level of attention includes alertness and the ability to focus on a stimulus; a second level is *selective attention*, which involves the flexibility to release attention from one stimulus and re-engage it on another. Lower-order attention processes are believed to be mediated by midbrain, parietal, and temporal cortical mechanisms, while more complex levels of attention are believed to be controlled by the frontal cortex (Rugle & Melamed, 1993). Researchers have found that impairments in frontally mediated executive functions are related to both ADHD (Douglas, 1984; Douglas & Parry, 1983; Weingartner et al., 1980) and substance abuse (Brandt et al., 1983; Grant et al., 1978). Neurological deficits therefore appear likely to be a contributing factor to the development of disorders involving an inhibitory deficit and a lack of behavioral restraint (e.g., ADHD, substance abuse, gambling), but more research is needed to understand the exact nature of their relationship.

An important question, however, is whether attention problems seen in adult substance users predate an addiction or appear as a result of using a substance. To address this issue, Rugle and Melamed (1993) compared control subjects with non–substance-abusing problem gamblers, and found that gamblers performed worse on higher-order attention measures and reported more childhood behaviors consistent with attention deficits. The authors suggest that attention deficits may be a risk factor for the development of addictive disorders.

Blum, Cull, Braverman, Chen, and Comings (1996) support a *reward-deficiency theory* that states that specific human genes are linked to biochemical reward and reinforcement mechanisms in the brain, which are in turn associated with impulsive or addictive behaviors (e.g., problem gambling, alcoholism, attention-deficient disorder). If a chemical imbalance occurs in the reward system, the brain may substitute craving and compulsive behaviors for satiation. Comings et al. (1996), for example, found that 50% of a sample of white problem gamblers had a genetic anomaly that interferes with the brain's reward process, implying that a deficiency in the brain's reward process could be one potential explanation for the development of impulsive or addictive behaviors, and the apparent comorbidity of ADHD and gambling behavior.

Very few studies have investigated the link between problem gambling and the presence of ADHD. Do causal gamblers and problem gamblers exhibit the same rate of ADHD, or do certain types of gamblers exhibit higher rates of ADHD? Does ADHD typically occur before the development of a gambling problem or afterwards? Do people with childhood ADHD have a more severe gambling problem than people who develop it later in life? These are important empirical questions that need to be addressed more fully in future research.

Narcissism

In general, a narcissistic individual has airs of self-assurance and deficient social conscience, and is interpersonally exploitive. The DSM-IV describes three personality clusters, with narcissistic personality disorder (NPD) included in the "dramatic cluster." Individuals in this cluster are often described as dramatic, emotional, and erratic; some characteristics include impulsivity, disinhibition, affective instability (e.g., marked shifts in mood in response to environmental stimuli), personal rejection, criticisms and ego-threat, and intolerance for frustration. The other personality disorders in this category are antisocial, borderline, and histrionic personality disorders.

The particular question that concerns us here is whether gamblers have a high incidence of narcissistic personality disorder. A number of researchers have explored the comorbidity of gambling and narcissistic personality disorder, and some studies found support for such a relationship. Black and Moyer (1998) studied individuals with problem gambling behavior and found that 20% of participants met the diagnostic criteria for narcissistic personality disorder. Similarly, Specker et al. (1996) studied problem gamblers and found that 25% of the subjects met criteria for an Axis II personality disorder (5% of the subjects had narcissistic personality disorder).

Blaszczynski and Steel (1998) conducted a very important study on personality disorders among problem gamblers. They found that a higher proportion of problem gamblers were found to be within the "dramatic" category of personality disorders. Forty-seven subjects (57.3%) were found to have narcissistic personality disorder. In addition, problem gamblers diagnosed with antisocial personality disorder or narcissistic personality disorder exhibited a greater severity of problem gambling. Further, subjects found to have at least one of the major personality disorders, including narcissistic personality disorder, were found to have heightened impulsivity scores. Subjects in the study met, on average, criteria for 4.6 DSM-III-R personality disorders, with 92% receiving a diagnosis of at least one such disorder. The authors note that "the higher levels of problem gambling displayed by those gamblers with narcissistic personality disorder suggests that narcissistic personality traits are also an important mediator of pathological gambling behaviors" (p. 67). This study provides substantial support for a relationship between problem gambling and narcissistic personality disorder.

However, more studies need to be conducted in this area of gambling research. Reich and Green (1991) and Stone (1993) both show that individuals with personality disorders commonly respond poorly to intervention strategies. An individual with narcissistic personality disorder has traits that may lead him or her to resist treatment, preferring instead to externalize blame on other individuals. Problem gamblers often exhibit similar characteristics, such as poor motivation for treatment, resistance in therapy, and externalization. Therapists need to be able to relate better and be more effective with such individuals.

Coping Skills

Engagement in a problematic impulsive behavior, such as gambling, is cued or stimulated by a triggering event, which may be internal (e.g., boredom or anxiety) or external (e.g., exposure to a situation wherein someone is engaging in the activity). Following this triggering event, an individual will either engage in successful or constructive coping, or use an escape avoidance coping response (i.e., gambling; McCormick, 1994). Folkman, Lazarus, Dunkel-Schetter, DeLongis, and Gruen (1986) argue that the coping efforts of individuals serve two functions: regulating distressing emotions (*emotion-focused coping*) and actively altering the stressful person–environment relationship (*problem-focused coping*). Problem-focused coping includes proactive problem-solving and conflict-resolution behaviors. Emotion-focused coping, on the other hand, involves behaviors and cognitions of escape or avoidance, and keeping one's feelings to oneself (Folkman, Chesney, Pollack, & Coates, 1993). The use of an escape avoidance coping response can create a relapse cycle, and the more a person passes through this cycle, the faster the cycle of engaging in the problematic impulsive behavior accelerates (McCormick, 1994).

Browne (1989) demonstrated that when card-playing poker players felt frustrated at work or at home, they felt a desire to gamble. Thus, when the gamblers were unable to deal with the stress in their environment, they opted to dispense with it through escape and distraction. When asking individuals about their gambling, Dickerson et al. (1996) found that gamblers began to play as a means to escape depressive feelings or to avoid dealing with frustration.

The *goodness-of-fit hypothesis* refers to the relationship between appraisal (perceived controllability of the stressor) and the coping strategy applied (Folkman, 1992). With respect to appraising a situation, Lazarus and Folkman (1984) have distinguished between primary and secondary appraisal. *Primary appraisal* occurs when the individual asks him- or herself whether the event is relevant to their well-being and, if so, what type of stressful event it is (loss, threat, or challenge). *Secondary appraisal* establishes whether the stressful event is within or beyond their personal control and what resources are available to manage it. Scannell, Quirk, Smith, Maddem, and Dickerson (2000) found that the lower the control over gambling, the greater the reliance on emotion-focused coping. In addition, Shepherd and Dickerson (2001) studied regular poker machine players and confirmed that players with low control over their gambling used more avoidance-focused coping strategies when facing a gambling loss situation. Further, they also adopted these strategies in controllable and uncontrollable loss situations unrelated to gambling. To a large extent, these findings confirm that, when gamblers feel a lack of control over a situation, they choose to rely on emotion-focused and avoidance-focused coping more frequently than on problem-focused coping.

Some researchers have suggested that avoidance-focused coping may be more related to certain stable characteristics of an individual than to contextual factors (Felton & Revenson, 1984; McCrae, 1984; Parkes, 1986). In support of this hypothesis, both trait anxiety (Endler & Parker, 1990) and neuroticism (McCrae & Costa, 1986; Vollrath, Torgersen, & Alnaes, 1995) have been found to be related to avoidance-focused coping. Shepherd and Dickerson (2001) hypothesize that emotion- and problem-focused coping are more situationally determined, while the use of avoidance-focused coping may be more strongly influenced by an individual's disposition. Further research is needed, however, before definitive conclusions about this distinction can be validly drawn.

It is unclear whether the use of avoidant-focused coping strategies is adaptive or maladaptive. There are findings that suggest that the use of avoidance-focused coping strategies is associated with increased distress and psychopathology (e.g., Vollrath et al., 1995). Holahan and Moos (1987) hypothesize that, in the initial phases of an overwhelming or unexpected event, such strategies have the short-term benefit of providing a period of time during which an individual can marshal resources. In the long run, however, the continual use of these types of strategies prevents an individual from dealing with the stress, and eventually leads to psychological dysfunction. Suls and Fletcher (1985) conducted a meta-analysis on coping studies and found that, while avoidance-type strategies do seem to offer short-term benefits, approach-type strategies are nevertheless more effective in the long run. Thus, whether using avoidance-type strategies is adaptive or maladaptive depends to a large extent on the frequency of use and the period of time.

When studying a problem gambler, it is useful to understand his or her repertoire of coping skills by looking at three factors: problem-solving skills, personal or emotional support sought, and escape/avoidance coping strategies. Problem gamblers may vary in how developed their problem-solving skills are, but even individuals with good problem-solving skills often do not know when it is appropriate to use problem-solving as a coping mechanism. In addition, most problem gamblers have poorly developed skills in seeking personal or emotional support, principally because frequent gambling often leads individuals to lie to and deceive those closest to them, thereby making it difficult to find support (McCormick, 1994). As McCormick (1994) explains, "A deficit in using emotional or personal support as a coping mechanism is particularly problematic for the pathological gambler who is often faced with internal emotional triggers" (pp. 80–81). Finally, problem gamblers may use a variety of escape/avoidance coping strategies, which often include other problematic impulsive behaviors (e.g., substance use), and may also include other avoidance mechanisms (e.g., lying, withdrawing from a situation, or procrastination; McCormick, 1994).

Shepherd and Dickerson (2001) believe that there is a paucity of empirical data to confirm or reject the significance of coping as a factor in the development of impaired control over gambling behavior and the subsequent management of its consequences. Along similar lines, Carver and Scheier (1994) further argue that the relation between coping and outcomes such as problem gambling is likely to be multidirectional rather than linear. Orford, Daniels, and Somers (1996) believe that there may exist an endogenous self-reinforcing cycle between profound loss, poor outcomes, and maladaptive coping strategies. Perhaps gambling is not the result of an avoidance-coping response, but is instead an avoidance-coping response to a troubled person-environment encounter (McCormick, 1994). Further research is needed in order to understand precisely how coping responses relate to the act of gambling.

Summary

Individual difference factors, such as anxiety and arousal, temperament, ADHD, narcissism, and coping skills may contribute to the development and maintenance of problem gambling behavior. In this chapter, we discussed each factor and its possible roles, but acknowledged that more research needs to be conducted in order to understand better this area of gambling.

Gambling can be seen as a way to moderate anxiety or arousal levels: In this view, problem gamblers engage in a larger amount of gambling behavior in order to alleviate levels of anxiety or arousal. Research does suggest that problem gamblers exhibit deficits in coping repertoires, have limited strategies, and lack flexibility in choosing an appropriate skill to deal with stressful situations. Problem gambling could therefore develop out of a person's inability to deal adaptively with abnormal levels of anxiety or arousal.

Temperament refers the usual mood or disposition of an individual. The avoidance or reduction of noxious physiological states or dysphoric moods also appears to be a major factor in the persistence in gambling. There is some support for a relationship between gambling and mood disorders, but some researchers suggest that the high prevalence of frequently reported mood disorders might just as well result from sampling bias, not from comorbidity. More empirical research is needed in this direction, especially because a relationship between gambling and mood disorders has very important clinical implications.

Some researchers have noted that problem gamblers exhibit higher rates of childhood attention-deficit hyperactivity disorder (ADHD) and adult ADHD. We discussed how neurological deficits could be a contributing factor to the development of disorders involving an inhibitory deficit and a lack of behavioral restraint (e.g., ADHD, substance abuse, gambling); understanding the exact nature and extent of the relationship still largely evades us. We also discussed how a deficiency in the brain's reward process may be one explanation for the development of impulsive or addictive behaviors, and the apparent comorbidity of ADHD and gambling behavior.

Someone who is narcissistic typically has airs of self-assurance and deficient social conscience, and is interpersonally exploitive. Narcissistic personality disorder is included in the "dramatic cluster" of the DSM-IV's Axis II personality disorders, and individuals included in it are often described as dramatic, emotional, and erratic, exhibiting characteristics such as impulsivity, disinhibition, affective instability, ego-threat, and intolerance for frustration. Some researchers have explored the comorbidity of gambling and narcissistic personality disorder, and the few studies conducted lend some support for such a relationship. More research is needed, however, particularly given the important clinical implications.

Engagement in a problematic impulsive behavior, such as gambling, is cued or stimulated by a triggering event. Following this triggering event, an individual will either engage in successful or constructive coping, or use an escape avoidance-coping response (i.e., gambling). Problem-focused coping includes proactive problem-solving and conflict resolution behaviors. Emotion-focused coping, on the other hand, involves behaviors and cognitions of escape or avoidance, and keeping one's feelings to oneself. The use of an escape avoidance-coping response can create a relapse cycle: the more a person passes through this cycle, the faster the cycle of engaging in the problematic impulsive behavior accelerates. When gamblers feel a lack of control over a situation, they may rely on emotion-focused and avoidance-focused coping more than on problem-focused coping. Fully understanding how coping responses relate to the act of gambling, however, awaits further research.

The development and maintenance of problem gambling is likely to be the result of multiple factors, all of which interact in a complex manner. Individual difference factors, such as anxiety and arousal, temperament, ADHD, narcissism, and coping skills may contribute in important ways. However, it is clear from the chapter that this area of gambling research is still not developed enough to draw any definitive conclusions about how individual difference factors interact with gambling behavior.

Chapter 6
Gambling

A Sociological Perspective

Lisa Cavion, Carol Wong, and Masood Zangeneh

For why is gambling a whit worse than any other method of acquiring money? How, for instance, is it worse than trade? True, out of a hundred persons, only one can win; yet what business is that of yours or of mine?

F. Dostoyevsky, The Gambler

Gambling is very much everyone's business, thanks to centuries of emotional ideological contestation, cycles of government condemnation and promotion, as well as licit and illicit commercialization. Although gambling is frequently portrayed as a series of risky decisions made by individuals, it is also a highly social activity, occurring in a particular historical context, following specific collective conventions, and exerting structurally mediated effects.

It would be ideologically simpler, perhaps, and most certainly easier, if one could individualize gambling, profit from it, and then turn it into a disease when it gets out of hand. A person's relationship with risk would then become an individual responsibility involving individual moral questions and resulting in individual repercussions. However, gambling is no less a field for the production and reproduction of society's unequal power relations than any other social activity, and its consequences and rewards are, therefore, unequally distributed in socially significant ways.

This chapter examines the development of modern gambling in North America, which now consists of a variety of commercial contexts for the wagering of money. As gambling has been legalized and institutionalized, its practices have changed from illegal and informal to regularized and consumer-oriented. This development has not affected all people in all of the same ways; the expansive capitalist program of late-20th century North America serves some citizens better than others, and this is as true in gambling as in other activities. Gender, ethnicity, social class, and economic status, among other variables, interact to determine the social and emotional roles that contemporary commercial gambling can play in people's lives. Gambling is very much our business, because society cannot have it any other way.

Lisa Cavion
Centre for Addiction and Mental Health, Canada

M. Zangeneh, A. Blaszczynski, N. Turner (eds.), *In the Pursuit of Winning.*
© Springer 2008

Vice to Virtue: Gambling Legalized and Legitimized

For the past 20 years, the trend in North America has been toward increasingly pro-gambling legislation, pro-gambling attitudes, and pro-gambling economic development policies (Abbott & Cramer, 1993; Morgan & Anderson, 1991; Roehl, 1999). These changes, resulting in large part from the two-pronged sponsorship of gambling by state and commercial interests, reflect and participate in the reconceptualization of gambling from vice to economically beneficial leisure activity. This has resulted in increased access to, awareness of, and participation in gambling behavior.

Gambling, even state-sponsored gambling, is not a recent phenomenon, of course; card games for money, charity raffles, and bingo halls have long been a part of North American social life. However, between 1860 and 1930, gambling was effectively officially abolished in the New World (Abt, Smith, & Christiansen, 1985). Gambling was seen as an ideologically insidious affront to the Puritan work ethic; it was believed to undermine faith in thrift, industry, and Providence, not to mention belief in the value of a dollar. It was condemned by psychiatrists, clergy, and some politicians as a road to financial ruin (Brenner, 1990). These attitudes have been transformed in the past few decades. Gambling is now praised as harmless fun and a financial savior by commercial interests and by (many more) politicians. "Our notion of what is immoral behavior has changed drastically," according to Yale law professor Steven Duek (quoted by the *Los Angeles Times*; reported in Newscan, January 21, 2000).

Gambling regulations, long a hodgepodge of federal statutes, state policies, and provincial commission statements, have always been the result of ideological and historical developments, rather than logical or moral ones (Skolnick & Dombrink, 1978). The increasing prominence of gambling in public life is due in part to liberalization of gambling laws in the latter half of the 20th century. The history of gambling laws consists of cycles of prohibition and promotion; we are now in the peak of a promotional upswing that began in the latter half of the 20th century. The first American state lottery occurred in 1963; in Canada, the major changes to the Criminal Code required to allow lotteries and other forms of gambling did not occur until 1969. By 1988, in the United States, commercial casino gambling was legal only in Nevada and New Jersey's Atlantic City. (Nevada, a bit of a rogue state, legalized casino gambling in 1931.) By 2000, however, some form of gambling was legal in 48 of the 50 U.S. states, with Utah and Hawaii the lone holdouts; 30 casinos had spread across the Canadian provinces and territories.

Of course, legalization is not the same as legitimization; while legalization is merely the formal act of a governmental decree, legitimization is the more gradual institutionalization of a behavior as it is inscribed into everyday life until it seems commonplace, if not inevitable. However, legalization is often a fairly important precursor to mainstream legitimacy for most behaviors, as it goes a long way toward removing their stigma. In addition, the proliferation of regulatory acts and their attendant administrative bodies (e.g., the Gaming Control Act and the Ontario Lottery and Gaming Corporation, respectively) speaks to the integration of gambling behavior into the official political imagination and practices of North American nations. The exercise of licensing and inspecting gambling operators and gambling-operator training institutes (e.g., the Academy of Casino Training, Mississippi or the Niagara College of Casino Training School) inscribes the bureaucracy of gambling into the everyday life of the civil service.

True legitimization, of course, requires participation outside of the officialdom of statutes and bureaucracy. One symptom of a practice's institutionalization is the volume of its presence in everyday life. The variety and prevalence of commercial forms of gambling testifies to their far-reaching social significance. Lotteries, break-tabs, and scratchcards are particularly important owing to their widespread availability in otherwise non-gambling oriented locations (e.g., corner stores). These forms of gambling have traditionally been the first to be legalized in most jurisdictions, and are frequently state-sponsored and controlled. Quick payoffs, low financial investment, and ease of play make them especially appealing to both providers and consumers. Further, their ubiquity and simplicity allow them to serve as "bait," normalizing it and making it more portable, geographically and culturally, than forms of gambling that require more substantial infrastructure (e.g., casinos, pari-mutuel wagering). In Canada, lotteries began as the federally sponsored Lotto-Canada in the 1970s; now both federal and provincial governments back and benefit from lotto revenues. Casinos are wildly popular in both Canada and the United States; in 1995 there were 154 million visits to American casinos. As elaborate, year-round, permanent installations run by licensed private corporations, casinos are believed to offer the greatest variety of entertainment and to contribute the most to the local economies that host them. Thirty-five percent of a total $8.1-billion Canadian dollars spent on gambling in 1998 was raised at casinos (Marshall, March 24, 2000). Another popular and profitable (and quite controversial) form of gambling is the video lottery terminal (VLT); introduced in the Canadian Atlantic provinces in 1990, VLTs are spreading quickly to other provinces. Despite concerns that they are the "crack cocaine of gambling" and despite referenda in Alberta leading to calls for their removal from local communities, VLTs contributed to 28% of the total Canadian gambling revenue in 1998 (Marshall, 2000).

Ubiquity contributes to legitimization by making a behavior an unremarkable element of people's lives. Gambling is now available on airline flights, and no trip on public transit would be complete without the cheerful Lotto-649 and Daily Keno "Winner Takes All" reminders. Commercial gambling opportunities are invariably accompanied by pro-gambling messages designed to promote these activities. The institutionalization of gambling can result from a surfeit of opportunities and communications either via an increase in the likelihood of participation in gambling activities, or by an alteration of attitudes toward gambling. Although gambling attitudes are undoubtedly becoming more positive in most samples, evidence for the connection between gambling availability and pro-gambling attitudes is equivocal. At least one study indicates that there is no relation between the length of time since the introduction of gambling into a community and positivity of attitudes (e.g., Giacopassi, Vandiver, & Stitt, 1997). It may be that shifts in gambling attitudes are due to more diffuse cultural changes in attitudes toward individual responsibility, chance, fate, and finances (as discussed later), rather than to the targeted effects of commercial gambling interests.

Regardless of the mechanism, it has been consistently found that regional differences in rates of gambling participation (and in difficulties with excessive gambling) are related to regional differences in gambling availability (Volberg, 1994). The introduction of gambling opportunities usually increases gambling behavior among local residents. Room, Turner, and Ialomiteanu (1999) found that Niagara Falls residents increased their participation in and expenditure on gambling a year after the opening of the local casino (for a similar study concerning the Hull Casino, see Jacques, Ladouceur, & Ferland, 2000).

Another important pathway to the legitimization of gambling has been through its financial impact; a fiscally healthy industry is a popular industry. Although figures are somewhat inconsistent, American spending on pari-mutuel wagering, lotteries, casinos, legal bookmaking, charitable gambling, and Native American reservation gambling has been reported to total $47.623 billion (U.S.) in 1996; in the same year, the industry paid $16.8 billion in taxes (Christiansen, 1998). The Canadian per capita average contribution to the gambling industries was $370 (CAN) in 1999 (Blackwell, June 22, 2001).

The financial viability of the gambling industries is a powerful incentive for commercial operators to reframe attitudes in a bid for true social legitimacy. This is particularly important in the United States, where gambling initiatives must meet public approval in a referendum. Tactics employed for public persuasion by pro-gambling forces, according to Preston, Bernhard, Hunter, and Bybee (1998), include stigma neutralization ("gambling is good!," to put it crudely), exceptionalizing ("this isn't gambling, it's family entertainment!"), and excusing ("gambling will serve economic need"). For instance, the argument for legalizing or expanding gambling may be framed in terms of a special gambling initiative dedicated to a noble purpose, such as senior citizen aid, support for the arts, or revitalization of a dying city; in terms of increasing employment, developing a lucrative tourist industry, or avoiding an increase in personal taxes; or in terms of serving a legitimate leisure market.

Gambling as a New Revenue Stream

There is a North American tradition of employing gambling for socially beneficial ends; many prominent universities, including Harvard, Yale, Princeton, and Rutgers were financed by specially authorized lotteries in the mid-18th century. Tens of thousands of licenses are issued in Canada every year for hundreds of thousands of charitable gambling events, and a striking number of Canadian nonprofit organizations are dependent on gambling revenues. Twenty-eight percent of 400 nonprofits participating in a Canada West Foundation study rated gambling grants as their number one funding source; 20% relied on gambling industry funds for more than half their annual revenues (Youngman, 1999).

Certainly the gambling industries provide more than their share to the collective purse. In addition to normal taxation (e.g., on corporate income, sales, real estate, etc.), which gambling industries pay at rates comparable to those of other industries, they also pay "gambling privilege taxes" for the right to conduct commercial games. These privilege fees amounted to $16.8 billion (U.S.) in 1996 (Christiansen, 1998). In Canada, 1995 figures revealed that net revenues to the government (i.e., purchases minus payouts) ranged from $626.6 million dollars, or 2.8% of net Provincial revenues in Ontario, to a low of $4.7 million dollars, or 0.2% of total revenue, in the Northwest Territories. By 2000, a record $9 billion per year was being sent to the provincial governments, a 230% increase since 1992; gambling contributed 3% to 4% of total government revenues in 6 provinces (Blackwell, June 22, 2001; Marshall, May 4, 2001).

It is perhaps not illogical that anti-gambling arguments in some states "would be widely perceived as arguments against the public good" (Preston et al., 1998, p. 188). However, "without sound numbers with which to quantify the costs" (Christiansen, 1998, p. 51) that accompany gambling, there are little hard data with which to make rational public policy decisions on economic grounds. Of course, it is possible that rational economic grounds are not really the point. Once a behavior is institutionalized, it becomes self-sustaining and self-justifying for governments, for gambling corporations, and for gamblers. Certainly, it seems unlikely that individual gamblers are acting in economic self-interest; the expected payoff for the gambler is always fixed at a loss to ensure that the house makes money. Some critics have argued that because North American governments are making money from their citizens' gambling activities, governments are too invested in protecting their revenue streams to make rational, critical policy.

An excellent example of this controversy has developed concerning the proliferation of video lottery terminals in Alberta, where the government has been accused of disguising odds payouts and of attempting to "disassociate itself from the resulting financial ruin of thousands of Alberta families ... [T]he Government addiction to the easy money needs to be treated" (Gibson, 1998, unpaginated).

The revenue needs of governments have, earlier in this century, proved to be the decisive factor in arguments to legalize gambling (Abt et al., 1985); however, the explosion of commercial gambling in the 1990s also coincided with a wider social shift toward increased fiscal responsibility on the part of governments and diminished expectations for corporate contributions through taxation. Governments are expected to deliver ever more urgently needed services while exercising intense fiscal restraint. In the 1950s, corporate taxes contributed almost one-quarter of federal tax revenue; by 1994 that source contributed less than one-tenth of the public interest's income. This suggests that governments that profit from gambling are also acting in the interests of the powerful corporate groups they license.

Gambling as Institutionalized Leisure

In tandem with diminished expectations for corporate funding of social programs has been the increasing dominance of corporate-provisioned leisure activity. One pays for entertainment at the movies, at home with cable television and Internet access, at theme parks, at shopping emporia, and on cruise ships. Gambling is presented as simply another form of pay-for-play leisure activity in which the house advantage is rationalized as the fee-for-service involved in any commercialized leisure transaction. The gambling industry has, historically, aggressively advanced this understanding of its activities. Advertising slogans such "have fun in the sun!" (for a 1950s casino destination; cited in Hess & Diller, 1951) continue with today's 'happiness is yelling bingo!' and with Las Vegas's dramatic self-reinvention as a "family-friendly" destination packed with theme parks, amusement rides, museums, and Disney-themed hotels. This framing of gambling in terms of mainstream social recreation is a rhetorical move that affiliates gambling with socially unstigmatized forms of leisure and makes financial losses seem expected, unremarkable, and even peripheral to gambling activity.

Treating gambling as "just harmless fun" expands yet another area of our lives to aggressive exploitation by commercial interests. "Institutional leisure has reduced our opportunities for genuine creative play . . . contemporary people are perpetually bored, dissatisfied, and looking for safe risks" (Politzer, Yesalis, & Hudak, 1992, p. 23). When these risks are made available by government-licensed corporate interests, public policy becomes complicit in feeding widespread cultural dissatisfaction. Economies of scale are an incentive to stimulate buying; if finances are being extracted from the public at too slow a rate, the government is able to stimulate directly or indirectly (in the case of licensing) both opportunity and desire to gamble by increasing the penetration of these commercialized forms of "risky" entertainment. Governmental and commercial interests form a power bloc in which the ability to

> determine the shape and dimensions of gambling markets is shifting from consumers to suppliers . . . the business of risk is replacing naturally occurring gambling behaviors with stimulated responses to programmed experiences designed to produce maximum losses from the maximum number of people. Gambling interests are thereby served, but at the costs of increasing the personal and social risks of gambling. (Abt et al., 1985, pp. 158, 174)

Powerful Agendas Rewarding Powerful People

Governmental catering to corporate and government welfare at the expense of rational examination of the citizens' best interests and, sometimes, of the popular will, is made easier by the use of media, public relations, and lobby groups to dominate public discourse and to relabel government and corporate interests as "community interests." Gambling corporations and governments have the financial wherewithal to distribute their messages widely, to advertise on billboards, television and newspapers, and to produce very "slick" promotional materials (Griffiths & Wood, 2001). An example is the 1981 movement to reconceptualize Atlantic City's gambling controls as "too strict" (discussed in Abt et al., 1985); media were observed to bury concerns about casino management under propagandistic headlines "camouflag[ing] the social implications of Big Gambling" (p. 147). In contrast, the public "has none of this apparatus of institutionalized power" (Abt et al., 1985, p. 148); the public has only the government—and the government, as we have seen, is in something of a conflict of interest.

It is perhaps unsurprising, of course, that interests occupying powerful social positions are able to advance their agendas. However, it is worth noting that these agendas triumph by ignoring and obscuring the social structure that they dominate. Benefits from gambling are unevenly distributed, and is reflected in people's subjective experiences. For instance, while a majority of "community leaders" (i.e., mayors, members of city council, members of the business, law enforcement, and the social services employee community) may hold favorable opinions about the social and economic impact of a local casino (Giacopassi, 1999), younger, female, less educated, and lower income individuals perceive more quality-of-life problems associated with casino gambling (Stitt, Nichols, & Giacopassi, 2000). Gambling expansions do not often live up to job-creation expectations. The jobs that are created tend to require less education, be lower-paid, part-time rather than full-, and employee rather than self-employed. In other words, although the expansion of gambling may create jobs, employees will remain marginal, with low control, low status, and low pay.

Interestingly, Scott's (2001) analysis of the expansion of gambling in Cyprus highlights the industry's connection with politically and economically marginal conditions inter- as well as intranationally. Cyprus is a small, island-bound nation boycotted by the United Nations and highly dependent on Turkey, its only source of both political recognition as well as post and telecommunications support. Cyprus's gambling industry is developing explosively, with 20 casinos having recently opened in its 3355 kilometer-square region. The island's economic marginality makes it eager to satisfy growing demands for casino gambling. Unfortunately, its economic dependence on tourists from elsewhere has undermined regulatory attempts while its isolation ensures that potential gambling-related problems are shifted into its borders and away from wealthier metropolitan centers. Although money does flow into Cyprus thanks to its casinos, "it is far from clear who is benefiting from these flows, and it seems likely that the gains to the public purse are extremely modest" (Scott, unpaginated, 2001). Casino licensees make a great deal of money by illegally reselling their licenses, and other hotel owners and restauranteurs complain that the casinos are being unfairly subsidized and monopolize scarce tourist flights; meanwhile, government quotas meant to encourage local employment are being ignored. In other words, casinos flourish in economically deprived conditions, but their development does not encourage reciprocal development in the marginal environments that they colonize so successfully.

Gambling cannot be analyzed without looking at the specific structural relations in which it occurs. In addition to international, macrostructural developments, gambling is strongly affected by the micropolitics of individual identities and practices. Gamblers are influenced by their economic and social characteristics, including gender, race and ethnicity, age, income, residence, religion, and comorbid disorders. Gambling poses different appeals and difficulties for different groups, and it frequently holds the greatest appeal—and the greatest risk—for marginalized and dislocated populations.

Gambling, Gamblers, and Demographic Variables

Gender

Gambling is traditionally understood as a male-dominated activity, for both adolescents (Adlaf & Ialomiteanu, 2000; Fisher, 1999; Ladouceur, Boudreault, Jacques, & Vitaro, 1999; Winters et al., 1993) and adults (Cox, Kwong, Michaud, & Enns, 2000). Male at-risk players outnumber their female counterparts by more than two to one (Hendriks, Meerkerk, Van Oers, & Garretsen, 1997). In the case of younger people, studies have shown an even greater sex difference, with ratios ranging from 4:1 (Ladouceur, Dube, & Bujold, 1994a; Lesieur & Klein, 1987) to a more recent 2.5:1 (Ladouceur et al., 1999).

However, Mark and Lesieur (1992) note that despite the predominance of male problem gamblers, most of the literature overlooks the role of gender in gambling situations. The relations between ideologies of masculinity and femininity as well as the respective structural and economic positions of men and women gamblers have been undertheorized. Studies have traditionally treated gambling as a unisex recreational and diversionary pursuit (Jacobs, 2000; Ohtsuka, Bruton, DeLuca, & Borg, 1997); however, "given the myriad differences between men's experience and that of women, research generated and executed by men cannot help but reflect men's reality while ignoring women's reality" (Mark & Lesieur, 1992, pp. 559). It is only within the last decade that studies have begun to explore female gambling—perhaps unsurprisingly, many of these have been inaugurated and supervised by female researchers (e.g., Crisp et al., 2000; Getty, Watson, & Frisch, 2000; Hing & Breen, 2001; Ohtsuka et al., 1997; Scannell, Quirk, Smith, Maddem & Dickerson, 2000b).

Gender consistently affects preference for game types (Hraba & Lee, 1996; Lindgren, Youngs, McDonald, Klenow, & Schriner, 1987). Whereas a higher percentage of males engage in nearly all forms of gambling, a higher percentage of females prefer bingo and casino gambling in a relatively safe, leisure-oriented environment (Gupta & Derevensky, 1998a; Hraba & Lee, 1996). Women also prefer legal over illegal gambling and wager less than men do (Lindgren et al., 1987; Mark & Lesieur, 1992). Adolescent gamblers also show gender differences in terms of preferred games (Derevensky & Gupta, 2000); while lottery-related games (lottos, pull tabs, and scratch tabs) appeal to both sexes equally, boys are more likely to gamble in traditional venues such as race tracks, to play cards or games of skill, and to bet with friends (Govoni, Rupcich, & Frisch, 1996; Moore & Ohtsuka, 1997). Interestingly, studies in England have found no gender differentiation among adolescent players of fruit (slot) machines, and it has been hypothesized that this is due to the relative social acceptability of fruit machines compared to other forms of gambling activities (Fisher, 1992).

Some of the gender differences among younger people can be explained by cognitive differences between the sexes. For example, male adolescents report higher levels of self-perceived gambling ability (Gupta & Derevensky, 1998a) and stronger illusions of control (Moore & Ohtsuka, 1999) than females. "The preferred games on which male juveniles gamble . . . tend to differ from those females play along a skill/knowledge to pure luck continuum" (Jacobs, 2000, p. 127). This phenomenon may also underlie the higher percentage of male gamblers of all ages.

There are also significant differences in the etiology of problem gambling between men and women. For women, disruptive gambling is more frequently related to frequent marriage and residential changes, childhood exposure to gambling, team lottery play, lack of a religious affiliation, and armed forces service, whereas alcohol consumption is a more significant predictor of men's problem gambling than women's (Hraba & Lee, 1996). Moreover, in terms of reasons for gambling, men more frequently report being reinforced by the thrill of winning, whereas women enjoy the escape from personal problems (Spunt, Dupont, Lesieur, Liberty, & Hunt, 1998). Our culture's highly dimorphic gender socialization intersects with gambling behavior. This is also suggested by studies indicating that women more often gamble as a result of traumatic events and interpersonal problems (Ladouceur et al., 1994a) and feel significantly guiltier about gambling than their male peers (see Lesieur & Blume, 1991b for a review). Further, a recent study (Getty et al., 2000) found that female Gambler's Anonymous (GA) members showgreater depression and reactive coping (i.e., brooding and ruminating over negative emotional experiences) than male GA participants. Many psychologists and feminist theorists have linked this pattern of dealing with life's difficulties to women's socialized perception of themselves as passive, reactive, and powerless, as well as to perceived and actual structural and economic differences in their ability to engage in active coping behavior (Ohtsuka et al., 1997; Stoppard, 2000). Far from being a unisex leisure pastime, in other words, gambling is a social field in which society's gender expectations for behavior are reproduced.

Several studies have suggested that, unlike other forms of psychological disorders, women are less likely than men to seek treatment for problems with gambling (Volberg, 1994). Mark and Lesieur (1992) proposed some reasons for this: (1) social services or clinicians do not usually screen for gambling behaviors among female clients and (2) gambling treatment programs usually cater to men and are ignorant of the needs of women. When female gamblers do seek treatment, however, they show different characteristics and concerns than their male counterparts (Crisp et al., 2000). Women seeking treatment are older, have less debt, and are more likely to be married, living with family, and have dependent children. In terms of concerns, female gamblers are more likely to report problems with their physical and interpersonal functioning, whereas male gamblers mostly report having external concerns such as employment and legal matters. Again, this female focus on interpersonal relationships seems to reflect traditional gender socialization.

Children and Adolescents

Studies of adolescents in the United States, Canada, and the United Kingdom suggest that most young people gamble to some degree (Fisher, 1993a; Winters, Stinchfield & Fulkerson, 1993) Like adults, the vast majority of adolescents who gamble do so socially (Fisher, 1993b) and come to no harm; however, a minority of young people will eventually gamble to excess (Griffiths, 1995). More importantly, prevalence estimates of problematic gambling have been found to be consistently higher among youngsters (4.4% to 7.4%; Shaffer & Hall, 1996) than among the general population (0.42% to 2.6%; Cox et al., 2000; Ladouceur, 1996). Gambling can begin at an early age (Fisher, 1993a; Ide-Simth & Lea, 1988; Shaffer & Hall, 1996), and there seems to be a link between the age at which a youth is initiated to gambling and the probability of becoming addicted (Fisher, 1993a; Griffiths, 1990a; Lesieur & Klein, 1987). Developmentally, it is less clear whether there is an absence of an age gradient among a young sample (Adlaf & Ialomiteanu, 2000; Ladouceur et al., 1999; Poulin, 2000) or different patterns of gambling behavior related to age. For example, Stinchfield (2000) found the foreseen result that older students gambled more often than younger students, possibly because of their higher level of income and experience in life. On the other hand, Gupta and Derevensky (1998a) found that grade 7 students had a higher rate of severe form of gambling than their grade 11 schoolmates, which can be explained by younger high school students' desire to imitate "older" students as a way to assert their identity (Griffiths, 1989). Future studies should look into both cross-sectional and longitudinal studies to shed light on this developmental dilemma.

Many investigators have showed a link between gambling and delinquent or antisocial behavior, such as high expenditures on gambling, poor academic achievement, truancy, lying, or the sale, possession, and use of addictive substances (e.g., cigarettes, alcohol, and drugs) (Fisher, 1993a, 1999; Griffiths, 1990b; Lesieur & Klein, 1987; Stinchfield, Cassuto, Winters, & Latimer, 1997; Vitaro, Ladouceur, & Bujold, 1996; Winters et al., 1993). Since access to gambling is prohibited by law for youth below a certain age in most jurisdictions, the use of fake identification or lying about one's age presents an independent risk factor for problem gambling (Poulin, 2000). Moreover, the likelihood of developing a gambling problem will probably be affected by the impact of liabilities (e.g., psychosocial risk factors) and assets, both material and social (Ladouceur et al., 1999). Like their adult peers, adolescents who are vulnerable to social marginalization on the basis of poverty, unemployment, or limited psychosocial skills are also more vulnerable to antisocial degrees of play (DiClemente, Story, & Murray, 2000).

As we can see, the vast majority of youth have had some experience with a gambling behavior; of this majority, most will become occasional gamblers. However, "adolescents who begin to emerge in recurrent gambling are not as protected by adequate coping skills, satisfaction, self-esteem, and source of income" (DiClemente et al., 2000, p. 311). Further research is still needed to look into this vulnerable group of people in our society.

Older Adults

Young people are not the only group that deserves our attention; older adults are also at risk of developing serious gambling problems. However, research on gambling-related behavior in older adults has been lacking. In 1976, Li and Smith (cited in McNeilly & Burke, 2000) suggested that chronological age was negatively related to the propensity for gambling. However, with the increased accessibility of gambling, this trend may be changing. Recently, McNeilly and Burke (2000) surveyed 315 older adults (aged 65+) and found that compared to community-dwelling adults, those who were sampled at gambling venues were more likely to report that they gambled more than they had intended, felt guilty about their gambling, argued over money and gambling, and borrowed money from a spouse or credit cards to gamble. Moreover, they also showed different reasons for gambling; the older adults who were sampled at gambling venues reported that they were more motivated to gamble as an avoidant coping behavior (e.g., as a means to relax, escape boredom, pass the time, and to get away for the day), whereas community-dwelling older adults were more likely to report that they gambled in the casino to meet new people.

McNeilly and Burke's (2000) study is only the opening chapter of this new field of research on older adults' gambling behavior. Further studies are called for to help us understand this increasingly precarious group of people being affected by gambling, and to introduce ways of assisting if they develop gambling problems. We have to remember that conventional treatments for adults may not be suitable for the older generation, and it is the job of our fellow scholars to investigate.

Socioeconomic Status

Gambling activity seems to be inversely related to socioeconomic status. Although it is sometimes reported that a greater proportion of people from higher socioeconomic classes gamble, lower income gamblers spend a greater proportion of their household income. For example, whereas households with a revenue of $80,000 spent 0.6% on gambling, those with less than $20,000 had an annual household spending of 2.3% on gambling—almost a four times as much as the higher-income group (Marshall, March 24, 2000; see also Abbott & Cramer, 1993; Kaplan, 1989; Suits, 1982). Most studies on lottery play around the world have shown that the working-class sector of the population, however it is defined for a given society, is overrepresented while those from the middle classes are underrepresented (Walker, 1985).

Recently, Lepage, Ladoucer, and Jacques (2000) studied 87 individuals who rely on community assistance for their survival and found that 12.6% met the criteria for problem gambling, a prevalence that is much greater than that of the general population. This suggests that there might be a strong correlation between living in poor socioeconomic conditions and problem gambling. At-risk players are also more likely to have a low income, to live alone and to be unemployed (Hendriks et al., 1997). In addition, problem gamblers are more likely to have lower education attainment, to live in a metropolitan area instead of an outlying suburban or rural area, and to experience residential instability (Hraba & Lee, 1996; Hraba, Mok, and Huff, 1990).

From the perspective of anomie theory (Merton, 1938), the lower income classes gravitate to gambling because their opportunities to live the good life are blocked elsewhere. Although these findings lend some support to sociological views on gambling that state that part of excessive or problematic gambling is rooted in a poor socioeconomic, deprived background, it is uncertain from the data whether these factors are causes, effects, or are otherwise related to at-risk gambling.

Religion

There is scant literature focusing on the role of religion in gambling behavior. Previous research suggests that high religiosity has a protective effect on other measures of mental health (e.g., Levin, 1994); it is unclear, however, whether this will generalize to measures of problem behaviors such as excessive gambling. Lesieur and Klein (1987) showed that affiliation to a dominant mainstream religion weakens the likelihood of disruptive gambling; while only 3% of Jewish, 5% of Catholic and 6% of Protestant students showed difficulties, this increased to 17% among students connected with no or an "Other" religion (e.g., Greek and Russian Orthodox, Muslim). Other research also shows that a lack of a religious affiliation (especially among women) or church attendance (Hraba et al., 1990; Hraba & Lee, 1996) predicts problem gambling. However, Hraba and colleagues report that although being Protestant is negatively correlated with gambling, being Catholic or Jewish is positively correlated with gambling behavior. Unfortunately, the small sample size for Jewish participants and limited information about the sample's social context make it unwise to generalize.

Ethnicity and Immigration

Studies in countries including New Zealand, the United States, China, France, German, Italy, Japan, and Russia show that cultural differences between nationalities are not significant in most cases, but rather that socioeconomic status within these cultures is a better predictor of problematic gambling behaviors (c.f. Morgan & Anderson, 1991, for discussion). Similarly, the gambling experiences of Canadian minority and immigrant populations seem to be related to stressors caused by marginalization from the mainstream and by processes of acculturation rather than to differences in population of origin.

Canadian ethnic communities face the stressful impacts of discrimination, poor housing, poor education, poverty, unemployment, and social isolation; all of these factors are known to lead to increased psychological and emotional difficulties. These stressors are exacerbated among immigrant populations, who are simultaneously experiencing the stresses of adapting to a new cultural environment. Immigration is commonplace in North America, especially in Canada, where the natural population increase would otherwise be negative if it were not compensated for by liberal immigration policies. The effects of immigration are particularly marked in Canada's urban centres, which are the points of entry and initial residence for most new arrivals. Canada's economy benefits from the influx of workers and consumers that immigration brings; many services are available to ease the acculturation process. However, the process of adaptation to a new cultural context is inevitably stressful, as linguistic barriers, changes in concepts of self and of community, struggles with finding housing, and new occupational status must be contended with.

Difficult transitions to new or marginalizing social systems may predispose individuals to problem gambling. Processes of resettlement expose ethnic populations to further risk of developing mental health problems, including problem gambling (Sundquist, 1994). With the exception of The Report on Gambling Activities and Related Issues among Clients of Multi-cultural Service Providers in Ontario (Faveri & Gainer, 1996), which found that at least 15% of their clients reported a gambling problem, there is little research into gambling behaviors among immigrant communities. However, extensive sociological research conducted in Canada demonstrates correlations between unemployment, language difficulties, cultural conflicts, and family violence as a result of immigration and settlement (Riutort & Small, 1985). The relationship between stressful environments and susceptibility to addictive behaviors may underlie the higher rates of gambling problems among marginalized and minority groups. Alexander's (2001) concept of dislocation, a lack of psychosocial integration following the loss or destruction of one's social matrix, may be applicable here. The First Nations populations in Canada and the United States have been highly dislocated by their historical relationships with the now-dominant European culture. These populations demonstrate extremely problematic levels of alcohol and drug use, as well as gambling behavior; the latter has been estimated as twice as prevalent among Aboriginal groups as among non-Native populations (e.g., Elia & Jacobs, 1993; Peacock, Day, & Peacock, 1999). Jurisdiction over gambling revenue and regulation has been hotly contested between state interests and First Nations groups, for whom it is simultaneously an element of larger claims for Aboriginal sovereignty and a means to access the financial resources of the dominant, non-Aboriginal culture. First Nations leaders in Canada and the United States argue that they have the right to establish gambling venues on reserves without government approval, based on their claim to sovereignty over tribal lands. However, 1985 Canadian Criminal Code amendments that granted provincial authorities full jurisdiction over gambling served to circumvent these claims, to some extent, in this country. Widely varying agreements have been reached between several provincial authorities and First Nations groups. In the United States, numerous legal challenges (e.g., Supreme Court 480 U.S. 202 [1987]) resulted in the creation of the 1988 Indian Gaming Regulatory Act, which establishes a national-level framework for regulating Aboriginal-run gambling. According to this act, gambling on Aboriginal lands is divided into three classes: Class I is traditional, largely noncommercial games; Class II is principally bingo activities; and Class III is the "everything else" of gambling that ranges from pari-mutuel wagering to slot machines to full-scale casinos. Aboriginal groups maintain independent control over Class I and II activities, while Class III activities are regulated by tribe–state compacts. Of the 561 federally recognized American Aboriginal tribal groups, 196 are involved in Class II or III gambling; 309 tribal gaming operations are spread across 29 states and generated 9.6 billion dollars in revenue in 1999 (National Indian Gaming Organization [NIGO], 2001). More than 120 casinos and 220 high-stakes bingo game facilities have since been established on Aboriginal land in 24 states, generating $5.7 billion in revenue in 1996. Much of this revenue remains within the Aboriginal groups that generated it (Christiansen, 1998) because tribes are not required to pay taxes on gambling revenues or on income taxes paid to resident Indian employees (Anders, 1998). They are, however, required by the Indian Gaming Regulatory Act to put revenues exclusively toward tribal government operations, the general welfare of the tribe and its members, and the support of tribal economic development; gambling revenues are therefore often important revenue streams for building houses, schools, daycare centers, and water systems, as well as maintaining drug and alcohol treatment programs, retirement programs, and college scholarships, such as the "Spirit Awards" sponsored by the National Indian Gaming Association. Given that more than half of all Native Americans in the United States have incomes below the poverty line, that reservation unemployment rates range from 45% to 80%, and that life-expectancy averages merely 47 years, the revenue and service boost gambling provides may appear "amid the shambles of the American welfare state . . . [as] an example of effective social legislation" (Christiansen, 1998, p. 41). However, gambling has not been an unambiguously positive addition to many reservations; in addition to the introduction of problem gambling into Aboriginal communities, conflict between states and between factions of tribal groups is frequently contentious, particularly concerning the initial introduction of gambling and the apportionment of gambling benefits. (The conflict between pro- and anti-gambling factions of Eastern Ontario Mohawk Nation members in the early 1990s was described as "bloody civil war" by Campbell and Smith, 1998, p. 25). Further, economic benefits are not necessarily as great as could be hoped; although Aboriginal gambling contributes 200,000 jobs to the American economy, a mere 25% of these are held by registered members of tribal communities (NIGO). Concerns have also been raised about the loss of sovereignty and distortion of Aboriginal traditions that result from the introduction of gambling. Tribal gambling may be regulated not only by the state but also by federal agencies including the National Indian Gaming Commission, the Interior Department, the Justice Department, the FBI, the IRS, the Secret Services, and the Treasury Department (NIGO). This raises the disturbing possibility that gambling further disempowers economically marginalized groups, becoming another form of colonization and cultural assimilation-through-regulation.

Unlike Native Americans, immigrant populations may also need to be educated about the nature of commercial gambling in their adopted home. Cultural differences between dominant and ethnic cultures also have an impact on help-seeking for difficulties with gambling. Fear of shaming one's family and a lack of culturally sensitive and first-language services are believed to be barriers for some ethnic populations, including Arabic and Korean immigrants to Anglo communities (reported in Purcell, April 21, 2000). Overall, ethnic community members have been found to have a higher threshold for the recognition of mental illness, to make less use of general mental health services, and to be less likely to stay in substance use treatment than the majority population does (McDonald & Steel, 1997). In particular, African American women have been generally less likely than white women to enter and to complete treatment (Messer, Clark, & Martin, 1996). Therapists will need to be trained to understand the system of values, rituals, and symbols of patient's culture, as well as the racial, cultural, and power-riddled aspects of mental health problems.

For instance, the Western philosophical view of "self" as a well-defined and distinct entity reflects a concept of the individual as an autonomous social agent. This contrasts sharply with the understanding of the "self" as held in some Asian, African, and Pacific cultures where clear boundaries do not exist between the organic and nonorganic, or the physical and mental. This results in different relationships to causality; whereas Western explanations tend to locate the cause of disorder within the individual psyche, other cultures may be more likely to consider independent somatic processes, supernatural forces, or social relations as the causes of mental illness. Differences in cultural approaches to discussions of personal or family problems and distrust of "mainstream" medicine may be misinterpreted as refusal of treatment or denial of the truth if these valid sociocultural differences are not acknowledged. Unfortunately, programs are often unable to sufficiently accommodate the specific needs of non-dominant groups (Browne, 1991; Mark & Lesieur, 1992; Volberg & Steadman, 1988).

Our current lack of knowledge and cultural sensitivity concerning problem gambling exposes the gap that is present in research on ethnic communities living in Canada, as well as in the United States. Very little research has been done on the effects of acculturation and the differences between Western culture and the cultures of the world. Clearly, there is an increased urgency for this research to be done as both gambling opportunities and levels of immigration to North American countries continue to rise.

Psychosocial Comorbidities of Problem Gambling

Psychological Comorbidity

There is substantial evidence of increased psychological disorder among problem gamblers as compared to groups from the general populations. Problem gamblers have greater incidences of affective disorders, especially depression (Beaudoin & Cox, 1999; Blaszczynski & McConaghy, 1988, 1989; Linden, Pope & Jonas, 1986). The directionality of the connection between gambling behavior and aversive affective states is unknown, but it has been suggested that gamblers may in fact be using gambling as a coping mechanism to relieve dysphoria (McCormick & Taber,

1988). Anxiety disorders are also common (e.g., phobias; Cunningham-Williams, Cottler, Compton, & Spitznagel, 1998). In addition to affective disorders, gamblers also show signs of Cluster B personality disorders (histrionic, borderline, and narcissistic), especially antisocial personality disorder (Blaszczynski, McConaghy, & Frankova, 1989; Blaszczynski & Steel, 1998; Cunningham-Williams et al., 1998; Graham & Lowenfeld, 1986).

There is also a general relationship between problem gambling and various types of addiction-like behavior. Drug and alcohol abusers have rates of at-risk or problem gambling ranging from 13% to 33%, several times higher than those among the general population (Cunningham-Williams et al., 2000; Hendriks et al., 1997; Lesieur, Blume, & Zoppa, 1986; Petry, 2000; Steinberg, Kosten & Rounsaville, 1992). Despite this, most substance abusers do not receive screening for or treatment of gambling problems. Within high-risk populations, the association of gambling problems with other substance abuse may represent a major, yet thus far overlooked, public health concern.

Suicide

Affective disorders are commonly linked with high suicide risk (e.g., Bostwick & Pankratz, 2000). Owing in part to the high rate of affective disorder associated with problem gambling, an alarming proportion of gamblers resort to attempting suicide to escape from their problems (Beaudoin & Cox, 1999; Blaszczynski & Maccallum, 2003; Lesieur, 1988; Moran, 1969; Zangeneh, 2005). The majority of suicidal gamblers are male, with a mean age of 40 years; most are unemployed or from less wealthy socioeconomic backgrounds (Blaszczynski & Farrell, 1998). Moreover, suicidal gamblers, compared to nonsuicidal gamblers, usually show greater severity of gambling problems, as evidenced by earlier onset of gambling behavior and related help-seeking, more frequent and expensive gambling behavior patterns, more relationship difficulties, and a greater likelihood of having committed offenses to support their gambling (Frank, Lester, & Wexler, 1991). Suicidal ideation and attempts are also problematic among gambling adolescents (Ladouceur et al., 1994a), and it has been suggested that younger gamblers are more likely to experience suicidal tendencies (McCormick et al., 1984). Ladouceur and colleague (1999) found that among adolescent problem gamblers, 46% have suicidal ideation and 25% have actually attempted suicide.

Family Disruption and Violence

Although numerous authors have noted the frequent existence of marital difficulties in problem gamblers (Lesieur, 1984; Lorenz, 1987), the existing body of knowledge regarding the spouses of problem gamblers is based, for the most part, solely on the wives of problem gamblers, and not the husbands. For example, Lorenz and Yaffee's

(1988) survey of Gamblers Anonymous and GamAnon members included financial, emotional, physical, and marital problems and sexual relationships as experienced by female spouses of male gamblers. Traditionally, the wife of a problem gambler has been viewed as a victim of her husband's behavior. Wives of problem gamblers report feelings of shame and embarrassment, reduced self-worth, and fear of the gambler. Further, a household with a problem gambler frequently experiences severe financial stresses. Politzer et al. (1992) state, "to obtain money to support gambling, pathological [sic] gamblers victimize those upon whom they depend for money and those who depend upon them for money" (p. 25). These effects are pervasive and long-lasting; Lorenz and Yaffee (1988) show that even after being assisted by GamAnon, marital recoveries seem to include only financial, and not familial, sexual or intimacy matters. Wives reflect a sense of anger and resentment even after couples have been in the GA/GamAnon program for many years. Moreover, Grodsky and Kogan (1985) stated that although the wives will occasionally be very protective of the husband and hide the problem, they usually are the ones who bring the problem to the attention of agencies.

Family violence, both emotional and physical, is emerging as another, deeply troubling, gambling-related social issue (Lesieur & Rosenthal, 1991). Unfortunately, while data on abuse are available, studies on the link between legal social pastimes and violent incidents are rare; a recent congressionally sponsored study of Atlantic City's gamblers found anecdotal reports linking problem gambling with domestic violence and child abuse, but was unable to produce a method to measure or establish the connection (reported in Arnold, May 5, 2000). Extensive research exists that links a range of addictive behavior with an increased likelihood of violence (Cochrane & Stopes-Roe, 1977; Lesieur & Rosenthal, 1991) In one study, 29% of spouses of gamblers reported having physically abusive husbands (Lesieur & Rosenthal, 1991). However, Lorenz (1981) reported that although they are recipients of the gambler's abuse, wives may also return that aggression, particularly when the abuse is directed at the children. In their study, four out of five gamblers who struck their children were in turn struck by their wives.

Women may also engage in problematic gambling behavior as an escape from family violence, as others might turn to drugs or alcohol. Studies reliably indicate that both physical and sexual abuse predispose women of all socioeconomic classes to higher levels of smoking, drinking, and other drug use, probably mediated by their higher rates of emotional and physical health problems (e.g., Browne, Salomon, & Bassuk, 1999). "Gambling [is] a means of escape from overwhelming problems" (Lesieur & Blume, 1991b, p. 184), including traumas of the past, abusive marital relationships, and loneliness.

Children

Children of gamblers are frequently verbally and/or physically abused by the gambler and also by the spouse of the gambler (Bland, Newman, Orn, and Stebelsky, 1993; Lorenz, 1981). Further, children of problem gamblers are more likely to grow up lacking life skills and coping mechanisms; Jacobs and colleagues (1989) found that these young people had inadequate stress management abilities, poor interpersonal relationships and diminished coping abilities, and that they were at great risk of developing health-threatening behaviors. Moreover, recently, Darbyshire, Oster, and Carrig (2001) revealed that children and young people who have gambling parents frequently experience great sense of loss, material, physical, and emotional.

Moreover, parents have a significant impact on their children's gambling behavior. They play an important role in initiating their offspring into gambling by playing with them. Surprisingly, some parents think that gambling with family members is a good family recreational activity and a majority of them report having bet money in company of their children and occasionally betting for their children (Ladouceur et al., 1998). There is evidence that early childhood experiences of gambling for money as a family activity may lead to gambling problems at a later age (Daghestani, Elenz, & Crayton, 1996). Several studies indicate that adolescents who have parents who gamble are more likely to become problem gamblers themselves (Fisher, 1999, 2000; Gupta & Derevensky, 1997; Ladouceur et al. 1999; Lesieur & Klein, 1987; Winters et al., 1993). Gupta and Derevensky (1998b) proposed that "it may not necessarily be the specific modelling of parental gambling that results in similar behaviors in their children, but rather the parental examples of having an addiction in order to cope with stressful situations" (p. 323).

Once their children develop gambling problems, parental reactions are often similar to those of gamblers' wives in that they are overprotective and continually bail out the gambler (Heineman, 1989). "As painful as it is to be the spouse of a compulsive [sic] gambler, it may be even more painful when the gambler is your child" (Heineman, p. 321). Most parents overestimate the age of children's first wagers and underestimate the probability that their own child has already gambled (Ladouceur, Jacques, Ferland, & Giroux, 1998). Because of fear of rejection by their children, parents may continue to lend money to their gambling children until they have reached their own limit with the gamblers (Lorenz, 1987).

The Sales Pitch: Gambling as Escape from Structural Marginalization

It is evident that socioeconomic and demographic factors are related to the presence and effects of gambling in people's lives. In any individual case, it is difficult, if not impossible, to ascertain whether particular social factors determine, mediate or simply correlate with gambling. Certainly, some of the appeal of gambling to marginalized or socially restricted groups, like the fact that it is an easily available source of pleasure and excitement, or that it provides a reinforcing subcultural sense of belonging, are not unique to gambling; these sources of appeal are shared with other commonly comorbid activities, such as drug use. This suggests that gambling may be one of a general constellation of coping behaviors employed by marginalized groups, or, less pejoratively, is one of a cluster of historically condemned behaviors more easily or openly adopted by groups with weaker affiliation to the dominant power structure.

Gambling, as an institution, has its own social rewards, including membership in a gambling subculture, whether as a veteran casino patron, swapping tips with new players; as an audience member for a lotto broadcast, sitting around a television with fellow hopefuls; or as a regular poker-player, hanging out with a friendly group. Gambling provides new peers, a social purpose, an identity, and a private language (Bloch, 1951; Ocean & Smith, 1993). In some contexts, particularly in the popular casino environments, gambling may allow the player to take on an exciting new social role, that of the adventuresome "high roller," who is accorded respect by others within the gambling environment. As mounting financial and time commitments increase the gambler's investment in the gambling milieu, it becomes increasingly difficult to redirect effort toward the world outside the gambling context—a world in which their gambling will probably serve as a source of stigma in addition to whatever self-concept difficulties they held before beginning to gamble. For groups such as women and minorities, gambling may be a temporary escape from victimization by social stereotypes, ensnarement by economic and social role pressures, or from intense guilt from their inability to measure up; however, because gambling is a stigmatized activity, it will in turn draw them further from where they feel they should be (Lesieur & Blume, 1991b).

Gambling as Capitalism's Solution to Capitalism's Problems

Gambling differs from other sources of anomie-regulation and subcultural identification in that it is, fundamentally, about the exchange of money. The rise of gambling to prominence as a commercialized and institutionalized leisure activity has been accompanied, in the past 20 years, by the retrenchment of government and corporate responsibility for citizens' economic well-being, as well as by the growth of the economic gap between upper- and lower-income North Americans. A survey sponsored by Primerica (www.primerica.com), a multinational financial corporation, tragically indicates that 25% of Americans believe that their best chance to build wealth for retirement is by playing the lottery; "those living paycheck to paycheck are even more likely to feel that way" (reported in *Love*, November 5, 1999). This suggests that the importance of gambling is not merely as one of many diverting leisure activities or compensatory lifestyle identities, but as a site for expression of the tensions between the ideological promises and practical effects of capitalist exchange relations, particularly among marginalized or disenfranchised groups.

Commercial gambling exists in an interesting relationship with the capitalist system that has spawned it. Our cultural emphasis on money as the key to success, power, and self-image has been called "the grand set-up" by Lesieur and Blume (1991) in their discussion of female problem gamblers. The North American version of capitalism relies on an ideology that emphasizes the value of rewarding work and the connection between merit and success, but its practice often fails to deliver return on effort in equitable ways. Gambling, because it combines the appearance of rebellion against the work ethic with a faint hope of succeeding on the (material) terms of the dominant classes, has been theorized as a "safety valve" for marginalized groups by some theorists; we suggest, however, that it would be more appropriately analyzed as a carnival-like behavior (c.f. Mikhail Bakhtin). Excessive, transgressive, it allows space for enjoyment and self-expression among groups marginalized by capitalism, but is also fundamentally co-opted by its commercialization.

Gambling can be fun, an enjoyable adrenaline-high, a risk, a rush. People may turn to gambling for escape from the constraints of social roles and/or stereotyping, lower income, and/or highly regularized employment where they have little control over their lives and little option of escape from the "routine and boredom characteristic of much modern industrial life" (Bloch, 1951, p. 217). The possibility of escape exists not only in the momentary fun of play, but also in the potential of a long-shot big win, the promise of permanent freedom from the crushing boredom of a constraining economic system. It is perhaps unsurprising that problem gamblers are often dissatisfied with their jobs (Politzer et al., 1992). With enough money, one never has to go back to the late-night clerk job with the oppressive manager; with enough money, one can reinvent oneself permanently.

Those most in need of reinventing themselves, of course, are generally those with the least ability to do so. Gambling promises an equal-opportunity "out" from social and economic constraints; "the belief that chance works equally in favor of each one of the contestants in a gambling venture sustains the hope for status or rewards, which the individual feels may not be achieved through conventional and acceptable channels" (Bloch, 1951, p. 218). In some ways, the gambler's reliance on chance, their "why not me, too?", is transgressive. Their insistence that they can and should be given something for nothing has historically been perceived as an affront to the capitalist relations insofar as it undermines the work ethic and exchange rationality.

> To many Americans, economists among them, fun is something people really should not have—because they should be working. Hard. In the Puritan worldview, money is work's reward, one sign of a virtuous life—not something to play with in a casino or to be accumulated through the chance operation of a lottery. (Christiansen, 1998, p. 42)

Interestingly, however, this form of transgression is exploited in two ways by commercial gambling organizations. First, the impulse to demand one's own shot at "being a winner" and to reject the ethos of work is cleverly used to spur gambling behavior. "Social class differences are explicitly recognized and exploited" in gambling advertisements (Hess & Diller, 1969, p. 26); lower-income and working-class gamblers have been observed to place a higher premium on "prestige" orientations (e.g., elaborate architecture, decorating, complimentary services, etc.) than do those from higher classes (Abt, Smith, & Christiansen, 1985). This is exploited by casinos' practice of "comping" players (i.e., providing free food, rooms, and services to make guests feel "special" and therefore more inclined to stay in the casino), as well as the use of "luck" and "wealth" as common lotto and scratchcard themes. A promotional e-mail from Windows Casino, an Internet gambling site, is particularly direct in its use of these appeals:

Tired of being a nobody?? Feeling like everyone is out to get you? Are You a loser? With Online Gambling, You CAN be a winner TODAY!! ... All day at work, sitting in your cubicle, not playing solitaire, instead you'll be playing hard-core casino blackjack!! (available online July 15, 2001)

A silent protest against work can be combined with a chance to win big, because winning big means never having to work again.

Interestingly, however, these beliefs in the neutrality of chance echo the beliefs in the neutrality of merit and effort that are at the core of capitalism's grand myths: that good, hard work is rewarded, regardless of the social identity of the worker, for instance, or that structural factors do not privilege some people over others. Both sets of beliefs serve to spur individual engagement with commercial systems, whether as gamblers or as workers, and both serve to obscure the systems' structural inequalities in access to resources. Messages of self-reliance and self-empowerment have become even more important as governments and corporations have adopted mantras of flexibility and disinvestment. Our narratives of admirable social behavior involve the triumph of individual merit and effort over whatever social and structural odds are in our way; our hero myths involve the all-nighter adventures of the start-up computer firm executive, the straight-talking, populist politician sweeping into Washington, a successful athlete pulling himself up from the slums. Gambling is similarly insistent on the individual's exceptionalism, his or her ability to triumph over the odds to achieve outstanding financial success while conveniently ignoring the house's overwhelming interest in frustrating and denying the very triumph that its existence promises. In this way, gambling is superficially transgressive while fundamentally echoing the mythological foundations and structural inequalities from which it promises escape.

Risking It All: Chance and Instability

Alexander (2001) has suggested that free-market capitalist societies produce universal dislocation in their members due to their lack of control over labor, land, money, and consumer goods:

At the end of the 20th century, for rich and poor alike, jobs disappear on short notice; communities are weak and unstable; people routinely change lovers, families, occupations, co-workers, technical skills, languages, nationalities, priests, therapists, spiritual beliefs and ideologies as their lives progress (unpaginated).

It seems inevitable that persons distanced from the mainstream by virtue of sex, ethnicity, migration, social class, or age will be even more vulnerable to further dislocation, as they frequently have fewer resources to insist on their right to develop and maintain empowering communities. Commercialized gambling offers a mainstream, governmentally sanctioned method of developing a "substitute lifestyle" (Alexander, 2001, unpaginated) and of simultaneously subverting and participating in the dominant culture's ideological orientations. It succeeds by offering a way of resolving the contradictions and anxieties inherent in occupying marginalized social positions. Lack of control over the invisible hand of the market is protested and reproduced through assertion that we are special, and blessed, before the equally invisible hand of chance. The orthodox ideology is that neither the market nor the numbers care a whit who and what we are, while the sociological trends—who gets to play, and who gets to win—speak very differently.

Conclusion

Contemporary people "appear to be perpetually bored, dissatisfied, and looking for safe risks" (Politzer et al., 1992, p. 20). As a product of an interaction between a gambler's psyche, the accessibility of gambling, and the social context in which the two interrelate, problem gambling reflects both the social positioning of gamblers and the institutional context of play. Gambling, particularly a heavy investment therein, can be read as symptomatic of the contradictions of late twentieth-century capitalism, in which we are alienated from both work and play. As commercially provided, "sanitized but dangerous" leisure activities gain in popularity, gambling entertainment banks on our sense of dissatisfaction and social exclusion.

The institutionalization of gambling as a legitimate, indeed, often state-sponsored, form of entertainment is thanks to the recent liberalization of gambling laws, the growth of commercial opportunities to gamble, and the dominance of the gambling industry's discourse in debates about its economic benefits. The incorporation of gambling into the cultural life of various communities offers socially disadvantaged groups a paradoxical field of play; as a form of rebellious risk-taking, it remains a potential outlet for dissatisfaction, while the fading stigma allows gambling to offer (potential) material and social means of participating more fully in a broader community. These possibilities, however, come at a high cost. Marginalized, minority, and dislocated groups are particularly at risk for engaging in excessive gambling activity. Compared to the general population, problem gamblers are more likely to be males under the age of 30 years who are unmarried or have marital/familial problems, belong to no religious group, or to a marginal one, and to depend more on community assistance for survival. They are also likely to be marginalized in other ways, frequently because of a comorbid psychological problem, substance use, or experiences of abuse and violence. Difficult transitions to new or marginalizing social systems also predispose individuals to excessive gambling.

Problem gambling seems to be more prevalent in "problem" communities, communities composed of people already marginalized and/or less well integrated into dominant social positions by virtue of their age, social class, psychiatric status, language abilities, marital status, or ethnic background. Adherence to dominant capitalist norms does not necessarily serve them, but gambling may provide the illusion that they can transcend their limitations to achieve the social and financial freedom believed to belong to dominant groups. As legal and economic changes encourage the spread and acceptance of gambling activities, these groups are more vulnerable to gambling-related social problems; their dissatisfaction can be made increasingly profitable for states and corporations who are willing to sell the possibility of rebellion through hedonistic risk-taking as well as integration through potential material benefits. It is unsurprising that social positions marginalized in capitalist society predisposes individuals to embrace behaviors promising a material "out" from a punitive system and a way to "beat the odds"; it is tragic, perhaps, that this leads to further incorporation into an exploitative system. We are all gamblers, of course, in some aspect of our lives—but when playing for cash it is always safer to bet on the house.

Chapter 7
A Critical Perspective on Gambling

A Sociohistorical Analysis

Amnon Jacob Suissa

Although gambling, in one form or another, has always been part of the human condition, the current enthusiasm for this kind of activity is hard for society to understand. Behavior that used to be considered as sin, vice, deviancy, and a racket is now understood as a disease, a psychiatric pathology tinged with loss of control or compulsion, for which abstinence is the only valid response if one wishes to be rid of the related dependency problems.

Governments present gambling as a legitimate form of entertainment, a catalyst for economic development, a source of revenue, and a tool for job creation. What was formerly a relatively stable social and economic reality, however, is now being questioned and debated by society; people now question the ultimate aim of government policies considered ambiguous and contradictory.

There appears to be a direct relationship between society's stance on gambling behavior and the occurrence of family and psychosocial problems. For example, the Quebec coroner's report confirms that there were 33 suicides linked to gambling activities in 1999. The last report of the Bureau du coroner du Québec in February 2004 shows 159 suicides directly linked to gambling within 10 years of exposure since the first suicide case registered in 1994. More than half of these suicides seem to be linked to video lottery terminals (VLTs) according to the written notes left by the suicide authors (Bureau du coroner du Québec, 2004). Among the most frequent risk factors identified are the presence of depression, significant financial debts, and relationship difficulties.

Such family dramas, which affect mainly so-called compulsive gamblers, have triggered a social debate not only in Quebec but also in the entire country, where the media and experts call on the government to fulfill its political and social responsibilities in this matter. These tragedies are in fact a symptom of a much more serious social malaise, as evidenced by the impressive increase in the number of citizens who call telephone help lines. In Quebec, since the opening of the first casino in 1993, more than 33,000 people have made use of the anonymous and confidential telephone listening, assistance, and referral service (Bilocq-Lebeau, Cantin and Hamel (2002); Jeu, 2000). It should be remembered that this service is funded

Amnon Jacob Suissa
University of Quebec in Ottawa, Canada

M. Zangeneh, A. Blaszczynski, N. Turner (eds.), *In the Pursuit of Winning.*
© Springer 2008

by Loto-Québec and its subsidiaries and provided by the Information and Referral Centre of Greater Montréal.

In this context, a number of government ministers have indicated their desire to address this complex problem. Briefly stated, the ministers' comments can be summarized as follows: Gambling has always existed historically, and Canada and other provinces, like many other governments, decided to exercise legal and institutional control over games of chance in order to avoid a historical error along the lines of the prohibition of alcohol and the concomitant rise of organized crime. Finally, it is acknowledged, albeit reluctantly, that certain types of gaming, such as Video Lottery Terminals (VLTs), create a larger number of compulsive gamblers, that the chances of winning are very slim, and that so-called compulsive gambling is primarily the responsibility of the person who has developed the dependency.

This finding raises social, political, and ethical questions about gambling behavior. Insofar as the governments marketing techniques, generally aimed at the weakest segments of society, are the same authorities who are in place to protect the population and the public interest, we are witnessing a double discourse colored by conflict of interest and certain fundamental contradictions that should be emphasized (Coram, 1997). Certain questions inevitably arise: What are the lessons we can learn from the history of gambling? What is the scale of the gambling phenomenon today? What bases does the government use to legitimize the current social discourse? Is there a consensus on what gambling addiction is? Are there real but unspoken issues surrounding this complex social problem? How much information do citizens really have about the psychosocial issues surrounding gambling?

Faced with these profound questions, we briefly survey the phenomenon of games of chance. Without claiming to cover all aspects, we limit ourselves to outlining certain major determinants, while favoring a critical psychosocial analysis. In this way, we hope to contribute to advancing the debate on the complex issue that gambling represents.

The Lessons of History: Some Benchmarks

Gambling—whether organized or otherwise, legal or not—has been present throughout human history. Certain retrospective studies of the development of gambling highlight that this activity has always been part of the human condition and forms part of the earliest knowledge we have on human behavior (Bybee, 1996; Castellani, 2000; Rychlak, 1992). Evidence of the popularity of gaming has been discovered in all cultures and societies. For example, the first version of the shell game was engraved on a wall of a cemetery vault in Egypt dated 2500 B.C.. Recent excavations in London revealed vestiges of dice games from 2000 years B.C.. In the 1st century B.C., the Chinese were already playing keno, and many cultures, including the Hebrews, Japanese, Indians, German tribes, Greeks, and Romans, left evidence of gaming.

The history of gambling legislation is another valuable source of information on landmarks that have influenced the current situation around the world.

According to Preston, Bernhard, Hunter, and Bybee (1998), governments have swung between promoting and prohibiting gambling, in cyclical fluctuations that have repeated throughout history and into the 20th century. From the gambling regulation commission in India in 321 B.C. to the modern legal infrastructure in place at the beginning of the third millennium, the debate over games of chance has always been topical.

In Europe, and particularly in France, royal lotteries were an important source of revenue. Under François I in 1539, they were applied to finance the state's debts; under Louis XIV, they were used to build churches. In England, the statutory decrees passed by Charles II in 1661 introduced regulations against the kinds of fraud or cheating associated with gambling. To promote the work ethic, England prohibited gambling in the 19th century. According to Munting (1996), the popular forms of gambling in the 20th century are most evident during the period between the two world wars, when the working classes saw them as a response to the difficult social and economic conditions in which they lived. To a certain extent, similar contexts prevailed in Italy, Spain, and most of Europe. However, it should be emphasized that, although certain European countries already had casinos, they were generally small, highly taxed, and reserved for the elite.

In China, the famous courtesan houses of Shanghai in the 19th and 20th centuries played a role fairly similar to that of the casini in Italy. Primarily attended by the male, urban Chinese elite, these houses were places where gambling played a predominant social role. Where brothels lived off the sale of sexual services, the courtesan houses derived the majority of their revenues from gambling sessions and banquets (Henriot, 1999).

On the other side of the Atlantic, the clash between supporters of the moral discourse, who intended to dissuade people from gambling, and those who preached economic development through games of chance was already clearly apparent in the North American colonies. The first laws and regulations in the new world were created by the Puritans, and consequently reflected the sacred values of the Protestant ethic. As early as 1660, bettors were punished in the colonies and subjected to public flogging. The authorities feared that, if people were able to become rich without working, the value of work would be undermined. From this point of view, reliance on fate and games with an arbitrary outcome was prohibited as being a violation of Holy Scripture. Until 1860, anti-gambling laws dominated most of the American states. However, a double standard became the norm. Thus, in 1889, Methodist ministers denounced the Louisiana State Lottery as evil, whereas other lotteries were allowed in order to build roads; revitalize cities and their public water supply systems; or make donations to the great universities, such as Harvard, Yale, Princeton, Rutgers, Kings College, and Dartmouth. On one hand, gaming was seen as a danger and a potential source of social disorder; on the other hand, accommodations and exceptions were granted depending on the circumstances and the power of the social and political actors involved.

This context is somewhat similar to that experienced in North America during Prohibition. On one hand, the Anti-Saloon League in the early 20th century was supported by major corporations, industries, jurists, and the mainly Protestant clergy who had promoted Prohibition. This movement carried out sophisticated, modern lobbying efforts to crystallize its strategic alliances in 1915. On the other hand, we find that the AAPA (Association Against the Prohibition Amendment), which opposed Prohibition, was formed only in 1926. This organization was financed by such companies as General Motors, DuPont Chemicals, American Telephone and Telegraph, Pacific Railroad, General Electric, Boeing Aircraft, and U.S. Steel. It was only in 1932, the worst year of the Great Depression, that Prohibition was repealed. The important point in the case of alcohol is that the working classes constituted a political, economic, and social force that skillfully exercised the powers they were granted in the "game of politics." Now, however, although the underprivileged classes are proportionately more affected by the psychosocial and economic problems related to gambling, they lack the political or social weight to impact the situation.

As for the anti-gambling movement, it was founded in 1890 and became more widespread in 1946. As an organization whose mission was to provide ideological legitimization for the legislative actions of governments, this movement succeeded in publicizing the idea that gambling should be prohibited and the population educated in other leisure activities. It should be recalled that, as with alcohol in Europe and North America during the same period, the interventions undertaken by governments in alliance with major corporations were primarily intended to control the actions of the working classes, who were seen as a labor force that had to be retained if industrialization was to continue successfully. As an illustration of this social control over the working classes, consider the significant number of police arrests in Manchester, where most files concerned members of the lower classes (Clapson, 1992).

It was not until the 20th century and the influence of psychoanalytic literature that the idea of gambling as a mental pathology emerged. It should be remembered that in the 1950s gambling was considered to be an illegal activity, with the emphasis being on law and religion. With the exception of the casinos in Las Vegas and certain Catholic churches, this type of discourse viewed gambling as a rational activity intentionally and consciously undertaken by the gambler. It was only with Bergler in 1936 and 1958 and Rosenthal in 1985 and 1987 that excessive gambling came to be considered as the expression of psychic masochism and an unconscious will to lose. In 1943, Edmund Bergler's article "The gambler: A misunderstood neurosis" appeared in the journal *Criminal Psychopathology* and marked the beginnings of a new conception of gambling; this landmark article stimulated several other publications that were also to become landmarks in the expansion of the medical model as applied to gambling. From the Freudian analysis of Dostoevsky to the psychodynamics of gambling, the 1940s and 1950s were to be characterized by the introduction of Bergler's line of thought, culminating with the appearance in 1958 of his classic book *The Psychology of Gambling*. Moving beyond the moral weakness generally associated with gamblers, Bergler defended the hypothesis that gamblers suffered from neurosis accompanied by an unconscious wish to lose, thereby situating this condition outside the framework of vice and sin. Understood as manifesting a psychological disease, gamblers gradually came to fill the role of sick people—Parsons' sick role (Parsons, 1975). As in the case of Jellinek and the social construction of alcoholism (Jellinek, 1960), we have seen a similar transformation of the labeling of pathological gambling as a disease of the mind.

It was only in 1931 that gaming was officially legalized in Nevada. It should be remembered that at the end of the 1920s, the Depression was a major factor behind the recourse to gambling as a strategy for getting through the financial crisis. Since then, the Nevada model has become the norm across North America and the rest of the world, through the implementation of laws and regulations designed to allow the creation of casinos and gaming rooms.

In 1957, Gamblers Anonymous was founded by two former gamblers in Los Angeles. Similar to the situation with alcoholism in North America and the foundation of Alcoholics Anonymous, this mutual-assistance movement received the support of the country's medical authorities. In 1972, the National Council on Problem Gambling was founded by Gamblers Anonymous with the cooperation of the medical profession, the clergy, lawyers' associations, and other leading authorities. It was in this context that the medical discourse associating dependency on gambling with a disease arose; in 1980, compulsive gambling was listed as a psychiatric disorder and pathology in the DSM- III (Diagnostic and Statistical Manual of Mental Disorders, Third Edition).

In summary, behavior that used to be considered as sin, vice, deviancy, and a racket is now understood as a disease, a psychiatric pathology tinged with loss of control or compulsion. Further, and insofar as a particular behavior is deemed to be socially undesirable or deviant by the groups of people who generally have the power to define what is socially acceptable and what is not, can we not say that the problem of so-called compulsive gambling is more of a social and historical construct than the product of an individual pathology?

The Scale of the Gambling Phenomenon: An Explosive Social Reality

In the field of gambling, one finds a widespread reform movement that is supported on two main pillars. On one hand, there is the currently dominant North American discourse associating gambling with a disease or pathology, which to some extent removes any responsibility from governments—it is all a matter of individual weakness. On the other hand, we see the social and institutional process of legalizing and socializing games of chance, which has become a major instrument of ideological legitimization for politicians, the private casino industry, and many native communities in North America. Some of these communities do not hesitate to speak of success in terms of opportunities, economic development and job creation, whereas others view gambling as a reason why families, communities, society, and even native identity break down.

In the past few decades, we have seen an unprecedented increase in access to legal forms of gambling in North America. The legalization of games of chance picked up steam mostly as the result of the legitimating of gambling as a socially acceptable leisure activity, and in response to budget cuts by federal governments and a decline in tax revenues at the provincial level. In Canada, the 1969 reform of the *Criminal Code* allowed provinces to legalize games of chance. In 1996, the report of the National Council of Welfare revealed that more than half of Canadians had gambled at least occasionally, with a significant number of people playing weekly (National Council of Welfare, 1996).

According to various sources, the amounts spent on gambling activities in Canada amount to between $20 and $30 billion, including $4.6 billion on lotteries; in the United States the amount of money legally invested in this industry has increased 3,000% in 20 years (Canadian Foundation on Compulsive Gambling, 1999, p. 12; Peacock et al., 1999, p. 7). In 1996 alone Americans spent $586.5 billion on gambling activities (Pasternak, 1997).

The last report by Azmier, Clemens, Dickey, Kelly, and Todosichuk (2001) updates very well the global portrait of the gambling industry. These authors demonstrate that the gross income from gambling in Canada is $9.040 billion, leaving a $5.561 billion net; these amounts will soon surpass the total revenue from the taxes on gas. The average loss by province and by adult is $491.00 in Manitoba, followed by Quebec with $475.00, and the lowest in Prince Edward Island, with $277.00. With its 14,700 VLT machines, Quebec occupies the first place in regard to income, with $553 million and 40% of the total number of VLT machines in the country, followed by Alberta with $525 million.

In terms of job creation, this increase is also reflected in an increase in the number of Canadians working in the industry, from 8262 in 1985 to 24,297 twelve years later. This context, which is perceived as favorable, led to casinos being opened across the country: in Ontario (Windsor, Orillia, Niagara Falls, Gloucester), Quebec (Montreal, Hull, Charlevoix), Nova Scotia (Halifax and Sydney), Manitoba (Winnipeg), Saskatchewan (Regina), and several native communities.

According to Topp and Charpentier (2000), Loto-Québec's 1998–1999 fiscal year posted record sales of more than $3 billion, with net income of $1.2 billion for the public purse. In a more recent portrait, the income for 2003 was $3.700 billion, where $1.800 billion of these revenues came from the sale of lottery tickets, $1.1 billion from VLTs, and $747 million from the casinos (Castonguay, 2004).

Although some economic benefit seems to result from the legal introduction of games of chance, many individuals, organizations, and communities oppose the proliferation of casinos, lotteries of all kinds, VLTs, and slot machines. For a variety of reasons, from religious beliefs to the negative social impacts on people who develop dependency problems, some people see the expansion of gaming spaces as government or private-sector exploitation of those least able to afford it or, as Eadington (1995) would say, a "tax on stupidity." Further, surveys carried out in the United States for some 30 years show that poor people invest a greater percentage of their income in lotteries and other types of gambling than the more prosperous (Brenner & Brenner, 1993).

There are also said to be negative consequences related to the dismantling of existing community networks and social and family ties, which may be reflected in the ever-increasing number of homeless people with a history of compulsive gambling (Castellani et al., 1996), psychiatric comorbidity, and attempted suicide (Black & Moyer, 1998). Young people, women, natives, and seniors are said to be the social groups most affected by the increase in and impact of gambling (Mandal & Vander Doelen, 1999; National Council of Welfare, 1996).

In addition, pathological gamblers in treatment are thought to be five to ten times more likely to have a comorbid alcohol or drug addiction compared with the general population (Daghestani, Elenz, & Crayton, 1996). From this perspective, an Alberta study revealed that 63.3% of compulsive gamblers were alcoholics, compared to 19% of the general population; in addition, 23.3% of people with a gambling problem were addicted to drugs, compared to 6.3% in the general population (Bland, Newman, Orr, and Stebelsky, 1993). Gaming intensity is also correlated with tobacco and alcohol abuse among young adults at university (Lesieur et al., 1991).

From an economic point of view, there is no doubt that games of chance represent an excellent investment for private financial groups that excel in social marketing and the promotion of gambling facilities presented as a unique opportunity for economic development and tourism. From a social and political point of view, however, some commentators view the current situation as a symptom of "political bankruptcy," insofar as no real debate has taken place concerning the ambiguous nature of the government's role, and the social dimensions of the phenomenon are placed on the back burner. In this regard, the study by Govoni (1998) on the impact of casinos on Windsor, Ontario, shows that psychosocial problems related to gambling have increased sharply in the last two decades. Thus, increased access to casinos explains the correlation with the increased prevalence of gambling dependency problems and of behaviors considered to be pathological. As early as 1976, a nationwide scientific study of gambling behavior in the United States demonstrated that, in Las Vegas, generalized access to various forms of gambling was reflected in a rate of gambling dependency three times higher than the national average (U.S. Commission on the Review of the National Policy Towards Gambling, 1976).

The Concept of Addiction: At the Heart of the Debate

Scientific studies of the prevalence of pathological gaming around the world are based on the use of two main tools to assess the scope of the phenomenon: the DSM-IV, the Diagnostic and Statistical Manual of Mental Disorders used by the American Psychiatric Association, and the SOGS, or South Oaks Gambling Screen. Today, these two instruments are the official references utilized when one wishes to evaluate situations of abuse and addiction in the world of gambling. Although they are able to provide certain information that is useful in understanding the personal situation of a particular client, these tools are still clearly incomplete and insufficient for diagnostic evaluation. For example, clients are always alone when they complete their questionnaires, and there are no questions about family context despite the belief that family context is an important marker in the dynamic surrounding the onset, continuance, and termination of gambling.

It should be noted that the SOGS was developed based on the criteria used by the American Psychiatric Association in the DSM-IV. Even though the revised version produced in 1991 incorporates the gambler's past and current problems into the criteria, the application of the tool will differ depending on context and environment. Thus, certain Canadian provinces, such as Quebec, prefer the original screen, while others, such as Ontario and Manitoba, opt for the revised one (National

Council of Welfare, 1996). Although there have been attempts to apply the SOGS to different cultural contexts, such as the Chinese (Blaszczynski, Huynh, Dumlao, and Farrell, 1998), Turkish (Duvarci, Varan, Coskumol, and Ersoy, 1997), or Cretan (Malaby, 1999) communities, it remains the case that the values attributed to the unpredictability, randomness, and arbitrariness of gambling are undeniably part of a specific cultural framework with its own historical and social milestones. One may therefore question the validity of these instruments at the international level, insofar as they take no account of the sociocultural contexts and values that are associated with the reasons, choices, and motives for using or abusing games of chance.

Lately, Ladouceur, Stinchfield, and Turner (2001) proposed the Canadian Problem Gambling Index in the hopes of developing a new and more meaningful measure of problem gambling for use in general population surveys. This tool will include more indicators of the social and environmental context of gambling and problem gambling behavior. Although there is a desire to complete a more global portrait of the gambling addiction process, we cannot say at this stage that the conception of gambling addiction is shifting from an individual pathology/excessive gaming to a multifactorial reality and to a psychosocial phenomenon. For example, while the governments are the principal actors in terms of institutions and structures that favor addiction behaviors, it is never considered as an active and producing factor in the prevalence and incidence of gambling abuse.

This lack of agreement concerning the concept of addiction in the definition and evaluation of drug addictions in general has an influence on studies of the prevalence of gambling. For example, some Canadian studies point out that adult participation in gaming activities declined between 1994 and 1998, as did the percentage of compulsive gamblers, from 5.4% to 4.8% (Alberta Alcohol and Drug Abuse Commission, 1994). On the other hand, the results of studies by the National Council of Welfare (1996) and Ladouceur (1996) show that, on the contrary, Alberta had the highest rate of problem (4%) and pathological gamblers (1.4%)—for a total of 5.4%—of any province in the country.

How are we to interpret these results, given that the prevalence rate for compulsive gamblers is recruited from precisely those persons who have developed psychosocial gambling dependency problems? Govoni's research (1998) provides a good illustration of the apparently contradictory fact that the number of problem gamblers increases in direct correlation with increased access to gambling. Thus, the proportion of the adult population in Windsor who had played games of chance increased from 66% before the casino was opened to 82% afterwards. Similarly, the Room, Turner, and Ialomiteau (1998) study on the Niagara region in Ontario confirmed the same trend: there was an increase in the number of compulsive gamblers and new social problems, owing mainly to increased access to casinos. Another paradox found by this study is that 75% of Niagara residents are in favor of retaining casinos, even though they know that this is creating social problems in their community. The same trend of results was revealed by the May 2001 referendum in New Brunswick, where the population decided—by a very slim margin (53% to 47%)—to retain VLTs in the province.

As for young people, research done in Canada and the United States reveals that between 9.9% and 14.2% of the adolescent population shows symptoms of problems related to gambling, with 4. 4% to 7.4% meeting the criteria for pathological gambling (Gupta & Derevensky, 1998a; Peacock, Day, & Peacock, 1999). In Canada, according to the report by the National Council of Welfare (1996), studies show that compulsive pathological gamblers are more likely to have started gambling at a younger age than noncompulsive gamblers. The studies conducted in Nova Scotia, Quebec, Ontario, and Alberta clearly reveal that the rate of compulsive and pathological gambling is higher among youths than in the adult population. In Quebec, a study on teen gambling revealed an alarming prevalence rate of 4% to 8%, with another 10% to 15% at risk for serious problems (Gupta & Derevensky, 1998b). This trend is confirmed by a number of other studies, including that of Ladouceur, Vitaro, and Arsenault (1998), in which prevalence rates are found to be higher in adolescents than in adults and are also shown to be linked to the abusive consumption of psychotropic substances.

Moreover, gaming addiction is not seen as part of a continuum; that is, a person may have periods of more or less intense addiction, in different circumstances and for different reasons. This basic element in the addiction cycle is well documented by Peele (1991, 2001), who found that people who are addicted at a certain time and place cease to be addicted at a different time and place.

According to this researcher, any powerful experience in which people can lose themselves can become the object of addiction. The result of this immersion is deterioration of the person's engagement with the rest of his life, which increases the person's dependence on the addictive object. On the opposite side, the disease dominant model of gambling posits that the addiction cycle is irreversible, with the idea being of a progressive worsening of the habit that requires treatment in order to stop the addiction. The 12-step ideology and model presented by Gamblers Anonymous reinforces this same progressive idea of deterioration that requires lifetime abstinence, acknowledgment of powerlessness over gambling, and submission to a higher power.

The Issue of Control and Abstinence Applied to Gambling

What We Can Learn from Cases Before the Courts

The issues of controlled gambling and abstinence have to be understood within a political framework in the field of addictions. The interesting thing about gambling is that, unlike other addictions, it does not involve the ingestion and consequently dependence upon, an external substance, such as cocaine, heroin, or alcohol. Because it is a behavior, and does not meet the standard definition of addiction, the DSM-IV officially categorizes this condition as an impulse control disorder. It is important to underline the fact that the diagnosis of pathological gambling is a list of symptoms. Once an individual is diagnosed, the complex etiology is forgotten and the problem is generally de-contextualized. From a brain disorder to a genetic/biological deficiency, the gambling abuse discourse is presented as a disease shaped by two central notions: loss of control and abstinence.

The management of cases before the courts reveals much about this heated debate. Unlike the situation with alcohol (Herscovitch, 1999; Suissa, 2002), the court cases involving gambling as illustrated by Castellani (2000) can be a good source of information and explanation of this complex issue.

In the case titled *United States vs. Torniero* (1983), Torniero was legally declared insane because he was a pathological gambler (i.e., chronically and progressively unable to resist impulses to gamble). He stole around $750,000 worth of jewelry, mainly for his gambling needs. Similar cases, like *United States vs. Lafferty* in Connecticut and *United States vs. Campanaro* in New Jersey, also called for a ruling of insanity. It was not until the case of *United States vs. Lewellyn* that this trend of ruling was challenged. While Lewellyn was found guilty of attempting to embezzle 17 million dollars, the court judges decided that there was not a sufficient causal relationship between his pathological gambling and the criminal activities.

> If Torniero had been arrested in 1979, his defense of insanity would have been impossible; it is only since 1980 that the DSM has included the category of gambling as pathology. Pathological gambling was also being used to assuage the severity of sentencing in both criminal and civil cases. As an example, instead of sentencing an individual to jail after he or she was convicted of felonies, the court put great weight on him or her to undergo medical treatment and to attend Gamblers Anonymous in order to recover from his illness. This shows us that the socioeconomical status of individual can be a major factor in the type of sentence that the courts may apply. If you are privileged on the social and economic level, the response will be more therapeutic than penal and also more private. For the same act, if you are under-privileged on the social and economical level, the response will be more penal than therapeutic and subject to a more public social response than a private one. (Suissa, 1998)

From the perspective of the law, there is also a direct conflict when we define gambling abuse as a disease because the law sees gambling more as a vice and not as a disease. Under the traditional view, individuals who gamble to excess are morally weak and deserving of a punishment; now the American law punishes individuals for being sick, for being victims of a disease they cannot control.

Alcoholism and Gambling: Some Similarities in Regard to Loss of Control

Inspired by the classical studies of Jellinek with alcoholism (Jellinek, 1960), four factors constitute the main arguments of the disease model in regard to loss of control:

1. Aimed to differentiate between alcoholics and non-alcoholics, gamblers and non-gamblers, several research results are not conclusive. By not conclusive, we mean the following central fact: when we put aside the substance or the gambling activity that is common to all the alcoholic and/or gambling abusers, we realize that the etiology of each individual's gambling addiction is unique.

2. The majority of people who develop an addiction toward alcohol or to gambling do it in a reactive manner (stress, low self-esteem, social isolation, depression, etc.). For example, the rates of alcohol consumption and gambling activities among elderly groups in their retirement period are rising while those for younger adults in their 20s were reduced significantly as they advanced in age. These examples illustrate that people can develop addictive behaviors during a certain period of their lives, but decide to change these same behaviors during other periods. We can then question the perspective of the progressive disease, as it militates against the strengths of people who can decide to change their life styles or behaviors.

3. Founded on the belief that when an alcoholic or a gambler reconsumes or replays, he or she cannot stop the process, the addiction activity being understood as an autonomous entity. In fact, by defending the idea that the potential relapse is the direct result of the disease condition, this permits us to evaluate the intentionality and the multiple choices in the decision process.

4. While abstinence is desirable, it becomes a real obstacle when it is a precondition to treatment. Research in Canada and in England supports the contention that abstinence at any price can on the contrary produce a psychosocial problem of adaptation (Suissa, 1998).

5. The value people attribute to their efforts as having a certain impact in the environment is very important to an understanding of the process of treatment. The internal/external control (i.e., locus of control) is a good explanation of the changing for good theory of Prochaska (2002). The people who continue to abuse psychotropic substances or gambling will be characterized more by an external control than an internal. In any case, environmental factors are far from being passive in the production of addictive behaviors.

To sum up, we should emphasize that the DSM-IV and SOGS do not refer to abusive gaming as an addiction phenomenon. It should also be noted that this concept itself is the topic of a major scientific and social debate, since scientists and other stakeholders—for example, government, corporate and professional authorities—are in disagreement. When one pays any attention to the conditions that allow a behavior to be designated as a pathology or a disease, one realizes that they change considerably depending on the social actors and power interests involved, as well as the historical, cultural, and social contexts (Peele, 1991; Room, 1995; Suissa, 1998, 2004a). From this perspective, gambling addiction cannot be reduced to an individual disorder of a psychological, pathological, or compulsive nature; rather, it is a complex multifactorial psychosocial phenomenon.

As Prochaska (2002) demonstrated in the stages of change in addictive behaviors, the perception of self-efficacy by the client is the best predictor of future behavior in high-risk situations. It also illustrates the fact that many people may develop addiction behaviors to gambling during a particular period of their lives and decide to change these behaviors at other times.

Some Markers for Empowering Persons, Their Families, and Social Network

Ausloos (1995) and Suissa (2004b) underline the sadly frequent difficulties that occur in intervention with families and their social practitioners and networks by proposing four parameters that favors the empowerment of persons seen in intervention: the competence, the pertinent information, the time, and the chaos/equifinality.

The Competence

The concept of competence invites us to deconstruct our social labels that associate generally behaviors in terms of difficulties, weaknesses, lack of skills, and deviance. The challenge of transferring power to people in vulnerable situations and crisis is possible, mainly by focusing on the competence. To the extent that it takes some competent skills to keep the psychosocial equilibrium in difficult conditions, sometimes chaotic ones, this postulate invites us to look more at the strengths instead of the weaknesses. Gamblers and their family and social networks change, not because we verbally interpreted their conflict, but because they experienced a possible replacement solution.

The Pertinent Information

This second parameter refers to the significant information that circulates within the family members while informing them about their own functioning. In other words, circulating the information among the family members by the clinicians and the practitioners cannot be limited to gather factual data about the gambler, it has also the challenge to let them discover certain pertinent information that they did not know about their relations before. As an example, a person who suffers from gambling can successfully hide his or her condition from his or her family members for a long time, sometimes during several years; when we see his loved ones during intervention, we can more activate the therapeutic process and psychosocial change becomes more possible.

The Time Factor

The way we live and perceive time differs strongly in cultures, contexts, and circumstances. In gambling, time is not the same for the gambler, his or her family members, and the therapist. If, for example, an individual's addiction to gambling developed over a 5-year span of time, it is unrealistic to think that it will take 21 or 28 days or 10 meetings to efficiently treat the gambling problem. Also, as we cannot objectively predict in advance the time required for a therapeutic process, can we say then that we should work more with the persons and not their symptoms or problems.

Chaos and Equifinality

The concept of chaos can be very useful in intervening with gamblers to the extent that the potential of creativity and unpredictability is infinite. While chaos is more associated with failure, alienation, and degradation, we have to see it also as a source of life, opportunity, and change. In the same logic, several ways can lead us to the same goal and vice versa. Many gamblers did develop their addiction for different reasons and many of them can find different solutions while sharing the same problem. This equifinality concept allows us to be more flexible with different categories of gamblers while focusing on their competences and the strengths of their social ties.

Conclusion and Perspective

In light of this chapter, we see that prevalence rates are increasing over time, relatively speaking, and that they are correlated with the number of years of exposure in the particular community: the greater the access to gambling, the higher the rate. We also see that, despite the impressive amount of research on gambling, the dominant approach to this condition is based on pathology, sidelining any macro-contextual explanatory factors of a political, historical, cultural, or psychosocial nature in constructing this discourse. Up to now, this definition has been the dominant explanation for the phenomenon of gambling.

Today, we question the results of the pathology/disease/impulsion disorder approach to the phenomenon of addictions. Like many other researchers, authors and practitioners, I share the following hypothesis: the more we label people as having or suffering from pathologies, the more we multiply their number; it is true with alcoholism and other addictions, it is true with gambling. This sad reality is the clear illustration of the governments' failure to find alternative solutions to the social problems in terms of how to integrate certain social categories and lifestyles considered undesirable and deviant to the social mainstream (Suissa, 2001a, 2004a). Contrary to the harm reduction approach, where people are seen as capable of exercising a certain control over their addictions, the American medical model represents the most dominant approach in regard to the issue of addictions and to gambling in particular. As an illustration, a review of 156 articles published in the *Journal of Gambling Studies* shows that the majority of the articles focused on the symptoms and etiology of the gambling as a pathology (Volberg, 1996).

In terms of social ties (Suissa, 2001b), we seriously question the AA and GA ideology as it produces certain social ties where pathology can be stopped but not cured, once a gambler always a gambler, your permanent disease condition is here to stay. While the AA self-help groups respond to basic needs in terms of breaking social isolation, providing support, active listening, and some solidarity, these organizations disseminate a certain conception of the human being, a conception where people are seen as incapable of exercising control over their lives even if they succeed in changing their life style or habits.

We also find that how gambling is used and perceived varies over time, referring to social reactions in the public arena which differ according to the social actors and social classes present and the economic, historical, and political context. We also see that, despite the impressive amount of research on gambling, the dominant approach to this condition is based on pathology, sidelining any macro-contextual explanatory factors of a political, historical, cultural, or psychosocial nature in constructing this discourse. In our day, this definition is the dominant explanation of the phenomenon of gambling. From this point of view, maybe we should think of gambling as a psychosocial problem that develops over time, rather than an individual and generally a permanent pathology.

One of the arguments that the governments have been making is that they take responsibility for investing in treatments or programs for people who have developed abusive behaviors; these treatments or programs include self-exclusion programs for problem gamblers, the training of competent practitioners, the removal of a thousand VLTs over 18 months in the case of Quebec, research, and the organization of prevention campaigns targeting youth by means of videos. Although these interventions are important, they are a drop in the bucket compared to the extent of the phenomenon and the reality of the related psychosocial and financial issues. It may well be said that the government is only reacting to existing problems and not preventing them. In the long term, we cannot reconcile the double standard and the ambiguity of the government's role as both gambling promoter and protector of the public, since this is a major obstacle to the implementation of an effective, ethical, and socially acceptable policy.

The question of the social costs should be also a serious concern. The last American research by Reutter (2003) demonstrates clearly that the social cost per person is $289.00 for an economic real benefit of $46.00. This economic adviser to ex-President Ronald Reagan estimates that there is a significant vacuum in the field of gambling and that it is imperative that we take in account these realities for the implementation of the appropriate policies in the future.

As for the history of alcoholism, the medical model of gambling is only beginning to exercise its influence and this is here to stay. From a pragmatic point of view, we can predict that the opportunities for gambling will rise and the potential of addicted gamblers will follow the same tendency.

In conclusion, we can say that the governments are evading part of their responsibilities insofar as they present this complex social problem as having its roots more in individual weakness than in collective failure, while governments themselves are the main operator of casinos and other forms of gambling. As long as these aspects of the matter are not questioned, we will continue to produce more and more so-called compulsive gamblers, and witness more and more cases of suicide, family violence, homelessness, and the other consequences of problem gambling. Finally, some intervention markers should be considered while working with gamblers and their networks. Treatments must include families and their social networks, the view that abstinence is not the best solution for everyone, and the opinion that counselors are and can the best mediators for empowerment and social change.

As Pfohl (1985) did say, deviants, in this case gamblers, exist only in relation to those who attempt to control them. If selling utopias can be good or necessary, we still have to assume the consequences.

Chapter 8
The Marketing of Gambling

Masood Zangeneh, Mark Griffiths, and Jonathan Parke

Since 1970, when the Criminal Code was amended to permit various forms of gambling activity in Canada, legalized gambling has grown to a multibillion-dollar industry (Canadian Centre on Substance Abuse, 1996). Similar patterns of growth have occurred in numerous countries around the world. The marketing of gambling is an important consideration for the Canadian government, as the revenue from gambling activities is touted as being important for the funding of social services. Effective marketing strategies are therefore employed in order to maintain this much-needed influx of revenue. Throughout this chapter, we focus on the marketing of gambling behind this multi-billion dollar industry.

Background

The legal forms of gambling in Canada have been successful because of marketing strategies that display thorough knowledge of the product and respond to changing customer needs. Knowledge of the product entails research into the demographic and geographic characteristics of its customers so that their particular tastes can be accommodated. Although it would be ideal from the viewpoint of gambling businesses if all customers could be satisfied, this is not possible; thus marketers tend to choose the most profitable customers to market their product to (Bowen, 1996). The gambling industry has always used various inducements, techniques, and ploys to attract new custom and to encourage people to gamble. An analysis of these methods shows that they fall mainly into two categories (see Griffiths, 1993, 1997). These are situational and structural characteristics. Situational characteristics are those characteristics that induce people to gamble in the first place. These characteristics are primarily features of the environment and can be considered the situational determinants of gambling. They include such things as the location of the gambling outlet, the number of gambling outlets in a specified area and the use of advertising in stimulating people to gamble (Cornish, 1978). These variables may be very important in

Masood Zangeneh
Centre for Research on Inner City Health, St. Michael's Hospital, Canada

M. Zangeneh, A. Blaszczynski, N. Turner (eds.), *In the Pursuit of Winning.*
© Springer 2008

the initial decision to gamble. Structural characteristics are those characteristics that manufacturers deliberately design into their products either to increase gambling or to facilitate continued gambling. These features are responsible for reinforcement, may satisfy gamblers' needs and may actually facilitate excessive gambling. Furthermore, they are independent of the gambler's psychological, physiological, or socioeconomic status.

Many casinos are successful as a result of performing their own "situational analyses," which include interviews or surveys with their clients to discern which segment of the population their casino is serving (Eade & Eade, 1997). Product assessment is also an important component of marketing plans. This process includes assessment of both the positive and negative attributes of the product in order to rectify any problems that may be present. As a result, marketers may decide to focus on attributes that may otherwise be overlooked or may not necessarily be thought of as desirable in an attempt to capture the interest of those who would not otherwise be interested in casino playing (Eade & Eade, 1997). Demographics are important in any marketing strategy, and in the case of gambling, it seems as though the demographics of gamblers has remained relatively constant over the evolution of gambling activities, even when taking into account variability across the wagers played by differing groups (Hsu, 1999). In gambling, knowledge of "the product and its customers" also includes knowledge of the psychology of gambling. The rest of this chapter briefly overviews the marketing of different types of gambling. There is obviously crossover in some marketing strategies, but most forms of gambling have particular marketing idiosyncrasies.

Racetracks

The oldest form of legal gambling in Canada is pari-mutuel gambling in the form of racetrack. This is where the winners divide the wagers placed by the losers, minus a percentage of the total kept by the race track (Mandal & Doelen, 1999). It could be argued that these racetracks market a certain "mystique" about them, and that it is associated with the glorious pasts of the wealthy "upper classes" who would assemble to watch the horses race hundreds of years ago. In this way, those who frequent racetracks may feel as though they are a step closer to the bourgeoisie, or upper echelons, and the attainment of their monetary goals. In addition, being in the presence of internationally reputed horses and drivers, and within the arenas where the "nobles would meet," allows gamblers to feel they are having a "taste of the good life" that may result from striking it rich at the tracks (Mandal & Doelen, 1999). In addition to the history behind the racetracks, they are also seen as venues with high entertainment value. Racetracks have, however, succumbed to the pressures of the other forms of gambling now allowed and do not figure as prominently in the current gambling culture in Canada.

Cornish (1978) also outlined a situational characteristic that, although not given an explicit name, could be described as "intrinsic association" and is important in racetrack gambling. Intrinsic association basically refers to the degree to which the gambling activity is associated with other interests and attractions. This would therefore include betting at a sporting event (e.g., a racetrack) at which the gambler would normally attend anyway. Another increasingly used marketing tactic is the introduction of newer forms of gambling alongside the traditional ones. For instance, in order to combat their decreased stake in gambling revenues, many racetracks have introduced slots machines and other electronic gambling machines (EGMs) to attract a wider range of patrons. The electronic games of chance were brought in to save the dying horse racing organization. The scheme appears to have worked well. Another marketing variation of this is "proximity play" (Griffiths & Parke, 2002). This could be described as participating in an activity as a consequence of it being located next to something else that the person is doing (e.g., being at the racetrack primarily to watch or bet on horses but going on to play a EGM instead).

Casinos

Casino gambling has expanded more rapidly than any other form of gambling in North America (Hsu, 1999). The basic objective of casino marketers is to invite patrons into the casino, to induce and maintain playing activity while in the casino, and to promote future casino visits (Eade, 1997). Thus, understanding *why* customers attend in large numbers to casinos has greatly assisted marketing strategists in their success. From a "situational characteristic" perspective, casinos are marketed as vacation destinations for those who would otherwise not have opportunities to be pampered and surrounded by wealth. This is reinforced in casino marketing, which also uses "incentives," such as free drinks and VIP service (Eade & Eade, 1997). In the United States, alcoholic drinks and free food may be brought to the table to keep the player playing. The payouts of the casino are sometimes advertised in order to attract those who wish to test the odds; however, individuals tend to interpret the results as indicating that winning is a sure thing. Amenities such as food and other incentives, including musical productions, promotions, and special sporting events, are also important in luring players (Eade & Eade, 1997). In the United Kingdom, research has also shown that a majority of slot machine arcades offer at least one alternative service (e.g., snack bar) in a bid to either attract new customers or to keep those already in the arcade as long as possible (Griffiths, 1994a).

When walking into a casino, a novice gambler is likely to be taken aback by the activity that abounds in the casino setting, for example, the flashing lights, the sound of coins hitting the payout trays, and the people laughing and enjoying themselves. These can be as exciting as the gambling activity itself and provide an enjoyable escape from everyday life. The atmosphere in a casino is one of excitement and activity that can produce a "psychological high" (Eade, 1997) and that can be entertaining enough on its own. The excitement of gambling in itself may also be enough to lure players repeatedly to improve their skills in the hopes of winning, for there are those who frequent the casinos simply to win. Further, a number of authors (e.g., Griffiths, 1993; Hess & Diller, 1969; White, 1989) argue that environmental sound effects are gambling inducers. Constant noise and sound in casinos gives the impression (1) of a noisy, fun, and exciting environment and (2) that winning is more common than losing (as you cannot hear the sound of losing!). However, these are very general effects that merely create an overall impression.

Slots are the most lucrative merchandising opportunity in many casinos and the bulk of promotion is spent on them. According to Greenlees (1988), the variables that are crucial to slot machine success are floor location, coin denomination, and payoff schedules of the machines. In casinos, restaurants are often positioned in the center so that customers have to pass the gaming area before *and* after they have eaten. Another strategy is to use deliberate circuitous paths to keep customers in the casino longer, the psychology being that if the patrons are in the casino longer they will spend more money. It is also worth noting that some forms of gambling (e.g., slot machines) are more profitable than others (e.g., table games) because they are much cheaper to operate. Table games, for example, require several trained dealers, pit bosses, and constant electronic surveillance. As a result, far more space in the casino is devoted to slot machines than to other forms of gambling in casinos. Nonetheless, casinos continue to offer table games to their customers. In addition, many advertisements for casino include images of table games. One reason is that casinos continue to offer the less profitable table games is that the presence of table games might make the casino seem more sophisticated or glamorous. It is hard to image anyone traveling a long distance for the opportunity to play a slot game; but high stakes poker or blackjack may attracts customers from around the world. In addition, the casino knows that some players want the added excitement of games that involve some skill (e.g., blackjack, poker) or a strong illusion of skill (e.g., craps). By including both types of games, the casino can appeal to a larger customer base.

Slot machine popularity may also be attributed to other factors, including the number and variety of machines and games available. Part of the reason is that slot games are easier to play (require no skill), the potential for large prizes, and offer very low minimum bets (as little as 5 cents per spin). These factors reduce consumer resistance to making an initial bet. The visual appeal, theme, and coordination of the machine's graphics with the casino are all designed to attract prospective players while hooking those already playing. In addition, the small monetary investment required of the player ensures that slot machines are less intimidating than tables, which can turn off potential players because of the added intimidation of the presence of a dealer and other players. Finally, there is a heightened anticipation of reward, due to the speed with which the transactions are completed (Eade & Eade, 1997) and weighted virtual reels that cause the winning symbol appear just off the payline much more often than it should by random chance (Turner & Horbay, 2004). Promotional strategies focus on the psychology of the slot players in terms of what may induce repeat plays, including the external features of the machines (i.e., how they look and sound), the perceived entertainment value, payback percentage, and the dollar amount of the jackpots and smaller payouts. External slot marketing, which occurs outside the casino, focuses on factors such as the size of the jackpots or the returns, anything in order to whet the appetite of the customers so they will enter the casino grounds to play. Internal slot marketing, on the other hand, sustains slot activity through slot merchandising and promotion (Eade & Eade, 1997). Other more specific marketing ploys that are used by the slot industry are examined in the next section.

Slot Machines and Other Electronic Gambling Machines

Slot machines were invented in the 1890s. Three reels were set in motion when a player pulled a lever (Turner & Horbay, 2004). Today slot machines and other electronic gambling machines are controlled by computers and the outcome is determined by a random number generator inside the machine. EGMs today are distributed around the world. In North America they are known as slot machines, or video lottery terminals (VLTs); in England they are known as fruit machines and in Australia they are called pokies. It is important to understand that EGMs actually describe a variety of games. The most common are slot type games in which reels spin and the player wins if the symbols on the different reels match. The second most common game is video poker, which is based on the card game. Slot games are games of pure random chance, but with video poker, players can use card skills to decrease their losses. VLTs are a particular type of electronic gambling machine that is generally located in bars rather than in casino and are multigame platforms that provide a choice of several different games to the player including video poker and two or three simulated slot games. They were originally called lottery terminal because the random numbers were determined remotely and distributed to the individual machines. This distinction may be important legally, but to the player a slot game on a VLT is essentially the same as a slot game located in a casino.

EGMs have been called the "crack cocaine of gambling" (Mandal & Vander Doelen, 1999) because of their addictive nature when used by those considered at risk for problem gambling. The high-speed operation of the EGMs occurs at a much faster pace than other forms of gambling, thus granting more plays per session and faster payoff times. Griffiths (1993, 1999a) claims that this feature of EGMs (i.e., event frequency) is one of the most important structural determinants of gambling. Logistically, some gambling activities (e.g., biweekly lotteries, football pools) have small event frequencies (i.e., there are only one or two draws a week). However, in many forms of gambling (e.g., slot machines, instant scratchcards), there are few constraints on repeated gambling, as limits are set only by how fast a person can scratch off the latex panel or how fast he or she can insert the next coin into the machine. The frequency of playing when linked with two other factors—the result of the gamble (win or loss) and the actual time until winnings are received— utilize psychological principles of learning (i.e., operant conditioning). Reinforcement occurs through presentation of a reward such as money. Schedules that present rewards intermittently have been shown to be most effective in facilitating high rates of response (i.e., excessive gambling; Moran, 1987; Skinner, 1953). Promoters appear to acknowledge the need to pay out winnings as quickly as possible, thus indicating that receiving winnings is seen by the gambling industry to act as an extrinsic reward for winners to continue gambling. In essence, games that offer a fast, arousing span of play, frequent wins, and the opportunity for rapid replay are associated with problem gambling (Griffiths, 1999a). The general rule is that the faster the event frequency, the more likely it is that the activity will cause gambling problems. Addictions are essentially about rewards and the speed of rewards. Therefore, the more potential rewards there are, the more problematic ("addictive") an activity is likely to be.

Another structural characteristic related aspect to operant conditioning is the psychology of the "near miss," which in EGMs can act as an intermediate reinforcer. A number of psychologists (e.g., Griffiths, 1991; Reid, 1986) have noted that near misses, that is, failures that are close to being successful, appear to encourage future play, inducing continued gambling. Some commercial gambling activities (particularly slot machines and scratchcard lotteries) are formulated and marketed to ensure a higher than chance frequency of near misses. At a behavioristic level, a near miss may have the same kind of conditioning effect on behavior as a success. For example, a slot machine's pay out line is horizontally located in the middle line of a 3 × 3 matrix. When three winning symbols are displayed, the jackpot is won and thus reinforces play. However, a near miss, such as two winning symbols and a third losing one just above or below the payline, is still strongly reinforcing at no extra expense to the machine's owner. Apparent near misses are also enhanced by virtual reel mapping (Turner & Horbay, 2004). Further, at an attributional level of analysis, the player is not constantly losing but constantly nearly winning (Griffiths, 1994b, 1999b).

Other recent innovations in slot machine design tap into the psychology of familiarity. Three areas that appear to have relevance are familiarity and its relationship to naming, appeal, and persuasion. These are briefly examined in turn.

Naming

According to Costa (1988), the names of slot machines are also important in impression formation. It is almost certainly the case that the names of slot machines themselves have little (if any) influence on gambling behavior. However, when tied in with more recent research on the psychology of familiarity (Griffiths & Dunbar, 1997), the names of machines do seem to be critically important—particularly in terms of gambling acquisition. It is now quite often the case that slot machines are named after a person, place, event, television show, or film. Not only is this something that is familiar to the slot machine player but may also be something that the potential players might like or affiliate themselves with. Table 8.1 highlights some examples of some very common UK slot machines. These are different from a simple naming effect in that they may encompass the whole play of the machine, including features, sound effects, and lighting effects.

Table 8.1 Some Common Examples of UK Slot Machines

Machine Name	Theme Genre
The Simpsons	US TV show
Friends	US TV show
Eastenders	UK TV show
Coronation Street	UK TV show
Only Fools and Horses	UK TV show
Gladiators	UK TV show
Blind Date	UK TV show
The Crystal Maze	UK TV show
Match of the Day	UK TV show
Sky Sports	UK TV show
The Flintstones (Viva Rock Vegas)	US Film
Indiana Jones	US Film
The Pink Panther	US/UK TV show / Film
Trivial Pursuit	Board game
Monopoly	Board game
Cluedo	Board game
Andy Capp	UK Newspaper cartoon strip
Hagar	UK Newspaper cartoon strip
Tetris	Videogame
Sonic the Hedgehog	Videogame
Mario Kart	Videogame

Familiarity and Appeal

The affiliation or familiarity of a machine can be very play-inducing. Why would a gambler play on one machine more than another if both had exactly the same chances of winning? Some speculative reasons include:

- *"Celebrity" endorsement*—If well know characters on *Coronation Street* endorse a game, a fan of the show might feel that it is a better machine than some of the others.
- *Trust*—with an international "quality" brand such as the American Sit com *Friends*, a player might think that they are unlikely to lose a lot of money. They might also think the jackpots are likely to be generous.
- *Experience*—long-time regular players of games such as tetris or fan of the Indiana Jones movies might think that knowledge can their knowledge will help them in the playing of the machine.
- *Fun*—it might simply be that a game named The Simpsons will be perceived as more fun and exciting. If the sound effects and features are novel, cute, and/or more humorous than other machines then the association with The Simpsons will have achieved its goal.

There are many cases similar to this one where it could be speculated that the slot machine becomes so much more inducing because it represents something that is special to the gambler (e.g., a special attachment that may in extreme circumstances provide "electronic friendship").

It is possible that familiarity is a very important aspect of why (for example) media-related slot machines have been more prominent over the last few years. The media theme may induce a "psycho-structural interaction" (Griffiths, 1993) and may result in repeated use. Consequently, if the themes are increasingly "familiar," an individual might be more likely to persevere with the complexities of a machine. Players may find it more enjoyable because they can easily interact with recognizable images they experience. Therefore, the use of familiar themes may have a very persuasive effect, leading to an increase in the number of people using them, and the money they spend. Although there are many other aspects that influence an individual's decision to gamble, the possible persuasive nature of the themes should not be underestimated. Therefore, an examination of the factors that may influence an individual's decision to gamble on slot machines is needed. These are overviewed in the next section.

Familiarity and Persuasion

Condry & Scheibe, (1989) outlined the stages in the persuasive process (as applied to advertisements), which can be adapted to the playing of EGMs. The framework constructed can be used to display the possible effectiveness of familiar themes in slot machine gambling. The stages in the persuasive process have been identified as exposure, attention, comprehension, yielding, retention, and decision to buy (Condry & Scheibe, 1989). Of the stages listed in the preceding text, the "decision to buy" is reinterpreted here as the decision to gamble. The following adaptation of this framework illustrates the point.

Exposure

For an advertisement to be effective, the individual must first be exposed to it. The same can be said for slot machines. Exposure of slot machines can occur at two levels. At the macro level, slot machines are endemic and can be found at a wide variety of outlets and are thus constantly exposed to the public. Second, at a micro level, machines within premises are placed so that they can easily be seen. For instance, in bars, they are usually found near doorways or close to the bar.

Attention

Even though many people may be exposed to the machine, very few may pay attention to it. Therefore, to gain the attention of an individual, manufacturers may use diverse and/or familiar sights and sounds to achieve this (e.g., the use of a TV show's theme tune, bright flashing lights, picture of a celebrity). In general, the tunes are repeated often enough to catch a person's attention, particularly when no one is playing on the machine.

Comprehension

When the individual is fully attentive, the message has to be comprehended and understood. Therefore, as far as slot machines are concerned, if a familiar theme is incorporated into the machine, the individual is more likely to comprehend that gambling may be socially acceptable because the images and sounds he or she sees and hears are familiar and likable.

Yielding

This is when the individual agrees with the message or claim made by the advertiser. When referring to slot machine gambling, if a familiar TV show theme is included in the design of the machine, the person may be more likely to accept fully (i.e., agree) that gambling is socially acceptable because he or she "likes" the images and sounds that are experienced.

Retention and Decision to Gamble

According to Condry and Scheibe (1989), these two final stages occur much later than when the individual is initially exposed to the advertisement. When in the shop, the person must recall the product that may have been advertised a long time previously, and decide whether to buy it. With regard to slot machine gambling, it is possible that the players may be instantly attracted to the machine because they are aware of immediately familiar images and sounds, leading to a much quicker decision to gamble. This point can be better illustrated with the following example.

Individuals may enter a bar, have a drink, and then notice the familiar tune of *The Simpsons* TV show coming from a slot machine not far from the bar. However, they decide not to gamble, because they have never done so before. The following day, they visit another public house, which has two slot machines adjacent to one another. Their "attention" is gained when they once again hear *The Simpsons* tune that they recognize. They "comprehend" that because this well-known and likable signature tune is incorporated into the machine, it is acceptable to take a closer look. They may believe that the gambling process involves a theme based around aspects associated with *The Simpsons* TV show, and because they are attracted to, and "agree" with the "message," they "yield" to the view that gambling on this particular slot machine is socially acceptable. This leads to the "decision to gamble."

This hypothesized example suggests that the decision to gamble may involve a number of stages and that familiarity appears to be the most important aspect. It would appear that familiarity not only promotes a skill orientation once a player has begun to gamble (Griffiths, 1994b) but may also be an important factor in a player's (or non-player's) initial decision to gamble. This line of thinking requires further research, as it is a potentially important factor in determining people's initial decision to gamble.

Electronic Gaming Machines as a Source of Revenue

Despite the potential for very excessive gambling, EGMs are still considered a practical source of revenue by governments, and can be found in any Canadian province with the exception of the Territories, which have no slots or EGMs (Mandal & Vander Doelen, 1999; Smith, 1997). They are unique forms of gambling in their use of credits instead of cash prizes, thus psychologically hiding the true amount being wagering from the player (this is also examined later in the section on Internet gambling). In some Canadian provinces, EGMs are found in many non-gambling locales, such as bars and convenience stores; as a result, the individual does not need to make a special trip to a traditional gambling venue in order to play. Such is the case in Quebec, Alberta, and Manitoba, where the provincial government relies heavily on EGM revenues. Other Canadian provinces with legal EGM operations, such as the Maritimes and Saskatchewan, have restricted EGM operation to licensed establishments after a protest over the staggering amount of under-aged youths with gambling problems (Mandal & Vander Doelen, 1999). Many EGMs are set up illegally, but owing to the sheer number of EGMs, and the time and effort investment required to lay charges against the proprietors, EGMs remain rampant across the country. Finally, most games found on EGMs do not require any skill, allowing anyone to play and potentially become hooked. Because of the growing population of computer-literate young people, there is a higher demand for increasingly sophisticated machines with more interaction and a greater perception of control (Mandal & Vander Doelen, 1999; Smith, 1997).

EGMs have shown reliable fiscal growth since their introduction into the economy. In some Canadian provinces, such as Alberta, revenue from EGMs has become the primary source of gambling profits for the government, whereas provinces that are not as reliant on EGM revenue have lower than average profits (Smith, 1997). Thus, it is not surprising that provincial governments are reluctant to give them up. Despite the evident economic profits, the majority of the voting public is vehemently opposed to EGMs in their community, as the social costs may be devastating (Smith, 1997). Some Canadian provinces have printed cautionary messages on the machines, much like cigarette packages, reminding patrons to play in moderation so that "the game remains a game" (Mandal & Vander Doelen, 1999), while other provinces print telephone numbers for gambling hotlines on the machines.

Internet Gambling

An emerging issue in gambling regulation is the question of how to regulate Internet gambling. Potentially, Internet gambling may be addictive as EGMs, owing to their savvy marketing on Web sites, flashy colors, and sounds. This, combined with the added comfort of being able to play from one's home, has meant that Internet gambling sites have made their mark on the international gambling scene. There are no international borders, nor are there any age restrictions on the players. Many would like to see Internet gambling banned, but its regulation has proven to be difficult; however, security measures have been suggested, such as specialized software for age verification and the implementation of online accounting system to prevent fraud (Mandal & Vander Doelen, 1999).

In many countries there appears to be a slow shift in gambling coming out of gambling environments and into the home and the workplace. Gambling is now an activity that can be done in traditional gambling environments (casinos, betting shops, bingo halls, amusement arcades, etc.), retail outlets (e.g., buying lottery tickets and scratchcards in supermarkets, playing slot machines in cafes and chip shops), and in the home or workplace (e.g., Internet gambling, interactive television gambling, telephone wagering). The type of environment may have implications for gambling acquisition, development, and maintenance. For instance, recent research on Internet gambling indicated that women may be more approving of this type of gambling because it is not performed in a "masculine" environment such as a betting shop (Griffiths, 2001). Further, online behaviors will usually occur in the familiar and comfortable environment of home or workplace, thus reducing the feeling of risk and allowing even more adventurous behavior that may or may not be potentially addictive.

> In marketing terms, one of the biggest issues about offering e-commerce services online is trust. If people know and trust the name, they are more likely to use that service. Reliability is also a related key factor. Consumers still have concerns about Internet security and may not be happy about putting their Internet details online. If there is a reliable offline branch nearby, it gives them an added sense of security (i.e., a psychological safety net). Lack of trust and security issues will continue to be the leading inhibitors of online gambling. Customers need assurance and compelling value propositions from trusted companies to overcome these concerns.

The key to the successful marketing of e-commerce activities such as Internet gambling is a good infrastructure that includes an integrated online and offline system. "Brick" companies can also share a lot of their infrastructure costs between the channels. It is easier to put an Internet front-end onto a good logistics operation than build the logistics from scratch. It is also easier to migrate an existing business to an online venture than setting up a new online business. This is what is driving established service providers into new channels. Companies cannot afford to treat their Web sites as separate entities from their main business. The online arm of the business needs to complement what is already done. Stand-alone Internet companies may have difficulties in getting their product off the ground and are unlikely to succeed through technology alone. America Online (AOL) became the largest Internet service provider in the United States by saturating the country with free CDs and floppy disks. This strategy appears to have worked, as AOL currently has almost one third of all the Internet users in the United States as customers. Internet gaming companies will begin to do the same, starting with the existing player database and expanding from there.

It is still very early days in the marketing of Internet gambling. Companies are beginning to use the brand and infrastructure they have and integrate new services into this. Internet gamblers will gravitate to recognized and trusted brand names.

Traditional gambling or non-gambling businesses with an established brand have a key advantage when they go online. Building a dominant Web gambling brand presence requires the investment of significant amounts of time and money. Depending upon how the issues of taxation and regulation are resolved, the eventual winners in the Internet gambling business may not initially report a profit. The pioneering gaming companies who build and successfully maintain Internet gambling will be at the forefront of a huge business. Americans alone spend 10 cents of every leisure dollar on gambling. The potential for online gambling is enormous. Companies that invest in the future by acquiring customers now to build a brand successfully (possibly losing money in the process) will almost certainly come to dominate Internet gambling.

Internet gambling companies also have many advantages in market exploitation. Web sites are known for their ability to log visitors. Tracking data can be used to compile customer profiles. Such data can tell companies exactly how customers are spending their time online. Companies can also use this information to help in the design of Web pages. It may also link up with existing customer databases and operating loyalty schemes. Companies that have one central repository for all their customer data have an advantage, as it can also be accessed by different parts of the business. The technology to sift and assess vast amounts of customer information already exists. Using sophisticated software, companies can tailor their service to the customer's known interests. However, companies that do this face the "seller's dilemma." Customers do not like companies building up personal profiles and details about them, yet paradoxically they still expect them to remember their preferences and have a detailed understanding of them as individual consumers.

There are potential concerns about the marketing of Internet gambling. Consumers provide information in many ways. Many consumers are unknowingly passing on information about themselves. The most common are:

- filling in online registration documents when a site is first visited
- sending e-mails to companies of interest
- browsing Web sites
- browsing of banner adverts
- playing sweepstakes in which people are encouraged to take part in a sweepstakes by looking at an advertisement and are then asked questions on behalf of the advertisers.

In many of these instances, customers (including Internet gamblers) can unwittingly be tracked by the use of "cookies" (small data files identifying the user, generated, then stored on their computer when a Web site is first visited). This all raises serious questions about the gradual erosion of online privacy. The Internet appears to have become an online information free-for-all where a customer's profile can be passed onto anyone else for a price. Although various laws give individuals the right to find out what information is held about them, this does not really address the issue that allows such information to be passed on in the first place. Customers are being profiled according to how they transact with service providers. There appears to be a big difference between consumers who trust brand names, want advice, and are keen to have personal contact with their suppliers, and people who want to gather their own information and deal as remotely as possible with service providers. This latter group are the ones most likely to turn to the new forms of electronic media. Another shift may come in the form of "permissive marketing" in which the consumer willingly gives information and grants permission for a business to make contact with them about their services. In return, they will expect that all information they receive will be highly relevant to them.

Finally, there is one other issue that can impact on money spent in online gambling and other gambling media. For most gamblers, the psychological value of money can be decreased through the use of money substitutes, for example, chips (in casino gambling), tokens and smart cards (in slot machine gambling), and e-cash (in internet gambling). Gambling with money substitutes such as chips suspend judgment. The "suspension of judgment" is a structural characteristic which temporarily disrupts the gambler's financial value system and potentially stimulates further gambling (Griffiths, 1993). This is well known by both those in commerce (people typically spend more on credit and debit cards because it is easier to spend money using plastic), and by the gambling industry. The abstract nature of these forms of payment means that gamblers may be less likely to consider the enormity of their losses (i.e., they do not physically have to hand over cash). These types of money substitute are often re-gambled without hesitation as the psychological value is much less than the real value. Evidence suggests that people gamble more using money substitutes than they would with real money (Griffiths, 1999a).

Lotteries

The marketing of lotteries in Canada has been successful because the lotteries have been designed to appeal to consumer tastes. Probabilities of winning something on most lotteries are fairly high in comparison with other gambling activities, although the chances of winning the jackpot are very small. It is therefore likely that the ordinary "social gambler" does not think about the actual probability of winning but relies on heuristic strategies for handling the available information. What most people will concentrate on is the amount that could be won rather than the probability of doing so. The general finding is that the greater the jackpot the more people will gamble. For instance, more lottery tickets are sold on "rollover" weeks because the potential jackpot is very large. The chances of winning a typical "6/49" lotto game are approximately 1 in 14 million. The UK mathematician Stewart (1996) has gone as far to say that the lotto-type games are a tribute to public innumeracy! Why then—given the huge odds against winning—do people persist with their dream of winning the elusive jackpot? Part of the popularity of lotteries in general is that they offer a low-cost chance of winning a very large jackpot prize (i.e., low prices, big prices). Without the huge jackpot, very few people would play (Shapira & Venezia, 1992). In fact, the combination of a large number of winning opportunities and a large grand prize is generally accepted as being the optimum lottery prize format (Douglas, 1995; Shapira & Venezia, 1992).

The importance of the big money prize and the marketing campaign surrounding lotteries was realized during the development of "lotto-mania" in the 1980s, when government lotteries' jackpots exploded. In early 1984, when the government's Lotto 6/49 jackpot grew to $14 million dollars, tickets were sold in unforeseen numbers as people lined up for hours in the cold to purchase lottery tickets (Vance, 1989). As mentioned in the preceding text, low ticket prices have also proven to be an important factor in deterring or attracting customers, since low pricing in conjunction with large money prizes has shown to surpass the importance of the odds of winning the particular game, which seem to be irrelevant in deterring or attracting players. Inexpensive tickets with unreasonable odds still sell better than more expensive tickets with better odds. Nevertheless, a range of odds and payoffs has been shown to be the most successful. The odds of winning the big prize are astronomical in a lottery, but the odds of winning the smaller prizes are feasible; thus, many people do not win the jackpot but will still win *something*. These smaller prizes are important in reinforcing the generation of hope, and the feeling of *almost* winning it big (Vance, 1989).

Numerous and highly accessible ticket outlets are important to ensure frequent opportunities to gamble, as well as numbered tickets to guarantee anonymity, have also been cited as important in attracting players (Vance, 1989). Increased participation has also been attributed to buyer participation through the selection of one's own numbers. Although it is statistically impossible to increase the chances of winning through the selection of one's own numbers, since the numbers are drawn by chance, the act of choosing one's own numbers allows for the perception of control. This is especially important to those individuals without control over many aspects of their lives, such as those in lower socioeconomic groups. In fact, a whole industry that includes psychics and mystics has emerged in response to the ideology of lucky numbers and how one can discover which numbers will help them win (Nibert, 2000).

According to Cornish (cited in Vance, 1989), some people have a greater tendency than others to be influenced by aspects of the promotion of lotteries and other forms of gambling, thus rendering them helpless when faced with an onslaught of advertising. In addition to this argument, Cornish highlights the importance of the situational characteristics of the lottery in making it so addictive. Potential players are compelled to purchase a ticket because of many factors identified as being conducive to overindulgence in gambling. The prizes offered, the low ticket price, odds, and so on are powerful when combined with clever advertising campaigns that further the prevalence of chance ideology in suggesting tendencies in vulnerable individuals (Vance, 1989).

There is little doubt that advertising and media coverage have been critical in the success (i.e., increased participation) of lottery. Not only are these forms of gambling heavily advertised on billboards, television, radio, and national newspapers, but the accessibility is so widespread that it is highly prominent in most shops. This means that activities such as the lottery are more salient, and are more commercially successful than other forms of gambling that do not have the same freedoms to advertise and/or have their own television show. There is also another contributory factor that is worth mentioning. Most studies on lottery play around the world have shown that the working class sector of the population is overrepresented and that people from the middle classes are underrepresented in lottery sales (Clotfelter & Cook, 1989). Since television viewing is greater in the working class sector, the impact of television-based marketing of lottery gambling may be heightened for this group. Further, a televised draw (which happens in nearly all countries) highlights the perceived simplicity of winning while at the same time players are unlikely to consider the huge number of losers who are watching (Walker, 1992).

Advertising campaigns are aggressively promoted by marketing agencies as well by lottery vendors. Vendors and advertising agencies are driven by profit to promote lotteries. Lottery ticket vendors take in a percentage of their ticket sales, as well as a small percentage of the jackpot if the winning ticket is sold from their store. Thus, everyone wants to be involved in the business of lotteries, and tickets can be bought almost anywhere. The advertising industry has benefited greatly from the increased public interest in lotteries partly because designing new tickets and games is their responsibility. The heightened interest in lotteries has been fueled in part by the exciting ad campaigns that proliferate the mass media (Nibert, 2000). In a continued effort to increase sales, lotteries are promoted through mass media advertising, in the same way as less controversial products. Therefore, lottery advertising slogans accentuate the positive (but less probable) aspects of the product, for example, the actuality of winning, with slogans such as "It could be you" and "Maybe just maybe." Other slogans such as "Everyone's a winner" emphasize the charitable contributions made through ticket sales and again reinforce the "winning fantasy."

The most important aspect of the success of gambling in Canada, especially lotteries, is the dissemination of "chance ideology," which consists of illusions of equal opportunity of personal success that are spread to the public through images in advertising. This ideology is more highly valued by lower-income members of society because of their limited material means, as they grasp onto any hope that may lead them to achieving their dreams of riches. The relationship between gambling and economic need is greatest when the wager is small and the publicity surrounding the game is high. Chance ideology is also highly valued by the middle-income earning class because of the illusive hope of reaching the threshold to wealth and achieving control over one's fate. The entertainment value brought about by the wager has also been cited as a means of bringing some excitement into the lives of the working class, for they may be looking for a means of escape from the monotony of their jobs (Vance, 1989).

General acceptance of social forces occurs because individuals have been brought up to believe in them. This perspective is useful in considering the conditions that facilitated the re-emergence of lotteries and other legal forms of gambling (Nibert, 2000). The images that form in people's minds after being exposed to ad campaigns for lotteries disguise the real lack of opportunity for many Canadians, thus halting the possible formation of a counter ideology to the prevalent chance ideology. The lower-income classes have complied with the prevailing class system partly because of the aggressive promotion of lotteries that are associated with the hope of winning the jackpot; realistically, however, winning the smaller cash prizes simply provides fleeting enjoyment and merely reinforces hope of winning a larger prize (Vance, 1989).

In the United Kingdom, the National Lottery operator (Camelot) have stated that their own "ingredients of success" are popular products, effective marketing, convenience of play, security of system, and efficiency of operation (Camelot, 1995). However, as we have seen there are other important maintenance factors including successful advertising and television coverage, widespread availability, and a general misunderstanding of probability theory. Another potential marketing factor that may be important in why lotteries have been so financially successful is "entrapment. Entrapment refers to a commitment to a goal that has not yet been reached. The basic premise is to get the person committed to the cause or product as soon as possible. Once a commitment is made, the nature of thought changes. To the converted (in this case the lottery ticket buyer), careful and considered analysis of the situation is likely to be minimal. Lotteries have one great advantage over many other forms of gambling in that many people pick exactly the same numbers each week. In the United Kingdom, a newspaper survey reported that 67% of people chose the same numbers each week (Crosbie, 1996). Of this figure, the survey reported that 30% chose their regular numbers after an initial random selection and 37% chose the same numbers each week based on birthday dates, house numbers, favorite numbers, and so forth. However, no details were given about demography of the participants or the sample size.

By picking the same numbers the person may become "entrapped" (Walker, 1992). Each week the player thinks they are coming closer to winning. The winning day is impossible to predict but should lottery players decide to stop and cut their losses, they are faced with the prospect that the very next week their numbers might come up. Players are thus entrapped and the entrapment become greater as the weeks go by. According to Walker (1992), people can reach a point where holidays cannot be taken unless arrangements are made for the weekly ticket to be completed and entered. The "entrapment" process has sometimes been referred to in the psychological literature as the "sunk cost bias" (Arkes & Blumer, 1985) and is essentially another "foot-in-the-door" technique (Freedman & Fraser, 1966).

Another tactic in selling products is to gain source credibility. In many countries, national lotteries gain this almost immediately in that they have full Government backing. Governments introduce new legislation and pave the way for advertising their lottery on all the broadcast media. To add further credibility, the draws are broadcast on prime-time television programs by respected TV companies. For instance, in the United Kingdom, the National Lottery draws are televised by the BBC (British Broadcasting Corporation)—itself an organization of international credibility. According to Pratkanis (1995) source credibility can be effective for two reasons. The first is that it leads to the processing of messages in a half-mindless state—either because the person is not motivated to think, does not have the time to consider, or lacks the abilities to understand the issues. Second, source credibility can stop questioning ("if the government backs it, then it must be all right").

Government lotteries are perceived as a new opportunity for economic advancement, particularly because of mass media legitimization of the lottery as a life-altering opportunity. In fact, playing the lottery is encouraged and often touted as a perfectly reasonable and rational means of achieving success (Nibert, 2000). The general theme in advertising lotteries seems to be that the acquisition of wealth is desirable and possible by all; that is, they propagate a sense of equal opportunity. Overconsumption has become a status symbol of the wealthy as a result of television shows, such as soap operas and *The Lifestyles of the Rich and Famous*, which have glamorized the indulgence of the wealthy (Nibert, 2000). As a result of the glamorization of indulgence in pop culture, the poor have been pushed further down the socially desirable scale, as those with lower incomes are deemed to be inferior to be remedied by the acquisition of wealth. Those with limited resources are to be pitied and those with much are to be adulated; thus, "lottery culture" has permeated. Movies such as *It Could Happen to You* reinforce ideologies of chance and equal opportunity in the public's mind by showing how positively one's life can change after winning the lottery (Nibert, 2000).

Chance ideology works best at enticing those whose possibility for personal success seems remote, as they are the most willing to incur the costs of "winning big" in order to reach their goals (Nibert, 2000). Groups that are lower in socioeconomic status are targeted for special promotion in government ad campaigns that promote the undesirability of work and validate dissatisfaction with one's employment, consequently providing hope that winning the lottery will enable one to quit their job. This ideology has spread as a result of low worker morale in many industries where the capitalistic work environment has become wearisome and inhospitable. Many individuals who find their job to be a degrading experience, as working conditions are worsened through mergers and downsizing to make room for new technologies, are left unfulfilled. Heavier workloads and loss of control has resulted in feelings of separation from one's final product; thus, it should come as no surprise that any escape from this drudgery would be welcomed (Nibert, 2000). Traditionally, those in lower socioeconomic areas of society would be the ones who are less willing to accept dominant class authority and try to enact change, but this possibility is greatly reduced by the images portrayed in lottery ads in which one can easily have a better life by simply purchasing a lottery ticket (Nibert, 2000).

Many Canadians live in varying degrees of depravity, evident in the relatively moderate rates of unemployment in some areas. The large amount of resources available suggests that an equal opportunity exists for everyone, but experience reveals that this may not always be the case. To compensate for their inability to act competitively in the job market, those in the lower socioeconomic classes are willing to accept compensation, such as unemployment insurance and social services. In addition, to some extent, the acceptance of the ideas proliferated through lottery ad campaigns simply provide an escape from the drudgery of everyday life. Thus, the most fundamental component of the allure of gambling seems to be this escape (Vance, 1989).

Concluding Remarks

It is imperative to investigate the marketing of gambling when attempting to understand why some individuals develop and maintain their problem gambling behavior. The legal forms of gambling in Canada are successful because of marketing strategies that display thorough knowledge of the product and respond to changing customer needs. Many casinos are so successful as a result of performing "situational analyses," which include interviews or surveys with their clients in order to discern which segment of the population their casino is serving. Product assessment is also an important component of marketing plans. It includes assessment of both the positive and negative attributes of the product in order to rectify any problems that may be present. We specifically analyzed racetracks, casinos, video lottery terminals (EGMs), Internet gambling, and lotteries, and the specific marketing strategies that make these types of gambling so alluring to the public.

By analyzing these different forms of gambling, it is clear that the marketing of gambling through the use of situational and structural characteristics have the potential to induce gambling regardless of the gambler's biological and/or psychological constitution. Further to this, some characteristics are capable of producing psychologically rewarding experiences even in financially losing situations (e.g., the psychology of the near miss on slot machines). The success of situational and structural marketing characteristics (where success is defined as an increase in gambling due to the characteristic) depends on the psychostructural and/or psychosituational interaction. As highlighted by Griffiths (1993) previously, the importance of such an approach to gambling is the possibility to pinpoint more accurately where an individual's psychological constitution is influencing gambling behavior. Such an approach also allows for psychologically context-specific explanations of gambling behavior rather than global explanations (such as "addictive personality").

The effectiveness of these methods suggests there is much to be learned about the psychology of gambling from an analysis of these characteristics, and how they may facilitate both social and (in some cases) excessive gambling. Excessive gambling that leads to addictions always results from an interaction and interplay between many factors including the person's biological and/or genetic predisposition, his or her psychological constitution, his or her social environment, and the nature of the activity itself. This latter factor is becoming more important as gambling activities become more technological (e.g., Internet gambling, mobile phone gambling, interactive CD ROM, etc.). The identification and examination of the marketing features of new forms of gambling need to be ongoing. Such research is needed to find ways of minimizing the impact that these activities could have for individuals susceptible to developing problem gambling behaviors. There are many further situational and structural characteristics not outlined in this chapter. Other factors and dimensions (external to the person themselves) that have been reported in the general gambling literature and summarized by Griffiths and Wood (2000) include:

- stake size (including issues around affordability, perceived value for money)
- event frequency (time gap between each gamble)
- amount of money lost in a given time period (important in chasing)
- prize structures (number and value of prizes)
- probability of winning (e.g., 1 in 14 million on the lottery)
- size of jackpot (e.g., over £1 million on the lottery)
- skill and pseudo-skill elements (actual or perceived)
- "near miss" opportunities (number of near winning situations)

- light and color effects (e.g., use of red lights on slot machines)
- sound effects (e.g., use of buzzers or musical tunes to indicate winning)
- social or asocial nature of the game (individual and/or group activity)
- accessibility (e.g., opening times, membership rules)
- accessibility (e.g., number of outlets)
- location of gambling establishment (out of town, next to workplace etc.)
- type of gambling establishment (e.g., betting shop, amusement arcade etc.)
- advertising (e.g., television commercials)
- the rules of the game

Each of these differences may have implications for the gambler's motivations and as a consequence the social impact of gambling. Although many of these gambling-inducing situational and structural characteristics are dependent on individual psychological factors (e.g., reinforcement), they are a direct result of the situational and structural characteristics and could not have influenced gambling behavior independently. It is for this reason, above all others, that marketing analysis using a situational and structural approach could be potentially useful.

Chapter 9
Religiosity and Gambling Rituals

Robert Grunfeld, Masood Zangeneh, and Lea Diakoloukas

We are currently facing an unprecedented explosion of gambling in the world, with adverse consequences for individuals and communities. The current phenomenon is a reflection of a dynamic interaction of historical and psychological factors. Traditionally, gambling originated from religious rituals and quests for spiritual experiences (Reith, 1999). The change in societal structure, from a communal pre-modern system to the modern society, has led to collective psychological changes, such as feelings of increased alienation, accompanied by losing a sense of direction or purpose in life, and a probabilistic mindset (Giddens, 1991). The macroscopic changes altered our cognitive landscape, reciprocally influencing macro and micro changes in our societies. As societies grew increasingly secular, states began to sponsor and support gambling activities. This further contributed to the movement of gambling away from religion and spirituality. Gambling in the modern era fulfills our desires for upward mobility, control, and ontological security. The powerful and problematic appeal of gambling must be understood from a holistic perspective, which includes macro- and microscopic interactions. This perspective integrates psychological, economic, societal, and historical factors in accounting for this complex modern phenomenon.

At the Beginning: Spirituality, Religion, and Rituals

Throughout the phylogenetic history of our species, spirituality, religion, and rituals have been central components of our lives. The relationship between spirituality, religion, and rituals is marked by its dynamic nature. Although the terms "religion" and "spirituality" are sometimes used interchangeably, there is a notable difference between the two. Religion is the application of spirituality, much like technology is the application of science (Grof, 2000).

Robert Grunfeld
Professional Advanced Services in Mental Health and Addiction, Canada

M. Zangeneh, A. Blaszczynski, N. Turner (eds.), *In the Pursuit of Winning.*
© Springer 2008

Spirituality constitutes a "deep personal experience," often associated with a personal quest to rediscover one's own essence. Grof (2000) describes this quest as involving an entry into a "holotropic state." According to Grof (2000), a holotropic state is marked by a life-changing spiritual event, which constitutes the person's reconnection with the Creative Principle. The gambling experience may also be a type of holotropic state. While the gambling literature contains historical evidence of the influence of spirituality on gambling practices, there is little to substantiate the role it plays in gambling behavior today. Studies demonstrate the historical, spiritual, and moral significance of gambling (David, 1962) but do not emphasize how these elements have influenced the modern day player. However, more recent studies (Higgins, 2002; **Turner,** Ialomiteanu, & Room, 1999) have established a closer link between religion and gambling activity. Higgens (2002) reports a strong positive correlation between church attendance and lottery tickets purchased. A possible confound in this line of research is the operational definition of gambling. This includes any game of chance where money is wagered. Previous research may not have included lottery games as a form of gambling activity, and therefore may not have obtained the same results as Higgens (2002).

Gambling also performs a function analogous to that of religion. Marx argued that religion has a very important function in people's lives by providing psychological solace for the fear of death and the uncertainty in life (Avineri, 1968). David (1962) claimed that gambling has deep roots in religious ritual and that "gambling is entangled in the rudimentary forms of spirituality." Freud (1927) viewed religion and gambling as providing people with a sense of control of their destiny, and suggested that gambling could thereby act as a substitute for religion. In fact, there is a correlation between gambling activity and religiosity (Turner et al., 1998). According to statistics published on church attendance, fewer than 30% of Las Vegas residents attend church more than one time per year, compared with the national church attendance of 44% (Swanbrow, 1997).

Synthesis of the Gambling Rituals

On a macroscopic level, religion, as an institution, propagates itself through specific rituals performed by followers. The structure and function of rituals are central to all religions, and rituals can take on many forms such as praying, eating, the way one is clothed, and participation in ceremonies. Ritual refers to a modified act, which was once a functional behavior that has exceeded its usefulness down the evolutionary path. It is also considered to be an action or a behavior performed in the hope of improving one's luck or destiny. Rituals solidify and propagate the doctrine of religion. The philosopher Zizek (1989) stated, "the way to believe in God is to begin, mechanically to pray." According to Zizek (1989), belief follows action. Gambling is a ritual that propagates its own doctrine. The action of gambling propagates the probabilistic mindset of our capitalistic society (Reith, 1999). Higgens (2002) studied religiosity and gambling through the observation of gambling behavior in the elderly, and concluded that, "It would not be at all farfetched to suggest that for some, gambling itself becomes a religion of sorts."

Changing World: From Traditional to Modern Society

The physical landscape of our world has undergone tremendous changes in the past 400 years. This has impacted our behavior and relations to other people and objects. These changes in behavior from pre-modernity to modernity are a reflection of the macroscopic changes in community structure; from small, communal, familial, self-contained villages or tribes to our modern industrial nation-states (Giddens, 1991). The community structure has been altered, which resulted in decreased social inter-action and social support amongst community members. In pre-modern society, the emphasis was placed at the level of the community, highlighting the importance of the community. In contrast, in modern society the emphasis on the community has been shifted to the level of the individual, a system that is appropriately referred to as individualism. The enthusiasm for the new freedom and individualism of modernity reached its peak during the Enlightenment period, which occurred in the 18th century in Europe and North America (Cassirer, 1955). The time period was marked by a supreme belief in rationality and a pure belief in God. This era was characterized by optimism as a result of a declining feudal system and the perception of increased freedom from tradition and hierarchy (Cassirer, 1955). However, this enthusiasm would not be long lasting. The ailments of modernity began to surface in the 19th century, documented by writers such as Nietzsche, who is famous for documenting the loss of ontological security or psychological solace of this time period. Onto-logical security is defined as a state of contentment, and feeling secure and safe in the world. Ontological security began to decline with the emergence of industrial nation-states and the feelings of alienation that would follow. Nietzsche described a world devoid of God and meaning, where the sense of order has been lost (Solomon, & Higgins, 2000). This void provided fertile ground for rituals that would provide ontological security and a sense of order in the universe.

Although our external environment underwent drastic changes, the microcosm of basic human desires has not changed fundamentally over the past millennia. The desire for ontological security continues to be a universal human need (Giddens, 1991). The breakdown of traditional, pre-modern society has contributed to a loss of ontological security, which has resulted in feelings of alienation. To compen-sate for this, people have been increasingly drawn to rituals that would fulfill that void. However, in the modern era, rituals are no longer under tribal or communal guidance (Giddens, 1991), which can create problems for many individuals, such as addictions and their financial and health consequences. Giddens (1991) identified this as a contributing factor to the explosion in gambling addiction observed today. However, it is important to note that addictions can arise under tribal and ritual guidance as well, but the rules and mores of modern society, which espouse freedom and individuality, have left many people without a sense of direction.

The Secularization and Decontextualization of Rituals

In modernity, many rituals have been removed from their traditional ideology. The macroscopic factors, modernity and capitalism, have contributed to the isolation of certain rituals and behaviors for the sole purpose of propagating the consumer mass market (Zizek, 1989). Even in our leisure time, we continue being consumers. This is also true for the gambling ritual, as the modern form of gambling serves the purpose of the overarching capitalistic ideology (Reith, 1999). The action of gambling propagates the capitalistic ideology and influences our own cognitive processes. Overindulgence in rituals would not have been possible in the pre-modern era, whereas now, drugs and gambling have been decontextualized and isolated rituals. The peyote ceremony of Native Americans is an example of such a traditional ritual. Shamans act as guides during the ritual, and individual consumption abuse of the sacred peyote cactus is unknown in those communities (Gottlieb, Todd, & Westlund, 1997). Although the ritual is a personal experience, external guidance and regulation is provided under a shared value system. This represents the structure of pre-modern community rituals. On the other hand, modernity is marked by extreme individualism and a decline in communality. The modern gambler is disconnected from other gamblers (Reith, 1999), and forms a membership in an artificial and commercially driven community, which fails to meet gamblers' physical and psychological needs.

Breeding a Risk-Taking Culture

To propagate capitalism, a culture of risk-taking needs to be present. Our consumer culture therefore encourages activities that reinforce the status quo of capitalism. It is therefore not surprising that our government encourages risk-taking, as is evident by the popularity of the investment market and gambling (Giddens, 1991). Taking risks and feeling bold are the natural components of gambling, and this bravery is reinforced by our culture through social praise and material rewards. In fact, gamblers may often report a feeling of "affirmation of the self" while engaged in gambling (Reith, 1999). While modern jobs are often unfulfilling, boring, or even meaningless, gamblers often lead a second life where they are able to attain higher social status in the gambling community. For example, a person may work anonymously on the assembly line during the day; however, at night that same person is a respected member in the racetrack community, noted for its expertise. This function of gambling is analogous to that of role-playing games (e.g., Dungeons & Dragons), which offers a similar escapism and possibly an opportunity to adopt a new identity (Ryan, 1997).

Gambling in the Traditional and Modern Era

Modern commercial gambling has its roots in sacred play and religious rituals. According to Greek mythology, at the beginning of the world the fate of humanity was decided in a gamble (Reith, 1999). The ancient Greeks believed that

Zeus, Poseidon, and Hades divided the world between themselves in a dice game. Archeological findings illustrate that many early human cultures engaged in cleromancy, the drawing of lots to ascertain the will of the gods (Reith, 1999). The shaman would pose a question that was of importance to the community (e.g., should we go to war with our rival tribe?), and the gods would give the answer during the game of chance. The shaman would toss sticks, arrows, or bones and the formation of the objects was then interpreted as the answer from the gods to certain questions (Reith, 1999). These sacred games functioned primarily as tools in the decision-making process of pre-modern communities. Through ritualistic gaming practices (e.g., "casting lots") people sought to discover life's intentions. Players attempted to appropriate the future by risking something of value. Shamans often repeated their questions (i.e., the game) until a desired answer was received from the gods (Fiery, 1999). The commitment to such practices was strong and many people felt secure that their spiritual ritual was effective in summoning the gods.

Such communication with the mystic, spiritual world was not viewed as autonomous to gambling (Reith, 1999). Gambling practices were often incorporated into spiritual rituals forming a union that shaped how society interpreted the world. This epistemology encompassed many facets of life and incorporated repetitive gambling rituals into daily living. Spirituality and gambling merged throughout the world and remained resistant to scrutiny until the early 20th century (Reith, 1999). This is an important illustration of the power of repetition (Reith, 1999), which will surface again in our discussion of modern gambling.

The philosophy of this early cleromancy is based on a deterministic view of the universe, where random events were regarded as sacred signs of the gods, instead of insignificant random occurrences. Skilled individuals, such as shamans, interpreted these signs. Cicero, a mysticism historian, argued that in all cultures, no matter how advanced, people believed in the presence of signs foretelling future events. This provided people a forum by which to attain a sense of control over events and further to disregard the notions of randomness and chance. These early sacred games soon developed into the precursor of modern gambling, as people would begin to place wagers on the outcome of the games. These early wagers were used primarily for entertainment purposes, and were regarded as a playful aspect of divination (Reith, 1999).

Most of our modern games of chance originated millennia ago, and even the most recent games were already present in the Middle Ages. Dice are the oldest game instruments and made their first appearance in 600 B.C.., where they were referred to as "astragali" (Reith, 1999). In India, dice were called coupons and were used in the divination of Ramala rituals and in gambling. The gambling ritual was highly respected in India, and philosopher, Duryodhama, wrote, "if we gamble the heavenly gate will be opened" (Reith, 1999). In Greek and Roman era, the racetrack and chariot races were among the most popular forms of gambling (Reith, 1999). These games marked the first serration of gambling and sacred games, as the races were not associated with divination but functioned merely for the purpose of entertainment. The popularity of this form of gambling made Emperor Theodosius very concerned about the welfare of his empire so that he banned all gambling activities in 396 A.D. (Israel, 2002).

The origin of lotteries can be traced back to games of lots in ancient Rome, where Caesar was the first to sell lots to his guests. Prizes were given at the end of the night for guests with winning tickets (Reith, 1999). Wining in lotteries is dependent on the possession of the right ticket, and still practiced in the same manner today. In the Roman Empire, the winner was regarded as having been favored by the gods. The winners of lotteries continue to be regarded as special and lucky in the 21st century. During the 16th century, large-scale lotteries in Venice were the source of funds for public projects. According to Reith (1999), at one point the French government dependent solely on lottery revenue when citizens refused to pay their taxes. In Britain, public lotteries paid for the London water supply and the settlement of the Jamestown colony (Reith, 1999).

Lotteries also functioned as a measure of preserving social order and satisfying the economic and material desires of the citizens. In 18th century Europe, mobility aspirations of citizens could not be satisfied by the structured, inflexible economic system at the time. Lotteries filled this gap, as they provided the opportunity for sudden wealth. It is therefore evident that lotteries have existed in a symbiotic relationship with the early capitalist system. However, the love affair with lotteries experienced a period of tumult in the 19th century, where in Britain they were seen as a disguised form of gambling and therefore an immoral activity. The British Lottery Act of 1823 led to a temporary ban on lotteries (Reith, 1999). However, in the late 20th century, many governments reverted back to gambling revenue to support public projects, education, and even health care (Politzer, Yesalis, & Hudak, 1992).

In the medieval period, the standard game of chance involved dice. However, in that period, the forerunner of casino craps, the "game of hazard," emerged in Europe and gained popularity, especially among soldiers (Reith, 1999). At that time, wagers became increasingly important to the game. Rich people would gamble with their gold, animals, and land. On the other hand, the poor would gamble with their freedom, and if they lost the game, they would become slave property for the winners. With such high stakes at risk, gambling started to become a constant preoccupation and obsession for many.

Initially, the Christian Church did not condemn these rituals, and there are even numerous references in the New Testament to the drawing of lots and other gambling activities. However, in the Middle Ages the Church perceived gambling as an immoral act and placed a ban on games of chance, which were labeled as pagan and immoral activities. This led to a very clear separation between religion and gambling, although the connection between gambling and spirituality continues to be a powerful force for many gamblers to this day (Reith, 1999).

The 17th century was marked by a renewed gambling explosion, brought forth by the emerging mercantile society and the growth of a money economy. This money economy provided a universal and standardized system of value, which opened the door for globalized, commercial gambling. Society was changing, and in 1695, the Bank of England started dealing in stocks and shares, at a time when market speculation was rampant (Reith, 1999).

The casino made its debut in the 19th century, where public rooms were designated solely for the purpose of gambling (Reith, 1999). As gambling was endowed with a sacred status in traditional society, both the casino and the divine halls of pre-modernity acted as designated spaces, separating the gambling sphere. The first gambling resorts started in Germany, with patrons mostly from the middle and lower middle class (Scarne, 1986).

The Change in Cognitive Landscape: Probabilistic Mindset

The macroscopic changes many societies underwent also altered our own mindset and perception of the world, cultivating a probabilistic worldview. The departure of games from divination started in the late 16th century in Italy, with the secularization of chance. The advent of statistics and the calculation of probabilities was introduced in 1550 by Cardano and further refined by Pascal (Reith, 1999). Cardano, an avid gambler and mathematician, used his own gambling experiences to derive calculations of the probabilities in dice throws.

By the 17th century, the separation between chance and religious beliefs was clearly evident. This occurred alongside the rise of mercantile capitalism, and it was also the beginning of scientific calculation of probability. The emergence of the mercantile capitalist society led to increased trading through marine routes. In this climate, insurance companies and speculative insurance emerged (Reith, 1999). Marine insurance was interested in new tools to calculate commercial and economic risks. Pascal was the first to develop the concept of "average." Chance and determinism were thereby secularized, and as a result determinism lost its religious meaning. Reith (1999) argues that the concept of chance was "tamed" by the association with statistical laws. In the ancient tradition, "chance" was not an autonomous category. It was associated with destiny and the will of the gods and there were no explicit theories of chance. By the 20th century "chance" had become an autonomous, secular category. Giddens (1991) argues that in the 20th century, the calculation of risk has become a part of our probabilistic mindset. It represents the basis for our decision-making, as we no longer rely on shamans and cleromancy to aid us.

Gambling and Mystical Thinking: Perceptions and Beliefs Constructs

Gambling rituals have enabled people to participate in the outcome of their fates (David, 1962). What developed was a belief that individuals could summon something larger then themselves. When we consider magical and religious beliefs in forces such as luck, omens, fate, destiny, and even control or skill, as aspects of an entire worldview, the motives of players described as laboring under an 'illusion of control' and other so-called 'irrational cognitions' becomes clearer (Reith, 1999). Such knowledge makes sense to the gambler and gambling outcomes (wins or losses) become "emotionally meaningful as signs of favour or disapproval" (Reith,

1999). Confirmation (success in achieving one's desired outcome) may be viewed as an additional illusion that is incorporated into the gambling ritual. This may in turn maintain the choice behavior (waging rituals) and solidify an individual's constructed beliefs. This confirmation is expressed in the form of repetition and constant quest for reassurance. In view of the invariable uncertainty and doubt surrounding gambling practice and the world in general, people adapt such behavior as a way of lessening their insecurities.

Henslin (1967) suggest that, "if magic is defined as the belief and /or practice in control over the object or event where there is no empirical connection between the gesture as a cause and the object or event as an effect, then players do believe in and practice magic." The spiritual component of gambling practice seems to be unique in that it may foster in the player a certainty that can exceed logic or reason. The odds of winning in a particular game are usually against the player; those individuals who place faith in prayer or resort to ritualistic behaviors, however, believe they are changing the odds in their favor, thus creating a false sense of security. "Once totally involved in gambling, the gambler may reach a mood of mystical experience and get a sense of transcendence or becoming one with (God)." This state may also encourage the person by creating an 'illusion' of power. Dismissal of the laws of probability is common for such gamblers, and the transference of faith in spiritual power and its law is familiar. This faith or belief in forces that improve the outcome of betting may appeal to a fascination with the supernatural and the power it possesses.

Although there is a distinction that can be made between gaming and praying, their similarity lies in the fact that their intended and anticipated outcomes are very similar. For example, individuals gambles with the mindset that, through their gambling practices, they can "see" patterns, make connections, and attribute the outcome to something that is within their control rather than purely random chance. According to recent research (Turner & Liu, 1999; Turner, Zangeneh, and Litman-Sharp, 2006b), a higher knowledge of randomness is associated with lesser risk of developing problem gambling. There seems to be present within players a perceived relationship between themselves and the supernatural forces that govern their fate.

Bergler (1970) discusses a "strange sensation" that allows the person to feel like the "executive agent" of something beyond human capacity. His findings demonstrate the belief that is representative of the player's mindset. Described are the "powers" or "forces" at play while entrenched in gambling rituals such as possession of power and influence over event. Historically, this notion was clearly understood (Reith, 1999), but it may be less apparent in present-day gambling rituals. The use of spiritual tools that present "mystical enlightenment" and a perceived advantage in gambling may inspire in people the same confidence and rationale that it once did. Modern-day gambling may be adapting mystic historical events into modern gambling systems that cannot tolerate or accommodate in the same way the person's dedication and faith.

The belief in the power of something larger then one's self, for instance the supernatural, may create in a person a sense of grandeur that leads him or her to take unprecedented risks when gambling. The religious belief that significant people in an individual's life who have died remain a presence in life may be interpreted by a gambler as an opportunity to seek guidance or make connections with spirits based on "signs" or "a feeling" from this higher entity. Accessed through the use of rituals, a deceased parent, for example, a person that has provided guidance in the past, may be called upon when gambling stakes are high, to protect the person from loss or indicate to them in some way the best course of action. This position may be derived from a belief that the spiritual world has the power to "affect" the gambling experience. Although the person's influence over outcome is limited, he or she appraises his or her chances of winning as great.

Similarities of Pre-Modern and Modern Gambling

Although many aspects of life and gambling have been altered as a consequence of the transition to modernity, several underlying similarities remain. However, there are also similarities in pre-modern versus modern gambling. In both the pre-modern and modern eras, the gambling experience can result in a distorted perception of space – time, which is the result of an altered state of consciousness and even a loss of sense of self. In addition, in both time periods, gambling takes place in designated spaces, where the gambling sphere is separated from the real world.

Even though the popularity of gambling spread through the entire society in the Middle Ages, class differences were still highly evident. For the aristocrats of the upper class, games of chance represented display of honor and dignity (Reith, 1999). The goal of gambling was not wining but to project a self-image of order and composure. Goffman (1967) claimed that "taking action or knowingly taking risks through means of gambling provides the participant the opportunity to demonstrate possession of some highly valued and respected character traits, such as presence of mind, coolness under high pressure, courage, daring and the ability to graciously accept either positive or negative outcomes of the action." The children of the rich were tutored in different card games and game etiquette. Social disputes were no longer settled by sword, but in games of chance, where civility and dignity ruled. However, the poor played solely to win and were more interested in games that provided an opportunity for upward mobility, such as lotteries. The lower class would often play in unsanitary and decrepit gaming clubs. This class stratification continues in modernity, as the working class is overrepresented in lottery playing and the middle and upper-class overrepresented in casino gambling (Reith, 1999).

Modern Gambling Epidemic

The dynamic interplay between microscopic and macroscopic factors has contributed to the modern gambling epidemic. The proliferation of legalized gambling in the United States has led to a 950% increase in wagers from 1974 to 1986, after adjusting for inflation (Politzer et al., 1992). In 1986, Americans wagered $167 billion, a figure that does not include illegal gambling. In 1986, state lotteries surpassed casinos in revenue for the first time ever. According to Politzer et al. (1992), the increased exposure to gambling opportunities has created a new group of pathological gamblers.

In modernity, gambling has been removed from context, and only the ritual has been isolated. Gambling thereby no longer constitutes a functional behavior, as the ritual is meaningless without doctrine and consequently does not satisfy the gambler. Indulgence in the behavior only creates a greater craving and desire to repeat the action. Gamblers, similarly to traditional shamans, repeat their questioning of fate until they receive the desired answer. However, unlike the shamans, gamblers do not have a right answer in mind and continue to play even after winning large amounts of money. As a result, modern gambling has become an isolated and individual experience.

The victims of the modern gambling epidemic have been examined using an epidemiological model (Politzer et al., 1992). This model investigates the interaction triad of the host (gambler), the agent (gambling action), and the environment (family, community, culture). The problem gambler is on average dissatisfied with current employment, highly stressed, depressed, and easily frustrated (AADAC, 1994). Work has lost meaning for the gambler, which is a common symptom in modernity among the general population. It is a common belief that the erosion of the Protestant work ethic in our culture is a contributing factor in the proliferation of gambling. According to this view, our society endorses immediate gratification and consumption, at the expense of a consistent long-term ethic of work. We are implicitly encouraged to live for the moment, regardless of the consequences.

The Gambling Institution in Capitalistic Society

Gambling is very prevalent in our society, and we may at times be unaware of the extent it has permeated our lives. In all forms of media from newspapers, radio, television, and the Internet, gambling is explicitly and implicitly endorsed in the form of raffles, radio quizzes, sports betting, lotteries, horse racing, and charity casinos. Lottery commercials are explicit in stating the purpose of lotteries, namely for the fulfillment of capitalistic aspirations in terms of upward mobility. This is echoed by the slogan of the Ontario Lottery 6/49, "Just imagine . . . the Freedom." In modernity, freedom is achieved through material gains and the road to heaven or that one big earthly win is via materialism.

Gambling, as an institution, performs various functions in our society, generating revenue, employing individuals, and as an institutional leisure activity (Reith, 1999). In addition, the gambling institution functions to decrease class tension, by providing the illusion of upward mobility (Reith, 1999). Through gambling, the ideology of capitalism is reinforced and the status quo is thereby maintained.

As citizens in modern, capitalistic societies, the primary purpose of our existence is consumption. People are trapped in an endless cycle of consumer behavior, and define themselves as consumers by identifying with tangible, material goods and services purchased. Zizek (1989) referred to this event as commodity fetishism, a type of capitalistic exchange where the mind becomes conditioned for material consumption. This process is analogous to a parasitic infestation of the mind, as commercials reinforce the consumer cycle, through continuous, flashing images of new products and fashion. Karl Marx observed that our class structure will result in tension as the privileged class will always be the envy of workers, which brews feelings of hostility and rebellion (Avineri, 1968). Freud (1927), like Marx, argued that the lower classes will attempt to free themselves from the shackles of poverty, and when this is not possible, discontent will persist. Gambling can be regarded as an opportunity for the poor and helpless to become wealthy and thereby become members of the privileged class. It is therefore in the state's best interest to endorse gambling establishment, in order to appease the population. In general, risk-taking is an encouraged activity in modern society. Giddens (1991) argued that the secular risk culture is synonymous with modernity. People are preoccupied with risk assessment, as our everyday life is characterized by risk. In this climate, where certainty and ontological security have been eroded, there are no guarantees and no risk-free behavior.

However, gamblers are not the only individuals in modernity who long for escapism and risk-taking. Modernity is marked by a perpetual boredom and dissatisfaction with one's work and life, leading people to look for "safe risks" to engage in (Reith, 1999). Researchers (Beaudoin & Cox, 1999; Turner, Zangeneh & Littman-Sharp, 2006) found that a subset of problem gamblers use gambling as a coping mechanism for depression. In doing so individuals contribute to the uncertainty of their state. The player views their success as being subject to individual control through a connection to higher forces. In short, "commercialized gambling offers to many people efficient means of enhanced self-esteem and gratification" (Rosecrance, 1988). Proposed is an underlying human tendency to seek and protect that which conceptually fits their schema. Whether it is personal control, coincidence, or unseen forces that are responsible for the positive outcome, the outcome of the game takes on a tangible quality that is construed and attributed to personal ability.

Virtually our entire global village is experiencing erosion of communal support and increased feelings of ontological insecurity. This has made an ever increasing number of people susceptible to finding psychological solace through gambling and the rituals they associate with this practice. In light of emerging theories concerning spirituality and gambling, explorations that reveal the true nature of gambling and its ritualistic and spiritual components will deepen knowledge and understanding of gambling behavior and amend portrayals of gamblers, their motivations, and the means by which they seek the "pot of gold" at the end of the rainbow.

Chapter 10
Buying a Risk

An Application of Insurance Law to Legal Gaming

G. E. Minchin

At first blush, it may not appear that gambling and insurance have much in common. To this age, the conservative stolidity of Lloyds of London seems to be a far cry from the glitter of gambling. In comparison, when opportunities to gamble were far more limited, the English Life Insurance Act of 1774 specifically made insurances on the lives of those whom one had no interest in, null and void, as gaming and wagering. The distinction between insurance and gaming was one that forced the Court to strive for adequate formulations to differentiate legitimate from illegitimate enterprises:

> If it is correctly called an insurance on life, then it is not without an interest within the meaning of the same statute; for, although Field had no vested interest in the property of Mrs. Smith which he could sell, still a promise to assign a devise which he expected would be a sufficient consideration to support a promise to pay for it, in a contract not under seal; and the purchaser of such an expected devise would have an interest so far as to prevent his policy being considered the gaming and wagering prohibited by the statute." *Cook v. Field* (1850) 15 QB 460 Lord Campbell CJ

Other attempts were made to cast gambling as outside the law of contract on the basis of its contingent nature, and because of the uncertainty inherent in the transaction. In *Thacker v. Hardy* (1878) 4 QBD 685 (CA) Cotton J. characterized the transaction as a contract void for uncertainty, stating that "The essence of gaming and wagering is that one party is to win and the other to lose upon a future event, which at the time of the contract is of an uncertain nature." The difficulty with this formulation is that the stock exchange transactions at issue in that case are very close to many forms of socially acceptable speculation that also involve profit or loss dependent upon future events. Besides insurance on an interest, legitimate speculation has included such instances as an indemnity policy for a proposed transatlantic cable in *Wilson v. Jones* (1867) LR 2 Exch 139, and providing a guaranteed cure for the flu in *Carlill v. Carbolic Smoke Ball Co.* (1892) 2 QB 484 (CA).

Ultimately the only coherent divide was that set out by McCardie J in *Barnett v. Sanker* (1925) 41 TLP 660:662, in which it was stated that:

G.E. Minchin
Barrister and Solicitor of the High Court, New Zealand

M. Zangeneh, A. Blaszczynski, N. Turner (eds.), *In the Pursuit of Winning.*
© Springer 2008

> If the parties meant that no legal bargain should be effected between them, and that there should be no right to demand a payment of differences except a moral right, the contract is a gaming contract. But if the parties intended to enter into a legal contract, which gave legal rights and imposed legal obligation, then the contract though it deals with speculative transactions was enforceable.

Clearly, this is a culture-specific divide rather than a principled distinction. It separates speculation from gambling on the basis of the social constructs that inform the transaction. This is not a criticism, as there is no other defining feature for the law to fix on. Given the subtly of such distinctions, what was fundamentally at issue was the nature of the transaction, that nature was categorized in terms of the value system of the ruling morality. While outside of the prevailing morality, gaming and wagering constituted illegal contracts that would not be enforced. Gambling was not contractual for the same reasons that arrangements between husband and wife are not contracts. Despite all the elements of contract being present in agreements between husband and wife, such agreements are simply not arrangements that our culture understands as entailing legal consequences, as held in the leading matrimonial case of *Balfour v. Balfour* (1919) 2 KB 571 (CA). Broadly, where a transaction, which involves mutual exchange, is perceived to be within the law, rights and obligations follow. Transactions that a culture considers to be outside the province of the law do not give rise to a legitimate expectation of remedies at law.

This was the divide between legitimate insurance and insurance as gaming and wagering, despite the essential components of risk and vulnerability being fundamentally the same in gambling and insurance, as the actuary is nothing other than a bookmaker without the plaid, and the underwriter a bigger bag. While genuine insurance policies and other forms of futures speculation were seen as legitimate business activities by society, and gambling was not, the divide provided legal remedies to one and withheld the operation of the law from the other. With the sanctification of gambling by the state, all such speculation must conform with consumer safeguards and legal principle. Arguably then, the principles of equity and the common law duties of utmost good faith, which apply in the context of insurance law, are directly applicable to the gambling construct.

Defining Features of Insurance Law

Two related features give shape to the distinctions that separate contract law at large from insurance law. These are vulnerability to risk, contingent upon an imbalance of information. Clearly, these are not absent from other areas of contract, but are central to insurance law, as one party is dependent on the other at different stages of the transaction, and so a trust reposes between them.

The other distinguishing feature, as most other contractual obligations are reciprocal, is the trilateral relation among the insurer, the insured, and the injured party. This is the feature that requires fairness to impose upon the insurer an obligation to treat the interests of the insured equally to its own. Otherwise, the insurer's subrogatory control of litigation could open the insured to personal liability beyond the policy. It is the ability of the insurer to maximize its position as a result of the relationship itself that is tempered by the imposition of the duty on the insurer to give equal priority to the interests of the insured. At bottom, it is the meeting of the minds and contractual intention on which this duty is founded. The intention of the insurer is to gain protection from liability, and it is the representation that the insurer will assume liability that induces the insured to pay the premiums. This understanding would be defeated if the insurer unfairly resisted claims within the policy limit and, in doing so, opened the insured to liability for damages in excess of the insured peril. The law, taking the representation of the fact, then imposes the burden of that representation on the insurer by way of a duty to act in accordance with the representation.

Outside of public policy considerations there is no trilateral relationship in the gaming construct. However, what is achieved by the imposition of this duty on insurers is the holding of the insurer to their representation and the effecting of the contract in the manner it was portrayed. It will be argued that similar considerations impel similar duties being placed on the gaming consortiums, which misrepresent the risk entailed.

Risk and Vulnerability

Historically, it was the vulnerability of insurers to underwriting an unknown risk that developed the duty incumbent on the insured to inform the insurer of all information in their possession that was material to the insured peril. It was this vulnerability and the prerequisite of trust that placed insurance in the *uberrimae fidei* class of contracts.

In the leading case of *Carter v. Boehm* (1766) 3 Burr. 97 ER 1162, Lord Mansfield held that:

> Insurance is a contract of speculation. The special facts upon which the contingent chance is to be computed lie most commonly in the knowledge of the assured only; the underwriter trusts to his representation, and proceeds upon confidence that he does not keep back any circumstances in his knowledge to mislead the underwriter into a belief that the circumstance does not exist. The keeping back such circumstance is a fraud, and therefore the policy is void. Although the suppression should happen through mistake, without any fraudulent intention, yet still the underwriter is deceived and the policy void, because the *risque* run is really different from the *risque* understood and intended to be run at the time of the agreement . . . The policy would be equally void against the underwriter if he concealed . . . Good faith forbids either party, by concealing what he privately knows, to draw the other into a bargain from his ignorance of the fact, and his believing the contrary.

It appears, on Lord Mansfield's analysis, that the principled basis of the action is largely in equity, and it is a form of estoppel by which it is a breach of trust to profit from another's misrepresentation. The basis of the agreement is that one "trusts to his representation, and proceeds upon confidence that he does not keep back any circumstances in his knowledge." The burden is on the parties to give an accurate representation of the risk; intent is not required, and an innocent misrepresentation suffices to void a policy "because the *risque* run is really different from the *risque* understood and intended to be run at the time of the agreement." Beyond this, good faith prevents either party drawing "the other into a bargain... by concealing what he privately knows." At common law, if the risk run is other than that intended, the contract would be void for uncertainty.

Monopolies of Information

Historically, the law tended to consider the duty as it lay on the insured, as it was the insured who had a monopoly of information in regard to the circumstance of the loss, but the duty of disclosure was always mutual. In *Banque Keyser Ullman SA v. Skandia (UK) Ins Co. Ltd* the English Court of Appeal held that:

> ... the duty falling upon the insurer must at least extend to disclosing all the facts known to him which were material either to the nature of the risk sought to be covered or the recoverability of a claim under the policy which a prudent insured would take into account in deciding whether or not to place the risk for which he seeks cover with that insurer."
> (1990) 1 QB 665, 772

This statement of the insurer's duty was accepted by Lord Bridge in the House of Lords, although the duty does not extend to providing the insured with such information, as cover could be obtained elsewhere at a lower premium. It would also be necessary for the insured to show that the nondisclosure induced the contract. Both parties share the obligations, which stem from the trust and the duty of good faith, as the objective of the law is to place parties on an "equal footing" *Greenhill v. Federal Insurance Co.* (1927) 1 KB 65, 76 (CA). What is central then to the contractual relationship is the imbalance of information, "as the underwriter knows nothing and the man who comes to him to insure knows everything" *Rozanes v. Bowen* (1928) vol. 31 LIL Rep 231. Good faith applies to all types of insurance, *Seaton v. Heath* (1899) 1 QB 782; however, the duty of utmost good faith does not rest on an implied term of the contract, but arises outside of it, as it is based in equity not contract, *The "Good Luck"* (1992) 1AC 233.

Society's transition from the heroic phase of capital accumulation to structural monopoly, in which the balance of power has swung to favor the insurer, has meant that the burden has swung from generally reposing with the insured to catch the insurer with all its technocratic access to information. Beneath this legal transition lies a sociological substrata that charts the law's protectionism as it swings from favoring the fledgling entrepreneurs of the 17th century to shielding the dwarfed individual of the 20th. As the economic muscle of the insurer must now be factored in to maintain equality, the law places a burden on the dominant party, which is an obligation to act fairly at all times. In *Ontario Inc. v. Lloyds* (2000) 184 DLR (4th) 687 (Ont CA), the Canadian court has allowed substantial punitive damages for serious breaches of this duty. In *Whiten v. Pilot Insurance Co.* (2002) 209 DLR (4th) 257 (SCC), where information in the hands of an insurer did not support the palpably weak affirmative defense of arson put forward by them, the Supreme Court of Canada upheld punitive damages. In *Whiten*, the jury had clearly thought that the defense had been maintained in bad faith and had severely disadvantaged a family, which had lost their home. In the majority, Justice Binnie described the insurer's breach of good faith as an "actionable wrong" that was independent of the contractual terms The extent of this duty of good faith is demonstrated by the Canadian Court's refusal to strike out pleadings that claimed an independent duty of good faith on an insurer's employees, *Spiers v. Zurich Insurance Co.* (1999) 45 OR (3d) 726. In an obiter comment it has been considered a breach of this duty to lure a customer into a contract, knowing there has been a nondisclosure that would obviate any claim, *Gate v. Sun Alliance Insurance Ltd.* (1995) 8 ANZ Ins Cas 75,806.

Misrepresentation

While in *Carter v. Boehm* it was held that even an innocent misrepresentation voided an insurance contract, that decision drew upon the precedents of maritime insurance, which has always been in a special category of insurance. It is now considered that the legal rationale for this burden is that maritime insurance contracts contain the implied term that all material representations had been made by the insured. General insurance law makes a distinction between a misrepresentation, which was careless or negligent, and one that results from innocent misapprehension not amounting to negligence. Negligent misrepresentation or misstatement that is detrimentally relied on may ground an action in tort for damages, as in *Hedley Byrne v. Heller* (1964) AC 465. Alternatively, rescission or statutory damages for misrepresentation may be available. Beyond common law relief, innocent misrepresentations in the insurance context are actionable in equity if: (1) it is a statement of fact, not opinion or law; (2) it is untrue or inaccurate; (3) it was material to the acceptance of the risk; (4) it is a statement of present fact, not as to the future; and (5) it must have induced the creation of the contract.

Fact, Not Opinion or Law

In regard to the distinction between fact and opinion, statements by those who are assumed to know the facts may be fixed by their status, so that their statements are deemed to be grounded on fact. What is pivotal here is whether the representor is holding himself out as someone who is authoritative and can be relied upon.

Untrue or Inaccurate

In regard to the accuracy of the statement, the law looks to the whole truth, and whether the statement reflects that. In *Aarons Reefs v. Twiss*, Lord Halsbury held:

It is said there is no specific allegation of fact which is proved to be false. Again I protest, as I have said, against that being the true test. I should say, taking the whole thing together, was there a false representation? I do not care by what means it was conveyed, by what trick or device or ambiguous language, all those are expedients by which fraudulent people seem to think they can escape from the real substance of the transaction. If by a number of statements, you intentionally give a false impression, and induce a person to act upon it, it is not the less false, although, it one takes each statement by itself, there may be difficulty in showing that any specific statement is untrue. (1896) AC 273:281

Materiality

In general terms, materiality is conditional on the misrepresentation being in regard to information that a prudent person would have wanted to be accurately informed of, prior to entering the contract.

Present, Not Future Fact

Any representation of facts *in futuro* is a promise, a statement of opinion, or a statement of intention. As equitable relief looks at all the conduct of the parties, statements as to the future can be construed as promissory warranties and as "basis of contract" clauses, as considered in the House of Lords decision in *Anderson v. Fitzgerald* (1853) 4 HL Cas 484. Statements of opinion or belief may be a representation of present fact where there is the implied representation that there is an honest expectation, on reasonable grounds, that events will transpire as forecast, *Bank Leuni le Israel v. Britain National Ins.* (1988) 1 Lloyds Rep 71:75. A statement as to future intention can be construed as a statement of present intention, as the present state of a man's mind is a fact like anything else. The Courts may favor such broad interpretations of *in futuro* facts where there is deceit, *Edgington v. Fitzmaurice* (1884) 29 Ch D 459 483.

Inducement

For the misrepresentation to be actionable, it must have induced the contract, in that it would not have been entered into had the truth been known, *St. Paul Fire & Marine Ins Co. (UK) v. McConnell Dowell* (1995) 2 Lloyds Rep 116:124–125.

Application of Insurance Principles to Gambling Law

Legally, gambling is almost a *terra nullis*. As an illegal activity, it has long been outside of the law and, as such, contracts of wagering were unenforceable. As Christian morality has been eclipsed by a market ideology, gambling has been sanctioned by the state and, indeed, embraced as a source of revenue. As a now lawful activity, it falls to be treated as any other exchange relationship, but has no body of precedent to define the rights and obligations that condition the transaction.

At civil law, where individuals may seek a remedy for the personal harm caused to them by legalized gambling, new duties of care require proximity; that is, a causative link and an absence of contraindicating policy considerations, *Anns v. Merton London Borough Council* (1978) AC 728. Beyond these two broad fields of inquiry, it is helpful to be able to analogize the extant duties recognized at law. It is maintained that such an analogy between insurance law and legal gambling is tenable.

Vulnerability and Risk

As gaming is nothing but risk, it could be argued that punters assume these risks and enter the construct knowing what they are in for. However, the comparison made here is with insurance law, which embodies *uberrimae fidei* duties, the highest class of obligations at law. As with gambling, a contract of insurance is a form of speculation. The terms or circumstance of either is the *risque* understood—the represented odds. What is at issue then, is whether the punters are on notice of the nature of the risk and the extent of their vulnerability. The promoters are also caught with this vulnerability.

By an application of insurance principles, a trust reposes on the parties to ensure that each is not deceived in this, and the risk intended to be run is known. Insurers utilize the most exacting actuaries and access detailed personal databanks to appraise their exposure to risk. Similarly, in calculating their exposure, gambling consortiums bring enormous resources and expertise to bear in determining the risk borne. Against this tour de force, the gamblers are effectively hamstrung or, more accurately, debrained. They can do nothing but trust to the whim of fate the lotteries or pokies; and, in the casino, skill is specifically prohibited on the part of the punter. Significantly, the gambling consortiums are increasingly promoting a steady shift away from forms of punting such as horse racing, where knowledge of forms and odds is of some assistance (if you have not been told which horse is going to win) to gambling opportunities where intelligence is an obstacle. This shift is not a fortuitous one, but is driven by the promotion of those outlets that direct the most predictable revenue streams back to the consortiums.

There is a marked imbalance of power in the gaming construct that is as great, if not greater, as that between a multinational insurance company and a private individual. Just as most individuals could not sustain the loss of their house or the consequences of a serious personal accident, so too gamblers who are out of control have to gamble more, if they are to have any hope of recovering their losses. It is this vulnerability and the potentiality for such dependency that arguably could ground the placing of a duty of care on gaming consortiums as applies at insurance law.

Monopolies of Information

Casinos routinely deprive customers of even knowing what time of day it is or even whether it is day or night, as casinos are designed to avoid revealing any indication of the passage of time, so as to keep the punters at the wheel. The enormous profits derived from licensed gambling enables the gaming consortiums to amass scientific and statistical data on the efficacy of various forms of gaming. Through psychological profiling, games are purveyed to their maximum effect. The pokies, which are the most profitable form of gambling, are the most sophisticated Skinner boxes known to man or, rather, known to the consortiums, as the design characteristics are never revealed to the punter. To paraphrase *Rozanes v. Bowen*, the casino knows everything and the man who comes to it to gamble knows nothing. Arguably, this imbalance opens the consortiums to a good faith duty to not conceal "what he privately knows, to draw the other into a bargain from his ignorance of the fact, and his believing the contrary," *Carter v. Boehm*.

Misrepresentation: Common Legal Remedies

Beyond breaches of good faith attaching to a duty not to conceal, misrepresentations that were careless or negligent could ground an action for damages in the tort of negligent misstatement, as in *Hedley Byrne v. Heller*. Innocent misrepresentation not shown to be culpable could be actionable if the Courts were persuaded that the special circumstances that pertain to maritime insurance law are applicable in the gambling construct. In *Carter v. Boehm*, it was held that even an innocent misrepresentation voided an insurance contract in the special category of maritime insurance. Important to this analysis, the special nature of maritime insurance was a consequence of the heightened risks involved and the difficulty of forensic determination of the cause of the loss. Arguably, similar considerations apply to gambling.

Misrepresentation: Equitable Relief

If analogies from the insurance context can be transposed to the gambling construct, then innocent misrepresentations may be actionable in equity if the standard criteria are met. In regard to truth, the legalization of gambling gives authoritative weight to the truth of the consortiums' assertions. As Lord Halsbury held in *Aarons Reefs v. Twiss*, the law looks to the whole truth and whether the statement reflects that. It is the impression given with which the consortiums are fixed. In regard to materiality, it is the information that a prudent person would have wanted to be accurately informed of that is at issue. That information would include the lethality of the machines in question, and the effect of alcohol on the anticipation/adrenaline reaction designed into the display.

As all forms of gambling are contingent on future events, all facts could be said to be *in futuro* as either a promise, a statement of opinion, or a statement of intention. However, as equitable relief looks at all the conduct of the parties, statements as to the future can be construed as promissory warranties, particularly where the implied representation is that there is an honest expectation, on reasonable grounds, that events will transpire as forecast, or where there is deceit. It would remain necessary for the misrepresentation to have actually induced the contract of gaming or wagering.

Conclusion

The same features of risk and vulnerability, and trust and representation characterize both the gambling and insurance constructs. As applies in insurance law, it is maintained that, in the gambling construct, it is the reliance on the representation that the transaction is a reasonable one that creates the trust. It follows then, that at civil law, purveyors of gambling opportunities could be fixed with the same duties of utmost good faith as apply in insurance law.

In the context of legislative control, this means placing a higher obligation on gambling agencies, both public and private, than that which accords to normal commercial transactions, such as are controlled by Fair Trading and Consumer Guarantees Acts. Given the level of vulnerability, gambling legislation should parallel legislation such as the Door-to-Door Sales Acts, which recognize similar vulnerabilities. The application of this higher threshold would recognize the common law principle that, in high-risk situations, the burden is on the person knowing the risk to inform the other of its extent. If this threshold applied, gambling consortiums would be bound by strict liability, as in this context even an innocent misrepresentation remains a fraud. At a minimum, it would be incumbent on gambling agencies to provide accurate information as to the risk customers undertake and not to conceal what they privately know.

Part II

Chapter 11
Cognitive Behavioral Therapy for Problem Gamblers

Malcolm Battersby, Jane Oakes, Barry Tolchard, Angus Forbes, and Rene Pols

The cognitive behavioral therapy (CBT) approach used within the unit for the treatment of problem gambling is based on the same principles used to treat clients with anxiety disorders and depression. This approach is based on the work of Isaac Marks (Marks, 1986) and was introduced by Battersby (Tolchard and Battersby, 2000) to South Australia in 1996. The service is part of the Break Even network funded by the South Australian government Department of Families and Communities and is integrated with the Mental Health Sciences postgraduate courses in cognitive–behavioral therapy for health professionals at Flinders University, Adelaide, Australia.

This chapter provides an outline of the theoretical framework, assessment process, specific treatment methods, and measurement of treatment outcomes of the Flinders Therapy Service for Problem Gamblers. A case example and outcome data are provided to demonstrate the treatment model and its effectiveness. An overview of treatment outcomes for problem gambling assessing different modalities is discussed.

Cognitive therapy is used initially to dispute irrational beliefs related to gambling, and to help recognize and modify the negative automatic thought processes that clients may have that can cause and maintain psychological distress. The behavioral approach aims to extinguish the client's urge to gamble. This treatment enables mastery over and elimination of the urge to gamble, which facilitates recovery both in gambling behavior and functional recovery in the person's life. Once mastery of the urge to gamble has occurred, secondary control measures become unnecessary. The treatment process is described in this chapter, with the main focus being on gaming machine addiction. This approach can be used for other forms of gambling such as horse race betting, casino games, and sports betting.

Malcolm Battersby
Flinders Therapy Service for Problem Gamblers, Australia

M. Zangeneh, A. Blaszczynski, N. Turner (eds.), *In the Pursuit of Winning.*
© Springer 2008

Overview of the Literature on Problem Gambling Treatment Outcomes

There are many approaches for the treatment of problem gambling. Reviews of the treatment of problem gambling have noted few randomized control trials, with the majority using cognitive and behavioral techniques. The lack of theoretical understanding of the etiology of problem gambling limits the ability to establish effective treatment programs. Relapse rates in the best programs are high. There is a need to define the therapist skills and knowledge that are needed for the effective treatment of gambling problems (Abbott, Volberg, Bellringer, & Reith, 2004).

Although there is an extensive literature on the treatment of pathological gambling, there are only a few studies that meet level IV evidence criteria. Two extensive reviews, one by Pallesen (Pallesen, Mitsem, Kvale, Johnsen, & Molde, 2005) and the recent Cochrane review (Oakley-Browne, Adams, & Mobberley, 2005), report that there have been only four randomized control trials (RCTs) of psychological treatments for pathological gambling. In the Cochrane Review, (Oakley-Browne et al., 2005) it was concluded that experimental interventions using behavioral and cognitive therapy were more efficacious than controls in the short term. Pallesen et al. were less restrictive than the Cochrane Review and reviewed some 37 papers. Both groups of authors concluded that behavioral interventions (imaginal desensitization) and cognitive–behavioral interventions were effective in the short term for the treatment of problem gambling. Pallesen et al. were more positive and considered that pathological gambling could be treated with favorable outcomes. The authors were critical of the research design and power of all the studies. Our review of the literature agrees with these findings, including:

- Low sample sizes and the failure to specify inclusion and exclusion criteria
- Inconsistent follow-up periods and outcomes
- Failure to use standardized measures for both problem gambling diagnostic criteria and outcome measures
- Outcome measures that vary from "controlled gambling" to abstinence.
- Inadequate long-term outcome data addressing lapse and abstinence
- Explanations as to why treatment is effective or ineffective
- Lack of clear definitions of controlled gambling and gambling relapse
- Inadequate or no measurement of the gambling urge

Much remains to be done in outcomes based treatment research.

The Flinders Therapy Service for Problem Gamblers

South Australia has a population of 1.5 million people, with 1 million living in the capital city Adelaide. Legalization of electronic gaming machines (EGMs) has made more than 12,000 machines available in many hotels, clubs, and the casino. South

Australia has a prevalence of 2 % to 3 % pathological gamblers (Delfabbro, 2005). The Flinders Therapy Service (http://som.flinders.edu.au/FUSA/CCTU/CARD%20 Index.htm) works closely with many of the other state-funded agencies of the Break Even Network that provide gambling rehabilitation (e.g., counseling and assistance with financial problems) and refer clients to the therapy service. Clients self-refer or are referred from other agencies, community, general practice, and mental health services. Since its establishment, in 1996 the unit has received more than 1000 referrals, increasing to an average of 200 new clients annually. For clients unable to attend face-to-face interviews, phone contact or videoconferencing is used to provide treatment and follow-up. Close affiliation with Flinders University enables students of the Mental Health Sciences courses to develop clinical competency in both the assessment and treatment of problem gambling and comorbid mental health disorders.

The Service Model

The service is staffed by a psychiatrist and therapists with a range of professional backgrounds including psychology, nursing, and social work. All therapists have both mental health and masters level qualifications in cognitive behavior therapy. Clients are provided with a screening interview that includes a detailed cognitive–behavioral analysis of their gambling. Clients who present with problem gambling (almost all have a diagnosis of pathological gambling as per the DSM-IV), and who are able to define their gambling problems in a problem statement and define end of treatment goals, are suitable for admission into the treatment program. Clients are assessed for any comorbid mental health problems such as alcohol dependence, anxiety disorders, and depression and treated appropriately.

The client is offered either a group or individual treatment program. The group program runs for 12 weeks. Approximately eight clients are allocated to each group that meets for 2 hours once a week. One-to-one treatment is offered to clients who prefer individual treatment, cannot attend a group session, or require more intensive therapist input. Individual treatment is conducted with 1-hour sessions weekly for up to 12 weeks. A 2-week in-patient program is offered to those who do not improve after a trial of an outpatient program or live in rural areas and do not have access to specialist therapy services, have complex comorbid conditions or suicidality, or lack housing and social supports.

When clients complete treatment they are offered a follow-up program to enable maintenance of their treatment gains and to continue to develop their relapse prevention strategies. Follow-up is conducted in a group format or individual sessions as required. Once clients feel confident that they have gained control over their gambling and have appropriate relapse prevention strategies in place, they often decline the offer of regular follow-up sessions but often agree to have outcome measures collected by phone at 3- to 6-month intervals.

Clients admitted to the inpatient program receive a multidisciplinary team approach, including a psychiatrist, cognitive behavioral therapist, pharmacist, nursing staff, social worker, and occupational therapist. If the client has a significant alcohol, benzodiazepine, or illicit drug dependence he or she undergoes withdrawal before commencing a treatment program. Comorbid conditions are managed as appropriate. Throughout the admission, clients are required to repeat a variety of behavioral tasks up to four times daily and use cognitive worksheets to document their negative thoughts throughout the day. Clients are discharged to outpatient follow-up. Their significant partner or relative is included to provide support and to participate in control of the client's finances.

Etiological Theories of Problem Gambling Underpinning the Treatment Model

Social Learning Theory

Social learning is the concept that individuals tend to copy and repeat behaviors they observe when the behaviors are followed by reinforcement. Bandura's "self efficacy" theory states that vicarious experiences are the typical way that human beings change and modeling can have as much impact as the direct experience. Voluntary behavior change depends on individual perceptions of how one has the ability to perform the behavior. This is clearly true for gambling behaviors, as such individuals who observe others gambling may be more likely to gamble them-selves. Gambling wins are discussed rather than gambling losses among family and friends. This provides a strong source of positive reinforcement for gambling behaviors.

Conditioning

Within a gambling setting there are many stimuli making the environment rewarding because of the excitement, arousal, and tension they create in the individual. These stimuli include pre-race and race sequences at the racetrack, flashing lights of a gaming machine, and the placing of a bet. The basic proposition is that gambling behavior is maintained by the winning and losing sequences within this operant conditioning paradigm with a variable interval schedule of reinforcement. The psy-chology of the near miss on a gaming machine has the ability to manipulate the gambler through the reinforcement of the gambling urge, a psychophysiological response with arousal features similar to anxiety.

There are clearly unconditioned and conditioned responses as well as operant learning that occur in this complex setting of stimuli (Griffiths & Parke, 2002). It has been demonstrated that the many structural characteristics of gaming machines have the potential to induce excessive gambling regardless of the gambler's biological and psychological makeup. Some of these structural characteristics are capable of providing psychologically rewarding experiences even in situations when the gambler is losing money (Griffiths, 1999). Some gambling activities have small event frequencies as they can be played only once or twice a week. Biweekly lottery draws are an example of this frequency. Gambling on gaming machines provides few limitations on repeating the gambling behavior as they can be played frequently and continuously. This structure allows for the systematic shaping of responses due to classical and operant-learning mechanisms that are highly efficient in generating repeated behavior by participants. This factor, combined with the result of the gamble, whether a win or a loss, and the actual time until winnings are received takes advantage of the psychological principles of operant conditioning (Griffiths 1999). The intermittent and unpredictable nature of the reward provides variable ratio (intermittent) reinforcement, a powerful method to increase the psychophysiological gambling urge.

Cognitive Theory

The development and maintenance of gambling problems can be equally well explained by an information-processing hypothesis whereby the gambling behavior is driven by erroneous perceptions with regard to various types of outcome expectancies. The cognitive approach has become an increasingly popular explanation for gambling problems, with its proponents interested in how perceptions and attributions can account for the continued engagement in self-harming behaviors (Ladouceur, Sylvian, Boutin, & Doucet, 2002). Cognitive theory thus provides a mediation model whereby both basic and complex emotional responses and behavior are principally governed by the perceptions, interpretations, and expectations that occur in any given context. Therefore, in cognitive therapy clients are required to develop an increasingly sophisticated understanding of their thoughts and belief structures as pertinent to gambling and other life situations. It is very rare to find clients with gambling problems who function adaptively in all other areas of life. Indeed, typically the gambling problem has emerged in the context of an inability to manage one or more areas of life. These problem areas tend to remain, and will often have worsened as the gambling problem becomes entrenched. Clearly therefore it is important to include a theory that might also explain and provide a means to address the range of dysfunctional behaviors with which problem gambling clients present.

In summary, social learning theory provides a model to explain why people begin gambling and achieve early reinforcement. Conditioning (behavioral) models explain the ongoing and increasing gambling behavior based on reinforcement of the urge to gamble. External triggers (money, advertisements, visual and auditory cues) as well as internal triggers (sadness loneliness, boredom, and anger) become conditioned stimuli that induce the urge to gamble that is relieved only by gambling. Cognitive theory, while not disputing the role of classical and operant conditioning processes, is focused more toward an explanation that describes gambling behaviors as developing due to the formation of inaccurate expectancies (e.g., about the likelihood of wins and losses, about one's ability to predict or control the outcome of a wager), and importantly through faulty assumptions about self-efficacy that are activated in gambling and other contexts (e.g., a priori assumptions that an individuals may apply about their capacity for self-control when gambling, or indeed low-efficacy assumptions applied in relation to the capacity to effectively manage various aversive situations).

Treatment Theory

The treatment model is based on the assumption that psycho-physiological gambling responses can be learned and can therefore be unlearned or extinguished. The principal process of extinguishing such responses is called habituation. Wolpe proposed that fear reduction could usually occur by the simultaneous presentation of anxiety-provoking stimuli and stimuli evoking a response antagonistic to anxiety (relaxation), provided the antagonistic response was the stronger of the two. To ensure that this occurred, the anxiety-provoking stimuli were presented in a graded way, in a hierarchy. Wolpe taught clients relaxation and then encouraged them to continue with a step-by-step approach along a hierarchy of their fearful triggers. During this time, they maintained relaxation in order to inhibit the fear response. Exposure to the stimuli was initially conducted in the live situation but was changed to imaginal exposure because it offered an easier approach for the client. This process of combining exposure with relaxation was called "systemic desensitisation." Wolpe believed that systematic desensitisation was responsible for the reduction of fear. A rapid form of exposure is called "flooding" or, in imagination, is called "implosion." Clients are encouraged to imagine themselves in their most frightening situations.

McConaghy (1980) argued that once pathological gambling behavior is established the central nervous system has built up a neuronal pattern beginning with the initial triggers provoking arousal to the completion of the act. If the person did not follow through with this behavior, a noxious state of tension would develop. The high levels of arousal experienced when triggered would produce a higher level of compulsive drive if not completed. Therefore attempts to avoid gambling produce feelings of tension, irritability, and depression. The trigger also elicits a total preoccupation to gamble. These sensations and preoccupations continue until the person is finally compelled to complete the gambling task by placing a bet. Once a bet has been placed, the person experiences a reduction in both physical and autonomic arousal as well as the arousal of his or her varying emotional states. This experience then acts as a negative reinforcer. By second-order conditioning the person has learned that the act of gambling reduced the tension and levels of discomfort experienced before placing the bet (McConaghy, 1980).

RATIONALE

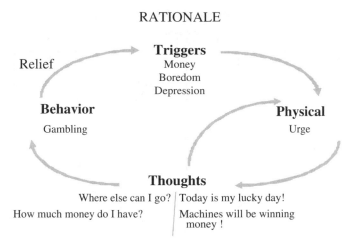

Fig. 11.1 Three-systems model of gambling urge creation

Exposure Rationale

Building on the work of Wolpe, Marks, and others (see Marks [1987], pp. 458–459) recognized that many behavioral treatments reduced anxiety through a process of continual exposure to the stimulus that is evoking the anxiety. Lang (1994) developed the "three systems model" of anxiety incorporating physiological, behavioral, and cognitive functioning. The model proposes that these three systems work generally in the same direction in response to triggers or cues that have been conditioned to anxiety. Treatment can focus on either or both the cognitive or behavioral component of the three systems. Empirical research for anxiety disorders has determined that the best outcomes are achieved when exposure is (1) graded, (2) repeated daily, (3) prolonged in each session until habituation occurs, and (4) focused, that is, distraction is minimized (Marks, 1987). In the same way, the treatment model developed by the Flinders service is based on the same three components of the gambling urge, which can be unlearned or deconditioned using exposure (see Fig. 11.1 for an example of the three-systems model for problem gambling).

Cognitive Therapy Rationale

While the exposure rationale provides a useful explanation to account for how a range of stimuli develop the properties of conditioned stimuli that have urge-provoking qualities, this rationale is of less use when attempting to explain many of the complex variations that can be observed with regard to individual differences in gambling behavior. Clearly not all persons exposed to the same gambling-related classical and operant conditioning contingencies will develop problem gambling

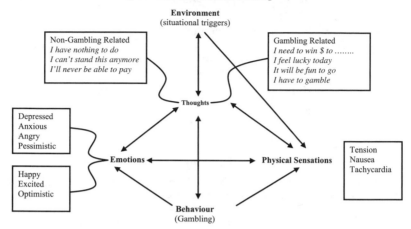

Fig. 11.2 Cognitive rationale of problem gambling

behaviors. It is here that a cognitive therapy rationale enables us to introduce the mediation model whereby the primary factor that determines the occurrence of gambling behavior is not "exposure to a trigger," but rather how the subject processes a wide range of information in any given situation. Figure 11.2 shows how the cognitive therapy rationale does accommodate classical conditioning in terms of the physical characteristics of the "urge," but indicates that the main process accounting for the performance of gambling behavior in any given context is centered on the expectations and beliefs of the individual.

Cognitive Behavior Therapy

A major emphasis in therapy is on the gambling urge being extinguished. The urge has to be extinguished, or clients are at an increased risk of a relapse. Using the behavioral (exposure) component of the three systems model, clients are asked to resist the gambling urge and expose themselves to the urge until it habituates (i.e., prolong the exposure). This model is based on the exposure and response prevention approach used for obsessive–compulsive disorder (Marks, 1987). Before being introduced to the exposure model, clients are assessed for the presence of erroneous beliefs regarding the likelihood of winning and their ability to influence the outcome. Where this is a problem, the client is taught to use a thought diary and then to challenge the erroneous beliefs in real-life situations. The client is encouraged to commence an exposure program as soon as possible.

The client will then no longer need to rely on avoidance strategies to prevent him or her from gambling. This means that at the completion of successful treatment, the client has mastery over the urge to gamble and can return to a normal lifestyle without modifying factors and avoidance strategies needing to be in place. Other

techniques are also incorporated into treatment including cognitive therapy addressing both erroneous beliefs related to gambling and depressed thoughts, which lead
to a depressed mood. Problem-solving strategies and relapse prevention techniques
are also taught as necessary in individual cases.

Cognitive behavioral psychotherapy includes:

- *Education*: The first step of therapy is to provide as much information about the
  client's condition as possible and to help the client understand when his or her
  experiences; feelings, and thoughts may be aggravating or alternatively helping
  the problem. To promote motivation to engage in treatment, clients must have
  a basic understanding of how their gambling problem may be helped using the
  therapy process, and this educational component must be extended to the client's
  family or others with whom they share a close relationship including work
  colleagues.
- *Coaching/guiding*: Within the cognitive behavioral psychotherapy framework,
  clients are empowered and allowed the opportunity to resolve their own problems
  without being told by a therapist what to do or not do. However, a certain amount
  of coaching or guiding is necessary, especially in the early sessions where the
  client is most vulnerable.
- *Homework*: One of the most important components of CBT is that clients continue to work on the problems addressed in therapy between sessions. This work
  is important to reinforce any cognitive or behavioral changes elicited during sessions.
- *Self-help/Self-treatment*: Combining all of the above, the basic principle of CBT
  is that the therapy is essentially providing a self-help framework for clients. Once
  they have learned the basic principles and there has been some noticeable change
  toward resolving the problem, clients are able with minimal support to go on to
  complete their own recovery.
- *Empowerment*: This whole process is designed to empower the clients. It is
  through this empowerment that most of the permanent changes will take place.
  One way to achieve empowerment is through the use of graded exposure, which
  by reducing the urge leads to greater degrees of control in their gambling. This
  control is strengthened as the client moves through the stages of exposure. Once
  this control is achieved, modifying factors and avoidance strategies are no longer
  required to stop the client from gambling.
- *Empirical*: CBT is based upon sound scientific research findings and is constantly
  being refined as techniques are modified in light of new research. Each client
  within therapy should be viewed as a single-case experimental design with outcomes being recorded throughout therapy.
- *Structured*: The client and therapist establish a framework for each session and an
  agenda is formed and worked on during the session. It is important not to make
  the agenda too long or too short; the momentum of progress needs to be maintained and this should be balanced at each step by allowing the client sufficient
  time for practice.
- *Problem focused*: As described, the client tackles problem(s) he or she has identified with the therapist. These problems are then dealt with in order of priority

determined by the client. The therapy process allows for new problems to be dealt with after negotiation between client and therapist.

- *Current*: The problem must be present at the time, or at least be determined to be present if certain avoidant actions of the client are stopped, for example, not visiting hotels, etc.
- *Goal directed*: The goals can be short, medium, or long term. Each week the client agrees to a set of between session goals based on the problem he or she has presented. Within therapy, the client will hopefully achieve the medium-term goals and go on to achieve the long-term goals while in follow-up. Measurement of progress toward achieving goals gives feedback to both the therapist and client, which in turn allows fine-tuning of treatment strategies. Ongoing measurement of progress toward achievement of goals also provides reinforcement of the process and acts as a reward for the client's effort, which in turn encourages the client to continue to work toward the next goal.
- *Client centered*: Within therapy, the emphasis should always be on what the client wishes to achieve. However, there are some constraints when using the CBT approach. These are, first, that the basic principles of therapy should be followed, and second, that the therapy remains client centered in that the work being asked of the client should not be too difficult to achieve. As a rule of thumb, the therapist should not expect a client to do something the therapist would not be prepared to do him- or herself. The client makes the decision as to what to do, not the therapist, yet the therapist must guide the client so that goals are not unrealistic and unachievable.
- *Collaborative*: As with the above comments, all aspects of the therapy process are done in conjunction with client and therapist. It is important that both parties here have ascertained agreement regarding the goals of therapy.

The Clinical Assessment

A course of therapy offered to a client is based on a detailed assessment so that the treatment approaches and skills to be learned are targeted to the individual's needs. A standardized semistructured interview called a cognitive behavioral assessment is used to look closely at the client's gambling behaviors and related problems. In addition, a psychiatric assessment including broad psychosocial issues and the patient's occupational, family, social, and cultural background is conducted. The cognitive behavioral assessment establishes the exact nature of the client's gambling problem. A behavioral analysis (sometimes called a "functional" analysis) is performed on the client's typical gambling pattern and takes into account the behaviors, cognitions, and physical sensations when a client is exposed to a gambling trigger and the consequences of this behavior. This detailed assessment helps to establish the treatment plan for the client. The assessment also identifies comorbid mental health conditions and includes an assessment of risk of harm to self or others.

Benzodiazepines and alcohol may reduce the client's anxiety and urges to gamble temporarily until the client is exposed to another gambling trigger. If the client is taking these substances, a withdrawal program should be considered before treatment can be commenced, as any new learning processes occurring during therapy while taking benzodiazepines will not be easily recalled when the drug is stopped. The urges to gamble would most likely return, as the habituation process to gambling triggers would not have been completed (Marks, 1987). Once the assessment has been completed and the problem thought to be suitable for CBT, the therapist provides a rationale for the development and treatment of the gambling problem. This is based on the three-systems model of problem gambling development and how this can be eliminated using exposure to gambling triggers, cognitive therapy, and lifestyle modifications.

Setting Up Treatment

In a subsequent session, the therapy program is established by developing an agreed problem statement and end of treatment goals (usually two). In addition, baseline outcome measures are taken (see later) and finally the initial homework tasks are agreed on. The problem and goals approach provides both an outcome measurement and motivational process by determining what the client wants from treatment. There is no mandated abstinence or controlled gambling goal. The problem and goal statements are rated by the client and therapist every 4 weeks, as are the standardized outcome measures.

CBT is based upon the "here and now" and works with the problem currently being exhibited. For example, the problem may be "....I have an uncontrollable urge to gamble on electronic gaming machines whenever I have money. I gamble at least 5 times a week and up to twice a day at times. This causes avoidance of hotels, not having access to money, relationship and financial problems and depression." Rated 0–8 on how much the problem affected daily activities: 8 = severe interference, 0 = no interference. This example describes a client with a current problem occurring several times per week. In this case, the therapist and client would have an observable problem to work on. An example of an individual goal may be "to be able to sit alone in a favorite gaming venue for a minimum of 1 hour twice a week, put $50.00 in the gaming machine and not gamble. To collect the money from the machine and leave without gambling." Rated 0–8 on current progress toward achieving this goal; 8 = no progress, 0 = complete success.

Treatment Sessions

Exposure

The principle focus of the exposure component is to enable the client to experience habituation to a gambling urge as soon as possible. Clients are encouraged to expose themselves to the situation or object that evokes the gambling urge, and for this to be repeated on a regular basis for a sufficient duration each time. Changing the behavioral component is an important variable that leads to the modification of the autonomic responses and thereafter eventually thoughts and attitudes about the situation follow. Ideally, these become congruent with the new behavior and physiological responses. When practicing exposure, engagement has to be emotional as well as physical; mere physical presence is not enough. Clients need to be focused on their urge and thoughts. There are a number of ways to minimize the response, including blocking, dissociation, discounting, ignoring, and distraction. The behavioral tasks must be graded sufficiently to ensure the client feels comfortable to fully engage in the task and not have to incorporate the previous blocking or distracting behaviors. Desensitization or flooding in fantasy, therapist accompanied exposure, and relaxation are rarely used.

The initial procedure, called imaginal exposure, is carried out with the therapist guiding the client through a scene. It is usually audiotaped. The client is instructed to imagine a typical gambling scenario. This is a graded experience, and the client is asked to rate his or her urge to gamble at regular intervals while verbalizing the scenario and stay with the urge until habituation occurs. The client gradually completes the scenario until eventually (in imagination) he or she is able to sit in front of their favorite gaming machine ready to press the play button without experiencing the urge.

Cognitive Therapy

For most clients this is introduced at an early stage of treatment. Clients need to understand that therapy will comprise a number of seemingly different yet complementary strategies, and this is explained by making use of the CBT rationale. As in most effective psychotherapy, clients need to be socialized to the model. With cognitive therapy, this involves an introduction to the view that one's behavior and emotions are only partially under the control of environmental factors, and that the more important determinant is how one perceives, interprets, and forms expectations. This introduction is achieved via the examination of various cause–effect situations, making use of a classic thought diary to demonstrate how cognitions are a primary influence of behavior and emotions. Considerable attention is also given to exploring how many thought processes occur quite automatically, but with conscious effort can be recognized and potentially modified. Clients are then taught how to identify and challenge both erroneous beliefs related to gambling and other dysfunctional thought processes that maintain depressed mood and various distressed states. Given this consideration, the cognitive therapy component is often done separately from the exposure tasks, as it would prevent clients from focusing on their desires to gamble.

Once the client has habituated to the urge, clients can then challenge the triggers for their urges to gamble and the negative thought patterns they may experience once the urge has been extinguished. Over the next 4 to 5 weeks, clients habituate to their urge to gamble using a variety of live tasks until their treatment goals are achieved. Clients complete tasks in their own homes at first, then at gambling venues with an increasing range of cues. These graded tasks slowly increase in difficulty as the client's urge begins to reduce and habituation has occurred. Clients are seen weekly and homework is reviewed and tasks regraded or new tasks agreed are on.

In summary, the main requirements for therapy are:

1. Client and therapist agree to define the problem in terms of observable behavior.
2. The behavior is current and predictable.
3. The client and therapist can agree on clear goals that relate to the client's handicaps.
4. The client understands and agrees to treatment.
5. There are no contraindications (e.g., psychosis, drug dependence, or depression).

Program Outcomes

Standardized Questionnaires

South Oaks Gambling Screen

The South Oaks Gambling Screen (Fig. 11.3) tool is a 20-item questionnaire based on DSM-III criteria for pathological gambling. It may be self-administered or administered by a health professional. Individuals scoring less than 3 are described as non-problem gamblers and those who score between 3 and 4 are potential problem gamblers. A score of 5 or higher is considered to indicate a probable pathological gambler (Lesieur & Blume, 1987).

Work and Social Adjustment (WASA) Scale

This generic measure of disability and handicap is a self-administered scale covering five areas of functioning on a scale of 0 to 40 (Fig. 11.6). The Work and

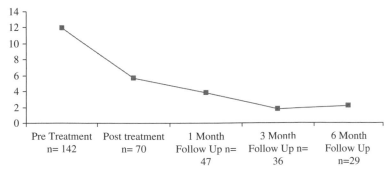

Fig. 11.3 South Oaks Gambling Screen (SOGS). Scores over 5 are considered probable pathological gamblers

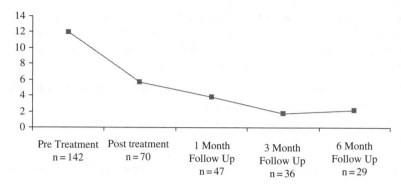

Fig. 11.4 Client-rated problem scores. Scoring of problem statement: Rated on how much the problem affects daily activities: 8 = severe interference, 0 = no interference

Social Adjustment Scale is a tool used to measure the disability and handicap in relation to work, home management, social leisure, private leisure, and family and relationships. It is an appropriate tool for those with both psychological and physical problems, because it describes the impact of problems on many aspects of an individual's life. This questionnaire measures the clients' own perceptions of their problems and how this impacts on their daily lives. It can be used as an indirect measure of success (Mundt, Marks, Shear, & Greist, 2002). The main advantages of this tool are that it is quick to use, applicable to a full range of severity, and has shown to be a sensitive measure over time.

Beck Depression Inventory

The Beck Depression Inventory (BDI) is a self-report questionnaire that provides cutoffs from depression into mild, moderate, and severe and is a validated and reliable measure of change over time. This is a 21-item self-rating scale scoring: 0–10

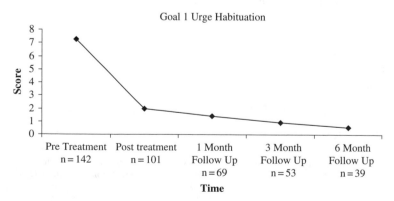

Fig. 11.5 Client-rated end of treatment goal 1. Scoring of goal statement: Rated on progress toward achieving this goal: 8 = no progress, 0 = complete success

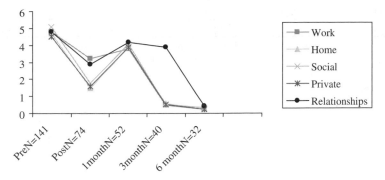

Fig. 11.6 Work and Social Adjustment Scale measure of functional ability and handicap in five areas. There was a similar reduction in the mean scores for both the Beck Depression and Anxiety scores. In all graphs, the drop in the mean score between pretreatment and completion of treatment was statistically significant ($p < 0.001$)

indicates no depression, 11–17 indicates mild depression, 18–23 indicates moderate depression, and 23 and above indicates severe depression (Beck, Ward, Mendelson, Mock, & Erbaugh, 1961).

Beck Anxiety Inventory

The Beck Anxiety Inventory (BAI) is a self-report questionnaire that provides severity cutoffs for anxiety into mild, moderate, and severe and is a validated and reliable measure of change over time. Scoring: 0–21 indicates low anxiety; 22–35 indicates moderate anxiety; 36–over indicates severe anxiety (Beck and Steer, 1990)

Problems and Goals

The aim of the problem and goal statement is for clients to describe as concisely as they are able what they perceive as their main problem and the specific and observable goals they wish to achieve in relation to the problem (Battersby, Ask, Reece, Markwick, & Collins, 2001). Problem statement scoring: rated 0–8 on how much the problem affected her daily activities: 8 = severe interference, 0 = no interference. Goal statement scoring: rated 0–8 on progress toward achieving this goal; 8 = no progress, 0 = complete success.

Client Outcomes

Table 11.1 represents consecutive clients who were registered ($N = 150$), completed treatment ($N = 123$), and were regularly followed-up between 1998 and 2004. The outcomes represent routine follow-up by clinicians and is not a research

Table 11.1 Client Flow Chart

Time Frame	Activity	Population	Percent (%)
Commencement of Program	Clients registered	150	
5–12 weeks later	Treatment completed	123	82
1-month follow-up		104	69
3-month follow-up		72	48
6-month follow-up		54	36

A summary of outcome measures for 150 clients is reported in Figs. 11.3 to 11.6. The numbers reported for each measure do not match with total numbers attending for treatment and follow-up, as not all clients completed all measures.

study. The follow-up process involves clients being encouraged to return for ongoing review but the clinic's resources do not allow clients to be actively pursued for data collection. Of the 123 clients who completed treatment, 54 (44%) attended 6-month follow-up. In addition, a further 55 were contacted by phone to determine non-gambling outcomes qualitatively. Of the treatment completers (123) at 6-month follow-up, 97 (79%) were in work, 9 (8%) had commenced studies, 3 (2%) had lapsed, and outcomes were unknown for 14 (11%). Hence of the 69 (56%) who did not attend for follow-up, the majority had returned to work or study and indicated that follow-up was unnecessary or impractical. There was a similar reduction in the mean scores for both the Beck Depression and Anxiety scores. In all graphs, the drop in the mean score between pre-treatment and completion of treatment was statistically significant ($p < 0.001$).

Case Study: "Melissa"

The following case describes the identification and treatment of a client assessed who was admitted to the psychiatric ward at Flinders Medical Centre following a significant suicide attempt. Melissa was a 40–year-old separated woman living in rental accommodation and employed as a shift worker at a local hotel. She was referred to The Flinders Therapy Service for problem gamblers by a trainee psychiatrist after a serious suicide attempt. This was in response to a significant loss of money due to gambling.

On clinical assessment, Melissa was diagnosed with pathological gambling. She stated her main problem was an uncontrollable urge to gamble whenever she had money. Her gambling history revealed that she gambled at least five times a week and at times up to twice daily on the electronic gambling machines. Melissa's total financial loss to gambling was approximately $70,000. She was gambling up to 70% of her total income. Melissa was screened for her suitability for CBT to address her problem gambling and depression. She was considered to be suitable and was offered treatment for her pathological gambling after discharge from hospital by one of the therapists at the unit.

Before the commencement of treatment the therapist assisted Melissa to formulate her own individual problem and end of treatment goal. These were rated throughout treatment and at follow-up.

Melissa's gambling problem statement: "When I have money I have an uncontrollable urge to gamble on the electronic gaming machines and eventually gamble. This results in financial and relationship problems, depression, avoidance of carrying money, and time alone." Rated 8 on how much the problem affected her daily activities: 8 = severe interference, 0 = no interference.

Melissa's goal statement: "*To save $75.00 per week and when my bills have been payed I will save this money towards a family caravan holiday at Christmas time.*" Rated 8 on progress toward achieving this goal; 8 = no progress, 0 = complete success.

Treatment was initially focused on her depression, using cognitive therapy addressing the negative thought patterns maintaining her depressed mood. It was noted that although her mood had lifted, her urges to gamble remained high. She attended weekly treatment sessions for 8 weeks in a group setting. Treatment involved graded exposure to her urges to gamble, cognitive therapy related to her erroneous beliefs about gambling, and relapse prevention strategies. Melissa completed her individual treatment goals at the end of the 8-week therapy course and was followed up over a 2-year period to ensure her treatment gains were maintained. She then moved to the country, where she bought a property with her new partner.

Results

Melissa's measures at assessment and follow-up over a 2-year period are described in Figs. 11.7, 11.8, and 11.9. The SOGS pretreatment, posttreatment, and 2-year follow-up scores are presented in Fig. 11.7. By mid-treatment Melissa's scores were in the nonclinical range. Melissa's problem and end of treatment goal scores are shown in Fig. 11.8. By mid-treatment her problem statement was rated as 0 out of 8. Her goal was achieved by mid-treatment. The 2-year follow-up showed that the

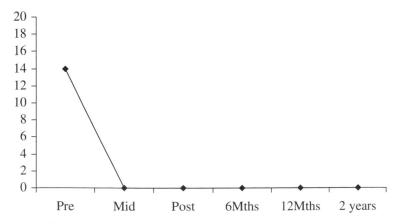

Fig. 11.7 SOGS scores pretreatment and up to 2-year follow-up

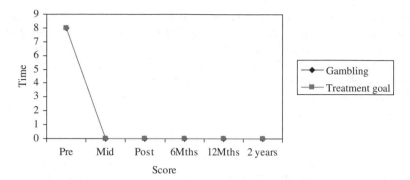

Fig. 11.8 Problem and goal scores pretreatment and up to 2-year follow-up. Beck Depression and Anxiety scores are shown in Fig. 11.9. By 1 month follow–up Melissa's scores were in the nonclinical range. Her depression score increased after a health scare at the 2-year follow-up

goal attainment was maintained. Beck depression and anxiety scores are shown in Fig. 11.9. By 1-month follow-up Melissa's scores were in the nonclinical range. Her depression score increased after a health scare at the 2-year follow-up.

This letter from a client after completing treatment provides a description of their perception of the treatment process.

Dear Jane,

I thought it was important to take the time and write you a few lines. The course around gambling is drawing to a close and I have to say the time has gone so quickly. Approximately 4 months ago, my life was a virtual mess. Although I remained employed and I had people who loved and cared about me I had to come to terms with the fact that I had a gambling problem. Not an easy thing when you're a relatively proud person, who has devoted their entire career to helping the sick, poor, and underprivileged.

From that very moment, I realized I took a "life changing" step toward determining my future path in life. I knew the next step for me was to seek help around my addiction, which is where your program comes into play.

I recall my 1st appointment for assessment was as daunting as it was exhilarating. For the 1st time in such a long time I felt in control of who I am and where I'm going. I think it's important for me to share with you and to let you all know how appreciative I am for the program you provide. As I write this, my mind reflects back to all I have managed to

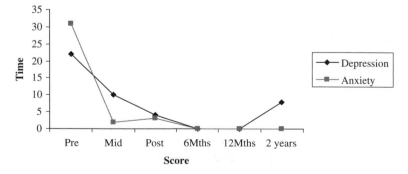

Fig. 11.9 Beck Depression and Anxiety scores over time

learn from your program. I wish to thank all of you for not only the content you provided, but also the manner in which it was conducted. Your program has provided me with tools and principles I can apply in all aspects of my life. Your method, although confronting and at times challenging, enables me to remain "grounded" in what was once this heavy "fog" called life. Thanks to your program and the hard work I have put in, I am actually living as opposed to merely existing.

I know I am not "cured" per say, but I am equipped and armed with powerful skills for the future. I have never subscribed to the adage "practice makes perfect", someone told me long ago "practice makes permanent." If you're taught the wrong thing or technique from the beginning and one continues to practice it, then it will eventually become permanent. In this case, I know if I practice the therapy principles and apply them. Over time it will remain permanent.

Thank you to all of you for assisting me in getting my life back.

Sincerely yours
Xxxxxxxxxxxxx

Chapter 12
Psychopharmacological Management of Pathological Gambling

Jon E. Grant, Suck Won Kim, and Marc N. Potenza

Although pathological gambling (PG) is relatively common and associated with significant distress and impairment (Argo & Black, 2004), little is known regarding effective pharmacotherapy for this disorder. The difficulty may stem from the inherent heterogeneity of PG (Blanco, Moreyra, Nunes, Saiz-Ruiz, & Ibanez, 2001) and the fact that several core psychopathologic domains could conceivably be targets for treatment: impulsivity (arousal), compulsivity (anxiety reduction), and addiction (symptoms of withdrawal) (Hollander, Kaplan, & Pallanti, 2004). In addition, neurobiological investigations of the etiology of PG have shown evidence of multiple system involvement (serotonergic, noradrenergic, and dopaminergic) (Shah, Potenza, & Eisen, 2004). High rates of psychiatric comorbidity with mood, anxiety, and substance use disorders (Bland, Newman, Orn, & Stebelsky, 1993; Ibanez et al., 2001; Linden, Pope, & Jonas, 1986) provide additional neuropsychopharmacological frameworks for treatment and add to the complexity of finding effective pharmacological interventions.

In contrast to drug addictions in which illicit drugs are used to induce pleasure, gamblers engage in a behavior to bring about excitement (Holden, 2001). The neural substrates of drug addictions have been well studied and include the ventral tegmental area (VTA) to nucleus accumbens (NA) mesolimbic circuit (Di Chiara & North, 1992; Hyman, 1993; Koob, 1992; Koob & Bloom, 1988). Illicit drugs often stimulate VTA neurons to release dopamine in the NA or block reuptake of dopamine within the NA (Kalivas & Volkow, 2005; Phillips & LePiane, 1980; Stewart, 1984; van Wolfswinkel & van Ree, 1985). This neurotransmission and subsequent neurochemical cascades within the NA and downstream effects in connected brain regions are believed to underlie feelings of pleasure, serving to reinforce the addictive behaviors. Although gamblers do not uniformly use illicit drugs, gambling, anticipated reward, or uncertainty associated with reward probability activates dopamine neurons within VTA which in turn triggers increased release of dopamine in NA (Fiorillo, Tobler, & Schultz, 2005; Schultz, 2002). Thus, similar neural substrates and chemical mechanisms appear involved in both drug addictions and non-drug addictions such as PG.

Jon E. Grant
University of Minnesota Medical School, United States of America

M. Zangeneh, A. Blaszczynski, N. Turner (eds.), *In the Pursuit of Winning*.
© Springer 2008

Consistent with the neurobiological findings described in the preceding text, pharmacological treatment strategies have targeted presumed region-specific dysfunctions. Low levels of the serotonin metabolite 5-hydroxyindole acetic acid (5-HIAA) and blunted serotonergic response within the ventromedial prefrontal cortex (vmPFC) have been associated with impulsive behaviors (Coccaro, 1996; Linnoila, Virkkunen, George, & Higley, 1993; Mehlman, Higley, & Faucher, 1995; Rogers et al., 1999; Virkkunen, Goldman, & Nielsen, 1995). Prefrontal glucose metabolism, especially within the orbitofrontal cortex (OFC), is inversely correlated with cerebrospinal fluid 5-HIAA levels. The processing of motivational drives and determination of object saliency involve the orbitofrontal and cingulate cortices (Bush et al., 2002; Jentsch & Taylor, 1999). The vmPFC includes the most ventral component of the anterior cingulate cortex and the medial portion of the OFC (Bechara, 2003). Disadvantageous decision-making as assessed by the Iowa Gambling Task has been observed both in individuals with stroke lesions in the vmPFC as well as in individuals with PG or substance use disorders (Bechara, 2003; Cavedini, Riboldi, Keller, D'Annucci, & Bellodi, 2002). As compared to control comparison subjects, individuals with PG demonstrate diminished activation of the vmPFC when viewing gambling-related videotapes or during prepotent response inhibition when performing the Stroop color–word interference task (Potenza et al., 2003a, 2003b). Individuals with PG also show relatively diminished activation of the vmPFC (and NA) during a simulated gambling task, and severity of gambling problem correlated inversely with signal intensity within these brain regions (Reuter et al., 2005). Together, the findings suggest that decreased serotonin function within vmPFC may engender disinhibition and contribute to PG. Thus, drugs targeting serotonin neurotransmission, such as serotonin reuptake inhibitors (SRIs), have been investigated in the treatment of PG.

Many SRIs have been shown to be efficacious in targeting symptoms of depression, obsessive–compulsive disorder, and anxiety. By extension, SRIs may be hypothesized to reduce context-specific obsessions or ruminations, such as gambling-related thoughts or gambling urges. Given that the overlap between PG and major depression in men has been found to be largely genetic in nature (Potenza, Xian, Shah, Scherrer, & Eisen, 2005), similar genes, and by extension similar biological pathways, may underlie PG and major depression. As such, medications helpful for treating one disorder may have efficacy for the other.

Another pharmacological treatment strategy has examined the opioid system that modulates dopamine function within the VTA–NA–OFC circuit. Mu-opioid receptor antagonists inhibit dopamine release in NA and ventral pallidum (VP) through the disinhibition of gamma-aminobutyric acid (GABA) input to the dopamine neurons in the VTA (Broekkamp & Phillips, 1979; Matthews & German, 1984; Phillips & LePiane, 1980; Stewart, 1984; van Wolfswinkel & van Ree, 1985). Thus, it was originally hypothesized that decreased dopamine in NA and motivation circuit would dampen excitement and cravings related to gambling behavior (Kim, 1998). Although modulation of drive and subsequent behavioral output by dopamine, endorphin, and GABA has been investigated, the specific mechanisms remain incompletely understood, particularly as related to PG (Kalivas & Barnes, 1993; Koob, 1992).

Other hypotheses concerning the pathophysiology of PG have resulted in different classes of medication being studied for PG. Antiepileptic agents enhance GABA function within the central nervous system and reduce neuronal firing rates. Selected agents in this class may reduce craving symptoms significantly (Hollander et al., 2004).

Although there are currently no existing medications approved by the Food and Drug Administration for the treatment of PG, multiple pharmacological interventions have been studied. This chapter reviews current pharmacological treatment strategies for PG, the neural substrates and transmitters that are proposed to underlie the symptoms of PG, and the rationales for applying various classes of psychotropic agents.

Antidepressants

Clomipramine (Anafranil)

Clomipramine, a preferential serotonin reuptake blocker that also inhibits norepinephrine reuptake, has demonstrated both antidepressant and anti-obsessional properties (Kaplan & Hollander, 2003). The first test of clomipramine in PG came from Hollander and colleagues, who reported a response to clomipramine in a single PG subject using a double-blind, placebo-controlled design (Hollander, Frenkel, Decaria, Trungold, & Stein, 1992). After receiving placebo for 10 weeks without a response, the woman reported a 90% improvement in gambling symptoms (using a measure assessing gambling urges, thoughts, and behavior) after being treated with 125 mg/day of clomipramine.

Clomipramine may result in multiple side effects such as dry mouth, constipation, blurred vision, sexual dysfunction, and weight gain. In addition, clomipramine may cause fine tremor and muscle twitching. Starting at a low dose such as 25 mg at night and slowly titrating the dose over several weeks to 150 to 250 mg/day reduces the likelihood of side effects. Clomipramine should not be used if a patient has a history of cardiac conduction disturbance or a central nervous system illness that might compromise memory. At 300 mg/day, clomipramine can cause seizures in about 2% of subjects. Clomipramine should not be used with medications such as fluoxetine or paroxetine that inhibit P450 isozymes, for they inhibit clomipramine hepatic metabolism and cause elevated serum clomipramine and desmethylated clomipramine levels. If it becomes necessary to use these medications in combination, serum clomipramine levels should be monitored frequently.

Fluvoxamine (Luvox)

Several studies have examined the efficacy of fluvoxamine in PG. In the first, Hollander and colleagues reported that 7 of 10 subjects treated for 8 weeks in a single-blind design responded (response was defined as "much improved" or "very much improved" based on the Clinical Global Impressions Scale and a 25% reduction in the total score on the Yale–Brown Obsessive–Compulsive Scale Modified for Pathological Gambling [PG-YBOCS]) (Hollander et al., 1998). In a double-blind, crossover study, 15 subjects entered a 7-day placebo lead-in phase, followed by 6 subjects continuing with placebo for 8 weeks and then fluvoxamine for an additional 8 weeks. Four subjects received the medication in the reverse order. Positive response (defined by the change on the Clinical Global Impressions Improvement Scale) was significantly greater for fluvoxamine (40.6%) compared to placebo (16.6%) (Hollander et al., 2000). Fluvoxamine did not differ from placebo when both phases were combined and the results were examined using the PG-YBOCS. Interpretation of the study is complicated, however, by a phase-order treatment interaction (i.e., the medication did not separate from placebo during the first phase but did in the second phase). In an independent double-blind placebo-controlled treatment study of fluvoxamine in PG, however, fluvoxamine did not demonstrate superiority to placebo, except in male subjects and younger subjects. The result of this study are complicated by high rates of treatment discontinuation and a high placebo response rate (59%) (Blanco, Petkova, Ibanez, & Saiz-Ruiz, 2002). Thus, the results are mixed with respect to the efficacy of fluvoxamine in the treatment of PG.

Although fluvoxamine is generally well tolerated, it may result in gastrointestinal distress, sedation, mild anxiety, headache, increased urinary frequency, and sexual dysfunction. Fluvoxamine is a potent P450 1A2 inhibitor, and drug–drug interactions should be considered before it is prescribed.

Paroxetine (Paxil)

Paroxetine has been studied in two double-blind, placebo-controlled studies. In the first single-site study, subjects were treated with paroxetine ($n = 20$) (20 mg/day to 60 mg/day) of placebo ($n = 21$) for 8 weeks (Kim, Grant, Adson, Shin, & Zaninelli, 2002). Paroxetine resulted in significantly greater reduction on several measures of PG severity (assessing gambling urges, thoughts, and behavior) after 6 weeks of treatment. In a 16-week multicenter double-blind study of paroxetine, however, no statistically significant differences were observed between paroxetine ($n = 21$) and placebo ($n = 24$) in terms of gambling urges, thoughts, or behavior (Grant et al., 2003). In this second study, a high placebo response rate was observed: at the end of the study, 48% of those assigned to placebo and 59% of those taking paroxetine were responders. Although paroxetine tends to be well tolerated, it may cause sedation, constipation, weight gain, headache, sexual dysfunction, and dry mouth. As with other antidepressants, warnings exist for the potential association between paroxetine and suicidal behaviors. Given the relatively short half-life of paroxetine, the potential for flu-like SRI discontinuation symptoms exist, particularly with abrupt cessation of high dosages of the drug.

Sertraline (Zoloft)

In a double-blind placebo-controlled study, 60 subjects with PG were treated for 6 months (Saiz-Ruiz et al., 2005). At the end of the study, 23 sertraline-treated subjects (74%) and 21 placebo-treated subjects (72%) were rated as responders based on a questionnaire assessing urges to gamble and gambling behavior. In this study, sertraline did not demonstrate superiority to placebo. Sertraline was well tolerated at doses between 50 mg/day and 150 mg/day.

Citalopram (Celexa)

In an open-label study, investigators tested the efficacy of citalopram in 15 subjects with PG (Zimmerman, Breen, & Posternak, 2002). With a mean dose of 34.7 mg/day, 13 subjects were rates as responders on the Clinical Global Impression scale ("much improved" or "very much improved"). The study, however, was not controlled and therefore how much improvement may have been due to a placebo response could not be examined. Citalopram is generally well tolerated, but may causes side effects similar to those of other antidepressants.

Escitalopram (Lexapro)

Escitalopram was recently studied in a 12-week open-label design of PG with comorbid anxiety (Grant & Potenza, in press). Of 13 subjects treated with a mean dose of 25.4 mg/day, 62% were considered responders in terms of both PG and anxiety symptoms. Four of six subjects who completed the study and were responders (defined as "very much improved" or "much improved" based on the Clinical Global Impressions Scale) were entered into an 8-week double-blind discontinuation. Of the three assigned to escitalopram, improvement continued for the next 8 weeks in all three cases, whereas both gambling symptoms and anxiety returned within 4 weeks for the subject assigned to placebo.

Bupropion (Wellbutrin)

In an open-label study, 10 patients with PG were given bupropion 100 mg/day for the first week, 200 mg/day for the second week, and 300 mg/day for the third week (Black, 2004). For the ensuing 5 weeks, subjects were maintained on 300 mg/day. Scores on the PG-YBOCS decreased from 20.3 at baseline to 8.8 at the end of the 8-week study ($p = 0.001$). Bupropion was well tolerated in this study, but may cause gastrointestinal distress, decrease in appetite, dizziness, dry mouth, increased sweating, trembling or shaking, and insomnia. Given the potential of bupropion to lower seizure threshold, its use is typically contraindicated in individuals with a history of a seizure disorder.

Nefazodone (Serzone)

Nefazodone, a mixed serotonin/norepinephrine reuptake inhibitor, was studied in an 8-week open-label trial involving 12 subjects with PG (Pallanti, Baldini Rossi, Sood, & Hollander, 2002). Although the lack of a placebo arm limits the critical evaluation of this medication, 9 (75%) of the 12 subjects were rated as responders based on gambling symptom improvement.

Case Vignette 1

C. L. is a 35-year-old man who came to the clinic for treatment of PG. C. L. has a 5-year history of casino gambling. He has not told anyone about his gambling, including his wife of 6 years. C. L. is employed by a reputable local company and he has not missed work due to gambling. Mounting credit card debt compelled him to seek treatment. C. L. feels guilty because he has not been honest with his wife and daughter. C. L. denied current or past history of chemical dependency. C. L. is physically healthy. During the interview, C. L. presented as a competent young married professional. On careful examination, however, he admits to feeling depressed and to having thoughts of suicide. C. L. has difficulty getting out of bed in the morning and his recreational activity has decreased significantly. C. L. also admitted that he has had depressive episodes in the past but there is no family history of depression. C. L. reports that his depression preceded his gambling behavior.

In accordance with C. L.'s wishes, his wife was not contacted. Citalopram 20 mg qam was initiated and was raised to 40 mg in the morning after 1 week. After 6 weeks, C. L. remained depressed and his gambling behavior had not changed. The citalopram dose was raised to 60 mg. Within 2 weeks of the dose increase, C. L. reported a dramatic improvement in his mood and his thoughts of gambling. He was able to stop going to the casino. C. L. began to play golf again and spent more time with his daughter and wife. Decreased libido and erectile dysfunction were treated with drug holidays and sildenafil.

Comments About Antidepressants

The results from these studies of antidepressants (Table 12.1) are mixed, with no positive, placebo-controlled study of an antidepressant in PG having been successfully reproduced. A number of important concepts in the use of antidepressants for PG, however, have emerged. First, as in the case vignette, it appears that the

Table 12.1 Trials of Antidepressant Medications in Pathological Gambling (PG)

Medication	Starting Doses	Effective Doses in PG Based on the Published Studies	Common Side Effects
Clomipramine	25 mg qhs	125 mg qd	Nausea, headache, restlessness, anxiety, insomnia, decreased libido, impotence, weight gain
Fluvoxamine	50–100 mg qam	100–250 mg qd	
Paroxetine	10–20 mg qam	40–60 mg qam	
Sertraline	25–50 mg qam	50–150 mg qam	
Citalopram	10–20 mg qam	30–60 mg qam	
Escitalopram	5–10 mg qam	20–30 mg qam	
Bupropion	100–150 mg qam	300 mg qd	Nausea, headache, restlessness, anxiety, insomnia, seizure risk
Nefazodone	100 mg bid	200 mg qd	Nausea, somnolence, potential liver failure

doses of antidepressants required to treat gambling symptoms are generally higher than required to treat depressive or anxiety symptoms. These findings are consistent with the findings noted in the treatment of obsessive–compulsive disorder. Second, in studies in which participants had few or no comorbid anxiety or depressive symptoms, antidepressant therapy remained effective in treating PG symptoms. This effect may be the result of serotonergic manipulation of the neural substrates that underlie impulsivity. One of the questions remaining from these studies, however, is whether the mixed results suggest that certain individuals with PG benefit more from antidepressant treatment than others. If so, can individuals with PG be accurately subtyped to target pharmacological interventions for maximize treatment response? We do not currently know whether antidepressants reduce gambling symptoms by reducing gambling-related thoughts, urges, or both. Therefore, more studies are needed to examine how these drugs help reduce gambling symptoms and who are more likely to respond to these interventions.

Mood Stabilizers

Case Vignette 2

A. D. is a 38-year-old lawyer who sought help for his gambling problem. Because of financial losses, lying about gambling, and missing family functions, A. D.'s gambling had resulted in severe problems in his marital relationship. The couple had started marital counseling, and A. D. was also receiving weekly individual psychotherapy. A. D. was gambling at least twice a week at a casino and reported $400,000 in gambling losses over the last 10 years. A. D. reported strong gambling urges that he could not control. A.D. denied significant medical or psychiatric disorders. A. D. denied a family history of mood disorders.

A. D.'s wife was invited to his visits, and his current clinical status and treatment plan were discussed. A. D.'s psychotherapist was also contacted and a mutually supportive treatment alliance was established. Re-examination of his clinical history with his wife revealed that A. D. had recurrent mood swings. A mood stabilizer, divalproate, was initiated. A. D. responded well to 1200 mg/day and has remained abstinent for the past 4 years.

Lithium Carbonate and Valproate

In a 14-week single-blind trial, lithium (n = 23) was compared to valproate (n = 19) in nonbipolar pathological gamblers (Pallanti, Quercioli, Sood, & Hollander, 2002). Both groups showed significant improvement in gambling symptoms without significant differences between groups. Lithium was also used to treat gambling symptoms in an open-label case series (n = 3) (Moskowitz, 1980). Using a mean dose of 1800 mg/day, three subjects with gambling symptoms and possible manic symptoms found lithium to be effective. The main effect was reduced euphoria associated with gambling.

In a recent double-blind, placebo-controlled study of 40 PG subjects with bipolar spectrum disorders, sustained release lithium carbonate was shown to be superior to placebo in reducing PG behavior (Hollander, Pallanti, Allen, Sood, & Baldini Rossi, 2005). Forty subjects who met criteria for bipolar type II, bipolar not otherwise specified, or cyclothymia, as well as PG, were assigned to either placebo (n = 22) or a staggered dose of oral lithium carbonate (n = 18) (therapeutic level defined as a blood level of 0.6 to 1.2 meq/liter) for 10 weeks. A majority (83%) of subjects in the treatment group displayed significant decreases in gambling urges, thoughts, and behaviors.

Carbamazepine (Tegretol)

A pathological gambler improved clinically (i.e., reduction in gambling behavior) after 12 weeks of single-blind treatment with carbamazepine (600 mg/day) (Haller & Hinterhuber, 1994). The same subject had been treated with placebo for the preceding 12 weeks (blinded to the subject) without significant beneficial effects. No significant side effects were noted in this case.

Topiramate (Topamax)

One study comparing topiramate to fluvoxamine in PG found that both agents were equally effective in controlling gambling symptoms (Dannon, Lowengrub, Gonopolski, Musin, & Kotler, 2005). The randomized, blind-rater comparison study

Table 12.2 Trials of Mood Stabilizer Medications in Pathological Gambling (PG)

Medication	Starting Doses	Usual Effective Doses in PG	Common Side Effects
Valproic acid	250 mg qhs	600–1500 mg qd	Nausea, diarrhea, somnolence. Hepatotoxicity and pancreatitis can occur but are rare.
Carbamazepine	200 mg qhs	600 mg qd	Drowsiness, dizziness, nausea, blurred vision. Acute renal failure and aplastic anemia can occur but are rare.
Lithium	300 mg qd	300–1800 mg qd	Fine tremor, nausea, diarrhea. Nephrotoxicity possible in chronic use.
Topiramate	25 mg qd	25–150 mg qd	Weight decrease, somnolence, anorexia, dizziness, difficulty with memory, kidney stones

assigned 31 males with PG to receive either topiramate (n = 15) or fluvoxamine (n = 16) for 12 weeks. Nine of the 12 (75%) topiramate completers reported full remission of gambling behavior, and three completers had a partial remission (some gambling thoughts, urges, or behavior remaining). Six of eight (75%) fluvoxamine completers reported a full remission, and the remaining two reported a partial remission.

Comments About Mood Stabilizers

Evidence suggests elevated rates of co-occurrence between PG and bipolar spectrum disorders (bipolar type I and II, bipolar not otherwise specified, and cyclothymia) (Argo & Black, 2004). In addition, some individuals with PG exhibit symptoms of subsyndromal mania. Individuals with bipolar disorder may demonstrate irrational financial behavior and impulsive behavior that resemble the symptoms of PG. In all of these instances, it appears that mood stabilizers may be effective in controlling gambling symptoms (Table 12.2). In addition, certain antiepileptic medications, such as topiramate, may reduce cravings and urges associated with addictive behaviors (Johnson et al., 2003) and may therefore be effective in reducing PG symptoms.

Opioid Receptor Antagonists

Case Vignette 3

H. D. is a 35-year-old single man who came to our clinic for treatment of severe gambling and drinking problems. His gambling problem started at age 17, a few years earlier than his drinking problem. He attended college and later established his own private business with an annual income of $140,000. Because of his gambling, however, mounting bank loans and credit card debts overwhelmed him, and eventually he had to declare personal bankruptcy. No family members knew about his gambling problem. Returning from the casino, he would often ponder whether life was worth living. Arriving home, he would experience substantial loneliness, anger, and despair. Over the course of a few years, his gambling and drinking urges completely preoccupied him. For the majority of every day, he thought about gambling. H. D. repeatedly attempted to stop gambling but was not successful.

H. D. had a family history of both gambling and drinking problems. H. D. denied other psychiatric problems or significant medical concerns. His baseline liver function tests were normal. H. D. was treated with naltrexone. H. D. developed nausea for the first four days for which he was treated with prochlorperazine (Compazine) 10 mg a day. Within 2 weeks, H. D. reported dramatic improvement in his gambling and drinking behaviors. Naltrexone treatment was discontinued after 2 years. His gambling and drinking behavior did not recur.

Naltrexone (ReVia) and Nalmefene

Because of the possible relationship of PG to addictive disorders, studies have examined the efficacy of opioid antagonists in the treatment of PG (Table 12.3). Crockford and el-Guebaly reported a patient with gambling and drinking problems who responded to 50 mg/day of naltrexone (Crockford & el-Guebaly, 1998).

A 12-week double-blind placebo-controlled naltrexone trial in 45 subjects with PG demonstrated superiority of active drug (n = 20) to placebo (n = 25) (Kim, Grant, Adson, & Shin, 2001a). Naltrexone (mean dose of 188 mg/day) was effective in reducing the frequency and intensity of gambling urges, as well gambling behavior. A separate analysis of subjects with at least moderate urges to gamble revealed that naltrexone was more effective in gamblers with more severe urges to gamble. The clinical use of naltrexone, however, is limited by significant side effects as well as the occurrence of liver enzyme elevations, especially in patients taking nonsteroidal anti-inflammatory drugs (Kim, Grant, Adson, & Remmel, 2001b). A recently completed multicenter study further demonstrated the efficacy of another opioid antagonist, nalmefene, in the treatment of PG. In a sample of 207 subjects, nalmefene demonstrated statistically significant improvement in gambling symp-

Table 12.3 Trials of Opioid Receptor Antagonist Medications in Pathological Gambling (PG)

Medication	Starting Doses	Usual Effective Doses in PG	Common Side Effects
Naltrexone	25 mg qd	50–200 mg/day	Nausea, loose stool, muscle cramps, insomnia, headaches, liver toxicity.
Nalmefene	5–10 mg qd	25–100 mg/day	Nausea, dizziness, insomnia, headaches, loose stool.

toms (several measures of gambling urges, thoughts, and behavior) compared to placebo in a 16-week double-blind trial (Grant et al., 2006).

Comments About Mu Opioid Antagonist

Opioid antagonists have been tested extensively in disorders, such as alcohol dependence, in which urges are prominent symptoms (Anton et al., 2004; O'Malley et al., 1996; Volpicelli, Alterman, Hayashida, & O'Brien, 1992). Opioid antagonists appear effective in reducing both the cravings and the pleasure associated with rewarding behaviors. Opioid antagonists work by blocking opioid receptors that process pleasure. In addition, these medications are hypothesized to work indirectly on dopamine and thereby affect the subjective experience of urges (Brahen, Capone, Wiechert, & Desiderio, 1977). Pleasure and urges are two core symptoms of some individuals with PG. Opioid antagonists may therefore be an effective treatment option in individuals with urges to gamble, in pathological gamblers with co-occurring alcohol use disorders, and possibly in individuals with PG and a family history of alcohol use disorders.

Summary

Physicians evaluating patients with PG should assess the circumstances that led them to seek help. In most psychiatric disorders, patients seek treatment because they are troubled by their symptoms. Patients with PG, however, continue to struggle with the desire to gamble and their need to stop gambling because of the mounting debts and other related problems. Thus, treatment adherence is often a problem. Once a treatment effect emerges, it becomes easier for the patient to comply with the treatment.

Physicians should remain alert to the correct diagnosis of PG. Gambling symptoms can be a part of a bipolar spectrum disorder, a response to depression or anxiety, or possibly secondary to dopamine agonist therapy in the case of Parkinson's disease (Stein & Grant, 2005). It is also crucial that clinicians pay attention to the underlying depression, anxiety, relationship problems, loneliness, or physical illnesses that can trigger a desire to gamble.

Physicians often need to apply drug combination treatment strategies to get the maximum treatment outcome and pay close attention to the emerging side effects. As the patient progresses to a stable clinical condition, clinicians should pay attention to how each individual is coping with life without gambling. Changes in relationships within the family, social life and recreational outlets should be closely watched and discussed with each patient. Patients may need psychotherapy referrals in some cases to address issues within the family and their own lives.

Pathological gambling, like other addictions, most likely has a complex etiology involving multiple factors—genetics, developmental issues, psychological issues— that appear to result in a heterogeneous neuropathology. As a medical problem, the option to use pharmacological management for PG appears appropriate in virtually all cases, depending of course on the wishes of the patient as well as medical contraindications to various pharmacotherapies. Effective behavioral treatments for PG are emerging, however, and should be considered in conjunction with pharmacotherapies.

Studies of PG suggest that there is potentially a neuropathological heterogeneity among individuals with PG and that heterogeneity may necessitate individually tailored treatment approaches. For example, there may be a subtype of PG that is more like an addiction, whereas other PG subtypes have more in common with other disorders such as obsessive–compulsive disorder or bipolar disorder. Those with a subtype of PG that is similar to addictions might respond preferentially to a pharmacological treatment targeting cravings. While these notions remain speculative and require additional studies to examine their appropriateness, one future direction for the treatment of PG may to better define subtypes of PG (using clinical symptomatology, neuroimaging, and pharmacogenetics) to guide pharmacological treatment selection.

Chapter 13
A Transpersonal Developmental Approach to Gambling Treatment

Gary Nixon and Jason Solowoniuk

It is the perspective of transpersonal psychology that all human beings are on a quest for wholeness, consciously or unconsciously. Some 80 years ago, Jung was heard making the remark that craving for alcohol was a low level spiritual thirst for wholeness and union with God (Leonard, 1989). Grof (1993) wrote of her own discovery that her alcohol addiction was a misguided thirst and quest for wholeness. From the perspective of transpersonal psychology, disordered gambling can also been understood to be a path paradoxically tread to recover lost elements of soul. With the plight of the gambler, we see a person who has not brought this quest for wholeness and individuation into conscious awareness (Singer, 1994). Instead, the gambler forsakes intuitive self-worth and takes a "short cut" to success by embracing the high roller motif and is subsequently seduced to chase fortune and fame at the hands of the Hero archetype (Leonard, 1989).

We will learn through this chapter that a transpersonal therapeutic approach calls for the gambler to become aware of his or her counterfeit quest for wholeness, and in recovery, authentically begin to search for meaning and purpose by working through the different developmental levels as set out in Wilber's spectrum of consciousness framework. Throughout the chapter, case studies and anecdotal accounts from past clients are used to better explain Wilber's levels of consciousness and archetypal theory, thereby providing an approach that will help clinicians work with disordered gamblers during their recovery process.

A Review of Transpersonal Psychology

Before we proceed further into the transpersonal approach to working with the problem gambler, it would be helpful to review the history and basic tenets of transpersonal psychology. As the founding father of the transpersonal psychology movement, Maslow (1971) delineated the higher or transcendent possibilities occurring at the further reaches of human nature. He suggested that, after a person satisfied physiological, safety, belongingness, and self-esteem needs, the next step inevitably led

Gary Nixon
University of Lethbridge, Canada

M. Zangeneh, A. Blaszczynski, N. Turner (eds.), *In the Pursuit of Winning.*
© Springer 2008

to the process of self-actualization. However, Maslow (1968, 1971) went one step further by establishing a need for self-transcendence within the process of becoming self-actualized. He called the impulse for self-transcendence a "meta-motivation" that is intrinsic to human nature. This necessitated, in his view, the development of a fourth psychology, transpersonal psychology. Extensive work has now been done in the area of transpersonal psychology in Western psychology (Assagioli, 1971; Cortwright, 1997; Grof, 1985, 1988; Hixon, 1978; Wade, 1996; Walsh & Vaughan, 1980, 1993; Washburn, 1988, 1994).

Over time, Cortwright (1997) observed that transpersonal psychology has shifted its emphasis to include not only the high end of human experience but also the personal realms and ordinary consciousness as well. We see this holistic approach including working with all realms of human existence with the works of the most prominent transpersonal philosopher, Ken Wilber (1977, 1986, 1990, 1995, 1997, 2000, 2006).

Wilber's spectrum of consciousness model mapped out 10 stages or levels in a developmental, structural, holarchical, systems-oriented format. Wilber (1986) initially synthesized the first six stages from cognitive, ego, moral, and object relations lines of development of conventional psychology represented by such theorists as Loevinger (1976), Piaget (1977), Kohlberg (1981), and the final four stages from Eastern and Western sources of contemplative development. Over time, in reaction to severe criticism and the need to be more comprehensive, Wilber (2000, 2006) has acknowledged limitations to conventional lines of development and integrated alternate perspectives such as Gilligan's work on female moral development (Gilligan, 1982), and the spiraling aspect of development through streams and waves rather than levels and lines captured in such theories as Kegan (1982), Susan Cook-Greuter (1990), and spiral dynamics set out by Beck and Cowan (1996), the latter theory heavily influencing Wilber's later work (Wilber, 2000, 2006).

Wilber's model is unique in that not only is it a developmental spectrum of pre-personal, personal, and transpersonal consciousness, it is also a spectrum of possible pathologies as developmental barriers can arise at each stage (Wilber, 1986). It is a model that allows us to integrate many of the Western psychologies and interventions. Originally, used for mental health issues (Wilber, 1986), it has now been applied to substance abuse issues (Nixon, 2001a), second-stage recovery (Nixon, 2005), hopelessness (Nixon, 2001b), and gambling issues (Nixon, 2003).

The first 10 stages of the developmental model will now be outlined along with corresponding pathologies and treatment interventions. We will see that each of these stages has implications in terms of gambling issues.

There are three phases of ego development: pre-personal, personal, and transpersonal.

Wilber's Transpersonal Model of Development

Pre-personal	Personal	Transpersonal
1. Sensoriphysical	4. Rule/role mind	7. Psychic
2. Phantasmic–emotional	5. Formal reflexive	8. Subtle
3. Rep-mind	6. Vision–logic	9. Casual
		10. Non-dual

Pre-Personal Stages

Sensoriphysical

The first three stages of development, each a pre-personal stage, are the sensoriphysical, phantasmic–emotional, and rep-mind (Wilber, 1986). The first stage, sensoriphysical, consists of matter, sensation, and perception. Pathologies at this level need to be treated with equally basic physiological interventions, as the primary point is to stabilize the person. In addictions, this typically means detox programs, but for gamblers this may consist of purely refraining from gambling or even taking the action to self-exclude oneself from a gaming venue altogether.

> I actually had plans to go in there and maybe play for five minutes before I completely barred myself. So I went in there, I had two loonies on me and I put them in and of course I lost. Then a lady came over and I told her what I wanted to do, I was almost a little embarrassed. I told her that I wanted to bar myself, I said this is probably a little unusual and she said: [Actually not at all!]. I had to stand in the corner and wait . . . I felt that the people were all looking at me and I thought to myself . . . They must think I have huge problems and I actually did.

Phantasmic–Emotional

The second stage, the phantasmic–emotional stage, is represented by the development of emotional boundaries to self (Wilber, 1986). Problems at this stage show up as a lack of cohesive self. The self treats the world as an extension of the self (narcissistic) or is constantly invaded by the world (borderline). Typical interventions focus on ego and self-structure building techniques such as object relations and psychoanalytic therapy. The core issue that epitomizes this level is that the self-structure of the gambler is split into parts. Each part seems to have its own personality and characteristics. On the one hand, winning will bring about a state euphoria, making him or her feel ecstatic, while on the other hand, losing will automatically bring about a sense of worthlessness, anger, and sometimes self-hate, all sheathed in the gambler's insistence that they should be winning.

> I figured I had to win, how could I not be winning, it's got to be time now and there was this lie in my head, keep going, you're going to win. The worse it gets the better the award will be, really sick, really suicidal, really scared. But the machine doesn't have a heart, it doesn't care, it doesn't know anything. It would talk me into things, like keep on playing your going to win this time. I was pathetic.

Clearly, the gambler who holds to a state of mind that is insistent and expects the gambling venue to disperse payment is exemplary of a regression to an infantile state in which the child believes that not only should he or she be doted upon, but his or her commands are to be fulfilled as if they were sacred promises. Therefore, during therapy the goal is help the gambler complete the separation–individuation phase, or in Jungian terms confront the internalized Devouring/Mother–Father, healing the split between the introjected "good me" and the "bad me" (Zweig & Wolfe, 1997).

Rep-Mind

The third developmental stage is rep–mind (Wilber, 1986). This stage represents the birth of the representational self. It is typified by the development of the individual's intrapsychic structures, that is, the id, ego, and superego. Problems at this level are experienced through psyche splits, due to issues that include inhibition, anxiety, obsession, guilt, and depression. Interventions focus on the intrapsychic resolution and uncovering techniques that bring back into awareness the split off parts that were repressed in childhood and thereafter contributing to a fragile identity (Jacoby, 1990). From the disordered gambler's perspective, gambling may at first appear to be the perfect panacea to healing the individual's wounds and symptoms that have occurred during this level of development. The rush of winning gives the gambler the illusionary fueling and subsequent increased sense of self-worth that is missing in the psyche.

> I had a lot of pain in my heart, low self-esteem; it was pure escape. So gambling made me feel empowered. I was in control, I was unique, it reminded me of movies of James Bond, the rogue, the voyeur, where I could go gambling and I was important. The world revolved around me, it was very consuming, it was a really nice escape from the doldrums of my life; the pain of my life.

Personal Stages

Rule/Role Mind

The pre-personal stages are followed by rule/role, formal-reflexive, and vision-logic stages of development and represent the mature ego developmental phase. The rule/role phase, Wilber's fourth stage of development and first personal stage, is highlighted by individual development of rules and roles to belong. A person's stance is becoming less narcissistic and more sociocentric (Wilber, 1986). Because problems at this level are experienced as a fear of losing face, losing one's role, and breaking the rules, typical interventions center on script pathology such as trans-actional analysis, family therapy, cognitive therapy, and narrative therapy. At this level, a person with gambling issues can have developed a whole set of unique roles and rules to support an addictive lifestyle.

From a Jungian standpoint, the rule/role developmental stage epitomizes the creation of the mask or persona that an individual creates as a result of becoming a civilized creature so as to the meet the requirements set forth by the collective society (Jung, 1959). Thus, the individual is often forced to find a middle ground between his or her instincts and the ego's demands to meet personal goals or maintain a sense of self that is appreciated by others and one that maintains a sense of self-worth (Jacobi, 1973). Therefore, the pathological gambler often adopts characteristics and personalities to meets the needs of both outer and inner worlds.

Gaming venues can provide the conditions (lights, action, and rush of winning) by which the archetypal image of the "hero" can manifest through intermixing and associating with the individual's personal unconscious and life environment, producing the necessary conditions to assert itself during gambling episodes (Jacobi, 1973; Judith, 1996). Therefore, with the hero's archetype's infinite reservoir of energy, the persona, regardless of its makeup is tempted to shed its mask for a seemingly new exciting lifestyle.

> I liked the casino; I was into the atmosphere and the people. I had really nice clothes and a great job, I had lots going for me, except I had a messed up attitude. You know, I was trying to be the bigshot. So the first night we played roulette, and the next weekend, and then it was every weekend, I ended up getting a name, I was the roulette Queen.

Formal–Reflexive

The next personal stage, and fifth overall, formal–reflexive, represents the development of the mature ego (Wilber, 1986). Persons at this level have a highly differentiated reflexive self-structure and have also developed the capacity to reason, assert themselves, and conceive of new possibilities for the future, based on their own desires, passions, and intellectual capacities. Therefore, during therapy, the underlying identity of an addict can be challenged. This challenge must be tailored so as to help the gambler sever the tie with the moneylender archetype (Leonard, 1989) who not only has assumed control over the psyche, but also supplies the necessary defense mechanisms to rationalize away extreme gambling behaviors (i.e., denial, displacement, projection, reaction formation, and sublimation) (Bollas, 1987).

> I went to the pub and all the machines were filled, so I went down to the Beidelberg and they were all disabled. So I decided to go home. I drove by the turn to my house and a little voice says to me: [Why don't you just ask God for a little help] and I could just feel my lower lip drop, because what it really comes down is do you really want to quit, cause if really don't want to quit, if really haven't had enough, nothing can convince you otherwise.

Vision–Logic

The following stage of development, the final personal stage and sixth overall, is the visionlogic or the existential stage. Here, the integrated body–mind confronts the reality of existence (Wilber, 1986). Thus, we see a concern for the overall meaning of life and a grappling with personal mortality and an effort to find the courage to be. This process can often be very tenuous, yet, nevertheless a critical developmental milestone that is sometimes reached during therapy, which exemplifies the climax of the existential stage of consciousness development (May, 1958; Yalom, 1980).

> Talk about going back into my room and not even knowing who I was at that point. Who was I? Like okay, so all the layers had been peeled off, I was like that little bulb sitting there saying: [I got to start . . . growing]. I was just this; I was very vulnerable; I think at that point I can actually say I was me. I was actually who I supposed to be, but I didn't know that yet. I needed to know that all these qualities were coming together. Out of all my years of recovery, gambling, having kids, doing all these things, that was the scariest moment, it was the moment of truth.

Transpersonal Ego–Transcendence Stages

Psychic

To this Western conventional scheme of development, Wilber (1986, 2000) also added psychic, subtle, causal, and the non-dual levels, which represent psycho–spiritual levels of transpersonal development integrated from Western and Eastern sources of introspective maturity. The first stage, beyond the mind–body integration of the existential level, and the seventh overall, is the "psychic" (Wilber, 1986). In this phase, cognitive and perceptual capacities, which used to be narrowly personal and individualistic, can expand to a more pluralistic and universal perspective. For a recovering person, there are many potential pitfalls at this stage of preliminary psycho–spiritual development, such as psychic inflation and "the dark night of the soul." People describe experiencing the high of the "pink cloud" syndrome of early recovery and then falling back into depression and sometimes relapse (Grof, 1993).

> I will never will forget my last day at treatment . . . I remember the head honcho, he wouldn't talk to me. He knew that I was a people person, it was a part of my addiction. So the last day, he grabbed me by the neck and takes me to the door. He's a big guy and he shakes my hand, he's like: [Congratulations]. It's six in the morning and we're up early. And then the door opens, the sun is coming up, eh. I will never forget how beautiful that was man . . . I could smell the winter air, and I could see the trees with no leafs, what a sense of freedom. But I am not there anymore; I can't carry on with my life until I come to grips with my self-image issue. I know that is my problem.

Subtle

The next transpersonal stage, and eighth overall, is the "subtle" and is referred to the level of the "saints" (Wilber, 1986). Here, subtle sounds, audible illuminations, and transcendent insight and absorption can be experienced. In certain traditions, such as Gnosticism and Hinduism, this is the stage of direct phenomenological apprehension of personal deity form (Wilber, 1986). This realm has also been referred to as pseudo-nirvana and refers to the realm of illumination, rapture, and transcendental insight (Goleman, 1988). Recovering persons can have wonderful transformational "white light" experiences at this level, yet struggle to integrate these experiences into everyday life.

> I phoned these missionaries and I called them over. I guess that in my mind I didn't know what else to do. I knew I needed to reach for God, but I knew that God was on Pluto and He did not love a wretch like me. Therefore, I needed a middleman so these two boys came over and they interviewed me and I was kind of weepy, and they came back about three days later. They were kind of stunned with the whole thing, this women spouting about her gambling problem. So, they came back and put there hands on my head and blessed me. I can still picture it, I remember them saying: [We bless you that you will be able to give your children what your mother never gave you]. I sat on the couch after they left and cried for two solid hours and I felt that love pouring through me. That love coming through there hands, and I felt for the first time in my life that God was with me. That god actually loved me and I could feel the presence of the spirit. With that one instance, I stayed clean and sober for one year.

Causal and Non-Dual

The next stage is the "causal." This level of the "stages" is the realization of the unmanifest source or transcendental ground of all the lesser structures (Wilber, 1986). In various traditions, it is referred to as the abyss, the void, and the formless (Wilber, 1986). People can prematurely experience this level of "cosmic consciousness" and struggle to integrate this "formless" awareness into everyday life. Losing one's attachment to the separate self and integrating all levels of existence leads to the final stage of "non-dual" living. At this level, the former disordered gambler is well aware that his or her gambling was nothing more than a desperate attempt at establishing a separate sense of self. Therefore, with this awareness the individual is able to accept him- or herself for who she or he is and find peace in just being.

> My buzz word today is acceptance, which is huge, accepting yourself for who you are and like coming to realize that there is nothing wrong with you, and who ever thought that, I thought there was. Really you are who you are, I don't have to do anything, um, I have come to that place, ah . . . wholeness. The connection with your heart, your soul, a connection to something bigger than you are, right!

Transpersonal Interventions

A large proportion of transpersonal psychology interventions focus on letting go of the egoic self, aiding the individual to experience the moment with clarity and stillness of a calm mind (Bayda, 2003 Kornfield, 1989; Tolle, 2003). This can take the form of working through the narcissistic wound and realizing that "I am not the answer." Therefore, the addict comes to realize that he or she actually betrayed Self and through the journey of recovery is intrinsically guided into working with inner darkness and emptiness she or he had previously escaped from, and making a return to find essence or ground of being (Almass, 1996). Techniques specifically employed during this process include developing "witness consciousness" (Kornfield, 1989; Krishnamurti, 1954; Ruskan, 2004), focusing on embracing the power of now (Tolle, 1996, 2003), or becoming aware of our tendency to split off from the present moment through our judging self (Nixon, 2005). Similarly, Katie (2002) developed a method of inquiry focusing on four questions, which helps the individual to burn through stories of victimhood and suffering. This method seeks to release the individual's attachment to the wound, bringing freshness to the mind and shutting the door to the harmful whispers of the past.

Jung (1959) demonstrated how people embrace unconscious motifs without conscious awareness and become victims of psychic inflation. With respect to a gambler, he or she may be seduced by the trickster archetype and feel that the self has managed to outwit the gambling establishment through special brilliance and cunningness. Ultimately, however, the individual gets lost in this unconscious grasping at specialness, and is then enslaved by the "demon" archetype, who unfortunately is the guardian of the addictive process (Leonard, 1989). With this process in mind, we will now fully explore the gambler's pursuit for wholeness and how transpersonal psychology with a special focus on Jungian psychology aids the disordered gambler to return to a life free from chaos, selfishness, and addiction.

The Counterfeit Hero's Journey of the Problem Gambler

Clinical case research has suggested that, in utilizing cognitive distortions, problem gamblers are unconsciously playing out unexamined myths (Campbell, 1968; Feinstein & Krippner, 1988; Jung, 1959; Leonard, 1989; May, 1991; Moore & Gillette, 1990; Pearson, 1989; Singer, 1994; von Franz, 1997). May (1991) has compared myths to the foundation of a house, where myths provide the basic structure in a person's life, but like the foundation of a house, usually go unexamined. That is, underlying cognitive distortions are largely unconscious mythic structures representing symbolic meanings bestowed upon actions, objects, and persons. For example, a gambler's behavior of chasing losses or gaming to gain notoriety must be explicitly interpreted in regards to the whole of the psyche's operating principles. Rather than seeing gambling as a mere occurrence, if understood and brought into awareness, it becomes a living experience that helps the individual to make a conscious choice instead of reacting to an insatiable personality complex (Carotenuto, 1985; Leonard, 1989).

As noted by Campbell (1968), who explored the hero's journey as a theme common to many different cultures, it is not surprising to find many gamblers unconsciously being pulled by this notion of becoming a hero. In literary accounts, Miliora (1997) noted the importance of the narcissistic fantasy of being a "winner" in the shared fantasies of gamblers. Nixon, Solowoniuk, and McGowan (2006) have recently described disordered gambling as "a counterfeit quest for wholeness," a spiraling into chaos through a three-stage process. The first stage consists of an initiation into the gambling environment and the conscious choice to try to become a hero through gambling. The second stage depicts gambling as a flight through psychic inflation and a vehicle in which gamblers believes they can gain financial freedom, ending in the manifestation of personality changes and a denial of the increasing dangers of frequent gambling. The final stage portrays how gamblers succumbed to the dangers of trying to become extraordinary. Nixon and Solowoniuk (2006) observed that at this final stage the gambler's shadow blackens all emotions and cognitions firmly become obsessed with gambling using whatever means available (see Fig. 13.1).

It is also important to realize that the counterfeit hero's journey of problem gambling coexists within one's sociocultural world. In this sphere, the individual is essentially at the mercy of "being in the world," especially in terms of today's sociocultural climate, where celebrities are the norm for whom a person is supposed to strive to or at least emulate. Andrews and Jackson (2001) remarked that, "What is new about contemporary culture is the scale with which variously celebrated individuals infuse and inform every facet of everyday existence" (p. 3). Hence, societies worldwide have forgotten that a true hero/heroine's role is to create a balance and

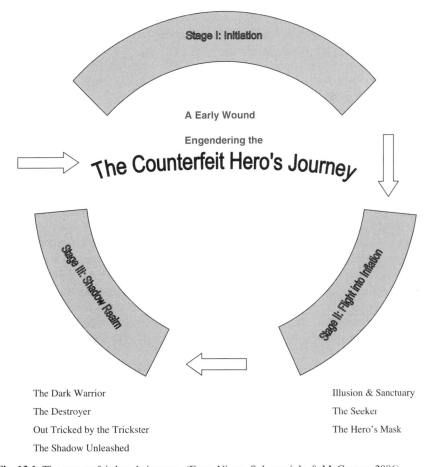

Fig. 13.1 The counterfeit hero's journey. (From Nixon, Solowoniuk, & McGowan, 2006)

establish harmony within a culture (Campbell, 1968). Consequently, when a society takes a hero to be a celebrity, an unreal image becomes symbolized and nowhere is their true achievement left to be valued or for that matter followed (Boorstin, 1992).

Interestingly, gambling research to date has typically relied on positivist constructions that abstract people out of the contexts in which gambling takes place (McGowan, Droessler, Nixon, & Grimshaw, 2000). To realize the seduction of the counterfeit hero's journey of gambling, one needs only to tune into the most recent reality TV to see the intense cultural pressure on people to be "extraordinary" in some way. The rising popularity of TV poker shows the attraction to larger than life "shrewd and cunning" poker players complete with appropriate costumes and dark sunglasses. Further, we live in a culture of adoration for larger-than-life athletic champions like Michael Jordan, Tiger Woods, Wayne Gretzky, and John Daley, to name a few. To be human and compassionate to others clearly is not good enough. One needs to be a star. Unfortunately, gambling offers a "quick fix" opportunity for stardom, and thus the counterfeit quest for wholeness through gambling offers a compelling opportunity to become just that, a celebrity, a seemingly real but not so authentic hero.

Archetypes

In succumbing to the shadow during the counterfeit quest, we are further introduced to the archetypes. The term "archetypal" or "archetype" can best be understood as storehouses of energy that coalesce around "abiding patterns in the human psyche that remain powerful and present overtime" (Pearson, 1989). According to Judith (1996), archetypes are symbolically represented by the "archetypal image." Archetypal images are icons, indexes, and categories that form into specific patterns over the years and become dynamic symbols based on interactions between the archetype and a particular culture (Singer, 1994). However, when an archetype is not fully integrated into the ego, the individual is then subject to illusion (Judith, 1997). This can occur when a pathological gambler's compulsion toward winning the big jackpot is not fused with the mature hero's understanding that he or she is not God, and that every adventure has an ending. For that reason, the pathological gambler's success is destined to be a failure (Judith, 1997; Leonard, 1989).

Leonard (1989) delineated 10 archetypes that appear to sit at the heart of the addictive process. Specifically, she formulated her theory of addiction and recovery around Jung's individuation process, and phenomenologically outlined a 10-stage development encounter with these archetypes: the hostage, moneylender, gambler, romantic, underground man, outlaw, trickster, madwoman, judge, and killer. Each archetype represents a phase in the addictive process, which once brought into consciousness, could be worked through and integrated in the psyche.

Thus, the mythic-archetypal journey is not about justifying gambling, placing blame, or merely offering a method for treatment. Rather it may be considered as a revolution toward understanding the process by which one becomes a pathological gambler as this journey is embedded in the lived experience of pathological gamblers themselves (Nixon & Solowoniuk, 2006). Once awareness of the counterfeit hero's journey is brought into awareness, a truly authentic recovery process can begin, where psychic inflation and narcissistic pathways of the counterfeit hero are recognized and released. As a result, true recovery takes place by metabolizing all the different developmental levels that disordered gambling brought to light, or those that have not been negotiated, but become available due to the recovery journey (Guntrip, 1971; Judith, 1997; Singer, 1994; Wilber, 1986). For example, a typical pattern is one in which gambling emerges through an orphan or wounded stage (Pearson, 1989). This is typically experienced at a basic emotional level, the phantasmic level, as presented in stage 2 of Wilber's (1986) Spectrum of Consciousness model. As we see in the following case study, true healing often means returning to a previous stage of development so as to work on the underlying pain that may have been the impetus for gambling. Over time, the disordered gambler in recovery opens his or her psyche to reality, gaining more awareness of the nature of the Self, as he or she climbs the ladder to greater freedom and authenticity.

A Case Study: Lynn's Desperate Hero's Journey of Gambling

Lynn is a 40-year-old wife and mother of two, who in the past has been a client of one of the authors. She entered counseling in desperation because her husband threatened her with a divorce if she continued to gamble. In her first session, she explained that her gambling had escalated in recent years and reported loving the feeling of being a "big shot," especially after receiving accolades from other gamblers and casino staff. She has recently fell victim to the chasing losses phase, and reported emptying out her children's college fund, not to mention, maxing out the couple's credit cards. She even reported skipping out on her family to gamble on Christmas Eve.

Level 1: Sensoriphysical: Treatment Alternatives

Wilber (1986) makes the point that to avoid an elevationalist perspective using the developmental model, counseling must begin at a basic level. It is evident from Lynn's reports that her gambling is out control. Therefore, the first task required is using the sensori–physical level to help Lynn explore strategies to avoid gambling venues as she reports that self-exclusion did not work. Lynn was referred to Gamblers Anonymous (GA), with the goal of giving her a place to find extra support and helping her realize that she is not alone in her battle with disordered gambling. A financial management program in cooperation with her husband is another option to keep her gambling in check, but Lynn may need a few counseling sessions first, before she feels she has the strength to disclose to her husband the extent of gambling problem.

Level 2: Phantasmic–Emotional: Returning to the Orphan's Wound

As the session progressed, an inquiry into the possible etiology of Lynn's gambling problem continued. Lynn reported growing up in a home that was split between being warm and inviting, which emanated from her father's presence, and one that reflected her cold, distant, and judgmental mother, who projected her own dismay in life and shadow issues onto Lynn.

> My mom was the type of person that money was power and if you had money you were somebody. So I was brought up with that in my head that if I only had five bucks in my wallet I was useless. You know, she also use to remind me, and I don't think I'm an ugly person, but I was always told by my mother that I was built like a brick shit house. That I never was going to amount to anything . . . So all of those things added up, to give me . . . I needed money to have security, to feel like I was somebody. Whereas, all I needed was somebody to say to me that I like you for who you are not what you got. So gambling was my way of feeling, I'm it. I think that was my downfall.

From a transpersonal perspective, Lynn's etiological basis for gambling can be understood, simply, as a seeking to quench a thirst. For Lynn, this thirst was in terms of trying to secure validation from her mother, which she believed would have given her a sense of love, support, and ground for existing here on Earth (Almass, 1996). However, this reportedly did not take place, and during her early 20s Lynn developed a feverish obsession with the casino, in particular the roulette wheel.

> We played roulette, didn't know what the hell I was doing and I am just watching people and I could feel my heart pounding. Then I was consistently back there. Me and my friends would go every weekend. This might sound really bad, but I have to tell you. Good looking blonde girls, you know, playing the scene having a great time, wearing the clothes, playing the part, like the big shot. I was getting a name . . . I was the roulette Queen, because there were some points I won so much money at roulette that people could not believe it. And my Dad was there and he said: [Can you lend me some money?] It was like who wants to marry a millionaire. I could have been throwing money up in the air; I won $6,300 that night.

Unbeknownst to Lynn, the big win phenomenon became an entryway into chaos and dismay; moreover, it also eventually dissipated her lack of self-worth, and covered up her emptiness (Almass, 1996). This "high roller" status led to an inflated sense of self. The therapist held off challenging the mask or persona for the time being, as regression too early on in recovery does not prepare the client to deal with the underlying emptiness that is at heart of the gambling cycle.

Thus, the integral work with Lynn did not begin until the third session, where Lynn was then guided to face the Orphan archetype that protected her ego from its impingement at the hands of her Devouring Mother. Here, Lynn reconnected with her loss of innocence and subsequent state of "not feeling good enough."

> I look back on it now, and think, (sobbing) God, why wasn't there someone back there then to help. She must have hated me; it must have been true hate. I have a little girl, if I talked to her the way my Mom talked to me . . . (Continuing to cry). She damaged me so much that I wanted her to be penalized, but sometimes I think she was right. I am a loser; I'm not going to amount to anything.

However, rather than just talking Lynn through her perceived deficiency, Lynn was invited to do something new. She was asked to just to sit in this pain with no judgment—no labels as to how bad her mother made her feel, just to sit and allow herself to experience the anger, rage, and sadness that boiled through her mind/body. Over the next couple of sessions, Lynn was guided to return to these feelings and began to learn that there was a pattern behind her "pain body" (Tolle, 1996, 2003). She became familiar with her anger, rage, and sadness, and instead of reacting, Lynn, learned to bring a kindness to these seemingly solid haunting apparitions (Batchelor, 2004; Kornfield, 1989). Although the reasons for the pain could not be undone, Lynn came to the conclusion that these feelings were fleeting. And as she was taught to breathe into and befriend her "demons," she became less attached to the wound, and the Orphan archetype's "need" to be heard decreased.

> I based my whole life on my looks, because I was always told by my Mom that you got to impress people so I never knew who I was. But now, don't get me wrong I still like things, fake nails, and stuff like that. But they're for me now, not for somebody to go: [Look at her]! I want them because I like them.

Level 3: Rep-Mind: Silencing the Critic

This work of releasing the underlying emotional pain and issues continued for the next few sessions. As Lynn became reconnected with the deep pain and sadness at the bottom of her being, it became clear that her internal saboteur would not seize its cries without a further inquiry, deconstruction, and transformation (Zweig & Wolfe, 1997). This brings us to level 3 of Wilber's model, which is characterized by the representational mind. Here, there are typical parts at conflict in the psyche, and with Lynn, like most of us, there is a huge critical self constantly berating and telling her that she not "good enough." So, at a simple level, we can see she has a very dominant superego that constantly discharges energy under the auspices of self-judgments. These judgments can lose their charge by a person fully experiencing the current that runs through the mind/body as he or she rises in consciousness. However, if this does not occur, it may necessary to drag the internal saboteur into the present moment through the experiential technique, know in Gestalt therapy as the empty chair (Perls, 1969).

Because of Lynn's confusion, the empty chair exercise was used to help Lynn understand the huge role of the critic in her psyche. The critic was not only a threat to her recovery program, but also the catalyst that affects the regulation and overall mind/body functioning within the psychic system (Jacobi, 1973). Thus, during the empty chair exercise, Lynn was guided to separate the interactions of the experiencing self from her critical self and give voice to both roles one at a time.

After inquiring into the nature of and strength of how Lynn's critical self carried a frequent chatter insisting that, "you should do this," and "you can't do that," and "you're not a good mom," Lynn was invited to set boundaries with the critical self. She later reported feeling empowered and gaining a sense of freedom from her internal saboteur.

> I have being realizing that I can't blame my Mom, which has been a big thing. I even wrote her a letter after this and said the relationship as Mother/Daughter was non-existent, but there is a possibility of building or spawning some sort of respect towards each other at a friendship level. I was becoming to see that I was not that child anymore, not that little person that made me feel weak. It's been hard, but it's nice to know that all these qualities are coming back together.

Level 4: Rule/Role: The Mythic Journey of Pursing Success

As the counseling work progressed, Lynn was able to examine the rules and roles she embraced in life. As Feinstein and Krippner (1988) asked, what has Lynn's mythic journey been like? Lynn was asked to talk about the family myths she grew up with. Using this as an investigatory tool, Lynn continued to disclose stories of needing to be a hero, and mentioned seeking attention from her friends in adolescence. In doing so, she reported in therapy that she would appease her friends by taking them out for lunch and also reported buying them lavish gifts. As she grew older and as her gambling continued into her mid-20s, she reports falling fallen victim to the caretaker archetype, where she would go out her way to help her family, be there for others, all while forsaking her own needs. Thus the casino provided her with a route to be alone, and offered her the opportunity to break away from the traditional role of being the dutiful mother and caregiver.

On the downside, fueled with the hero's war cry and insurgence of power, Lynn's gambling grew out of control, and finally came to a halting end at the demands of her husband. As therapy continued, Lynn became to realize that she no longer needed to get her self-worth from being a good mother per se, the smiling daughter-in-law, nor be the perfect wife. However, working through the rule/role stage can be a difficult and tumultuous time, not only for the client, but also for the spouse or significant other.

> I wanted to have perfect marriage, you know. I think I set myself up for one very high expectation. So my marriage has been a big adjustment in the past month, because all of sudden Jim is saying: [I don't know who you are anymore, because I feel like I'm walking on thin ice. I can't talk to you about your gambling because it is still a sore spot]. And I replied, give me some time! You know, and then I got mad and said, don't do the shit with me because I know what I should have done, but I didn't do it. So, I think am I really learning to stand up for myself for the first time in my life. And that was very difficult for Jim, because he is looking at this woman who he used to be able say: [Do this, get me that]. Yeah, but now I am not going to be the silent housekeeper or have friends over to play out this image.

Levels 5 and 6: Formal–Reflexive and Existential: Finding a New Identity and Meaning

As Lynn progressed in therapy, she moved close to an encounter with the deeper aspects of herself. This naturally leads us to the identity stage (level 5) and the existential level (level 6), whereupon Lynn began to inquire into the meaning and purpose of her life. During this time, the counselor may be required to follow up such an examination by posing the question "Who am I?" This question is often answered with a solemn "I don't know," and a further push can sometimes lead the client to question the nature of his or her existence and self-hood itself.

> It's like being a little bulb and you vulnerable, but there is a voice saying I got to start growing. I think at this point I can actually say I'm starting to become me. Sometimes I don't know who I am supposed to be and out of all my years gambling, having kids, doing all these things, this is one of the scariest moment. It's like the moment of truth.

During this period of therapy, clients are sometimes tempted to return to gambling, thus short-circuiting the identity building and seeking process. It is the experience of the authors that relapse is often a part of solidifying the recovery process as it brings to the surface issues that therapy bypassed or did not uncover. In addition, from a Jungian perspective, the therapist should inquire into the nature of the relapse, looking for possible signs of the trickster, who can carries both destructive powers and healing potions (Jung, 1959). Relapse maybe indicative of an unmetabolized desire to still seek fame and fortune through gambling. Thus, the therapist may need to return to earlier levels of development to make sure narcissistic pathogens and pathways have been fully brought to the surface. Similarly, from a level 6 existential perspective, the anxiety of not knowing who one is, may be too great for the gambler and so a return to a gambling identity may provide a sense of familiarity, and, as well, the energy to flush anxiety from the psychic system through gambling may prove to be attractive.

Paradoxically, Jung (1959) would suggest that we need to tap into the creative juices of the trickster, and look to settle the hero's passion for notoriety by seeking alternative means. Lynn was able to do just this, at first embarking on becoming a motivational speaker, but later deciding she needed a stable income. A month later, Lynn returned to therapy in a delighted mood and had engineered a plan to go to college. She reported feeling a sense of purpose while filling out the necessary documents for acceptance into a social work program, and remarked that her journey through gambling "was an emotional roll coaster, so now to just be, it's weird, and sometimes hard to just be there, but I'm grateful for allowing myself to go through it, it changed my life."

Thus, as Frankl (1985) observed, the search for meaning is key in modern day life. For Lynn, it appeared that the search for authenticity, meaning, and purpose came from making her counterfeit journey not only conscious, but also transformational, leading her to new sense of self that enabled her to embrace a life free of disordered gambling and to start a new mission in life.

Level 7 and Beyond: Psycho–Spiritual Work

The counseling work to date has taken about 10 sessions, and while Lynn reported being ecstatic about her new life and the sense of purpose, she was warned to not become too inflated and fall victim to the shadow's back door ingenuity. Here, the individual can exchange a gambling addiction for a pseudo-spiritual path bent on solving all of the world's problems. Interestingly, spirituality is not something covered much in the GA 12-step program. To make the dangers of psychic inflation more real, Lynn was introduced to the concept of "spiritual materialism" in which the dangers of treating spiritual experiences like a new bank account was explained (Trungpa, 1973). It was also explained that long-term recovery has its up and downs and that eventually the recovering individual will experience a "plateau effect," which does not necessarily mean that new life goals are without substance or greater spiritual practice is without meaning.

Similarly, as Almaas (1996) pointed out with his work on the transformation of narcissism, it is important to recognize that we often can fall prey to our narcissistic needs of wanting to be validated by externalized others. To Lynn, this seemed fairly obvious. Her gambling served as a narcissistic pursuit to gain validation from others, while at the same time finding a pseudo-"nirvana" by a high roller at the casino. Therefore, the final sessions with Lynn were used to help Lynn to sit and experience the ordinariness of everyday existence. For Lynn, she was able to get in touch "with the weirdness of being" and she realized that it was okay to not have to strive to be something she was not.

At this level of consciousness development, clients sometimes apprehend and come to understand that their gambling addiction was actually a self-betrayal

(Almass, 1996; Carotenuto, 1996). Despite the environments they were brought up in or conditions that took place thereafter, they may gain the insight that their attachment to their wound was actually the ego's striving to maintain dominance in the psyche. Therefore, gambling is just a means to solidify the ego's insistence on being heard, and together with the power of the hero archetype, which at the deepest level is just numinous energy projected into an ideal image, a false path is trodden upon for the sake of the ego. Hence, with such a realization, Lynn was able to settle in being, and continues to do psycho–spiritual work including consolidating identity issues of level 5, existential issues of level 6, and beginning spirituality issues of level 7. It was her hope that over time she would progress to experiencing more of the ego-transcendent phases such as the subtle level 8 and the causal level 9. Meanwhile, today, she is committed to obtaining a social work degree, but more importantly, is living a life free from disordered gambling.

Limitations

It is important when considering such an approach that the reader or clinician be aware of the various assumptions and concepts that underlie a transpersonal model of gambling pathology and treatment. For instance, within the case study offered, the reader is presented with a number of subjective states experienced by the gambler, and the psychological methods used to understand these states are presented in a transpersonal psychological lens and appear at times to be absolute statements of how to interpret the gambler's dilemma. Thus it is important to realize that there are limitations to adopting the transpersonal treatment approach.

A primary limitation is the proposition that there are developmental stages beyond the adult ego, which involve experiences with phenomena considered to lie outside the boundaries of the self (Kasprow & Scotton, 1999). In healthy individuals, these developmental stages can stimulate dormant human qualities, such as altruism, creativity, intuitive wisdom, and a "knowing" that the universe is basically good and trustworthy. However, for individuals who possibly may be lacking healthy ego structures, such experiences may lead to identity confusion, fragmentation, or a host of other possible crisis (Kasprow & Scotton, 1999). Thus, the clinician must be aware of these possible manifestations, but more importantly, it must be noted that it is not always possible to determine who lacks healthy ego structures.

Other limitations of this approach include a significant therapeutic time requirement to work through the developmental phases, not to mention a certain necessary client affinity for intellectual language. The transpersonal developmental approach also relies heavily on insight, requiring the client to process issues at levels that may not fit his or her personality structure, all of which may not match the client's presenting issues or goals for therapy (Schwartz, 2007). Lastly, transpersonal psychology, in addition to being criticized for its highly abstract underpinnings, has at its core a deeply spiritual bias, which limits its applicability and popularity for secular clients (Carrier & Mitchell, 2007).

Despite these limitations, there still exists a potent transformational opportunity when adopting a transpersonal perspective. This approach assumes that the client's gambling is purposive in nature, and by treating it as such, the therapist acts on equal footing with his or her client, with the knowledge that climbing the levels to embracing a higher consciousness is not without its pitfalls, shortcoming, and barriers. As a result, if treatment is understood from this perspective, the gambler has the opportunity to gain a sense of authenticity, freedom, and human dignity that comes from transcending the ego and embracing deeper aspects of being.

Chapter 14
How Science Can "Think" About Gamblers Anonymous

Peter Ferentzy and Wayne Skinner

Claiming to have been founded in the 1950s, though some have contested its account of its origins (Browne, 1994; Sagarin, 1969), Gamblers Anonymous (GA) is a mutual aid fellowship modeled on Alcoholics Anonymous (AA). Yet GA has its own unique culture of recovery, rendering it quite different from AA and other 12-step societies. A key difference emanates from the overwhelming financial difficulties many problem gamblers are forced to deal with, and GA takes it on itself to counsel members on these matters and even on legal challenges. GA can be viewed as a culture of recovery, where members internalize sets of beliefs and participate in practices that include diagnosing gambling problems without professional assistance, combining spiritual and financial conceptions of integrity, and taking their GA-based precepts such as greater humility and a rejection of self-centeredness into the world around them.

GA has a long tradition, and at least in North America, is probably the most frequent "intervention" that people with gambling problems employ (Viets & Miller, 1997). Yet as scientific discourse on problem gambling increases, the attention to GA has not increased progressively but seems to wax and wane. Arguably, GA received more direct attention than ever between 1985 and 1994 (Brown, 1985, 1986, 1987a, 1987b, 1987c, 1987d; Browne, 1991, 1994; Lesieur, 1990a; Stewart & Brown, 1988; Turner & Saunders, 1990). It is possible that professionals and scientists are disinclined to pay attention to GA, seeing it on the one hand as an informal and uncontrolled set of practices and on the other as founded on dubious and nonrational principles. While the perception may be accurate, we argue that this is precisely why a narrow conception of "science" may be insufficient for a deeper understanding of fellowships such as GA. In fairness, one may add that GA has often posed barriers preventing scientists from engaging with it, and thus has itself contributed to this phenomenon. That, however, is not the topic of this discussion.

One modern perception involves the division of human endeavor into art versus science: the first as mainly subjective, the second as (in principle) purely rational. This mindset can produce questions such as "is political theory an art or a science?", with answers normally hinging upon one's perception of the relative importance

Peter Ferentzy
Centre for Addiction and Mental Health, Canada

M. Zangeneh, A. Blaszczynski, N. Turner (eds.), *In the Pursuit of Winning.*
© Springer 2008

of subjectivity versus objectivity to that endeavor. Many would say it is a bit of both. Rarely is the polarization of art versus science questioned: why must political theory (or sociology for that matter) be either? Yet this hard distinction is relatively recent and, as current usage of words still indicates, trades and crafts were once called "arts" (the practitioners are still called artisans). Isaac Newton himself was engaged in "philosophy of nature," later to be called "physics." Yet to this day philosophy, purportedly the epitome of rational discourse, is classified by universities under the heading of "Arts." We argue that rigid conceptions of rationality and subjectivity often leave little room for a seemingly old-fashioned endeavor: thinking. The latter can, in practice, never be reduced to strict scientific criteria or to unadulterated expressions of one's emotions. Heidegger (1968) once made the lofty pronouncement: "Science does not think" (p. 8). Despite potential objections, many researchers have some experience with this: thinking is done before a project when defining parameters and choosing the right instruments, and it is done after, when drawing conclusions from the accumulated data, but during the actual process of investigation the instruments do the "thinking"—a moment at which even the most astute researcher becomes little more than a glorified technician. Our purpose is not to belittle a process that has proven to yield valuable results, nor is it to undermine the creative thinking often exhibited by researchers during the moments of the process when they are permitted to think, but to identify an absence in the process that could help to explain the gap between "science" and "objects" such as AA and GA which, we argue, can fall outside the purview of accepted scientific methods.

The discussion that follows is divided into two major sections. The first is an analysis of AA, and refers to works of some notable scholars on how that organization is inconsistent with modern sensibilities regarding themes such as individuality, professional authority, and, above all, rationality. Many of the points raised are political, and we discuss how AA presents a challenge to the ways in which we Westerners have governed ourselves over the last two centuries. While not everything said about AA should be presumed to apply to GA, much of it can, and our need to rely on AA studies simply emphasizes the need for GA itself to be studied on its own with similar considerations in mind. The second section is essentially a discussion of current literature on GA, and one text on AA, with an emphasis on questions raised in the first. Throughout both sections, we emphasize the need for direct, nonjudgmental observation of GA—without the "benefit" of a host of instruments.

Mutual Aid and the Limits of Scientism

In many ways, current perspectives and approaches to GA are best understood in the broader context of mutual aid in general. These informal—and arguably anti-intellectual—societies can irk scientific and modernist sensibilities. The contemporary scientific view of AA finds exemplary expression in Charles Bufe's (1991) *Alcoholics Anonymous: Cult or Cure?* The title itself reveals the predicament this 70-year-old movement faces when gazed upon by hyperrational minds. Bufe's criticisms (1991) of AA can be organized around two themes: its religiosity (which provides the cultish qualities), and the lack of empirical evidence of its effectiveness as a therapy for alcoholism. In summarizing the first point, Bufe (1991) says: "Is Alcoholic Anonymous a cult? No, though it does have dangerous cult-like tendencies. The ideological system of AA is that of a cult: AA is religiously oriented, self-absorbed, irrational, dogmatic, insists on the submission of the individual to the will of God, and views itself as the exclusive holder of truth (at least in regard to the treatment of alcoholism)" (p. 101). Regarding its effectiveness, Bufe (1991) suggests the evidence is not supportive, but adds that AA might be a good match for a narrow band of clients among the heterogeneous array of people needing help with drinking problems. "Is AA totally useless as a treatment for Alcoholism? Perhaps not. One of the current trends in alcoholism treatment is "client matching". . . Since AA inspires fanatical loyalty in certain members, it would be surprising if AA wasn't an appropriate treatment method for certain alcoholics..." (Bufe, 1991, p. 112).

Further complicating the scientific take on AA are recent studies, of which Project MATCH (1997) is an exemplar. It found that facilitated 12-step interventions were as effective overall as were the more science-based cognitive and motivational interventions. Indeed, in cases of alcohol dependence uncomplicated by comorbidities, the 12-step intervention was marginally more effective than the others. This raises the specter that it might be science itself that ends up endorsing an intervention model that is at odds with the rationality of scientism.

As will be apparent in the second section, studies of GA have tended to revolve around evaluation, either of its effectiveness or its recovery culture. Yet if Bufe's critique of AA is exemplary of an "orthodox" scientific perspective, there are other lines of research, slender and less common, that take issue with the way we see the world in the modern age. And 12-step societies such AA and GA can be viewed as addressing issues, personal problems, as well as questions related to meaning, that modernity has generated but has not been able to address.

More than 30 years ago, Gregory Bateson (1972) published "The Cybernetics of Self: A Theory of Alcoholism," wherein he argues that the conventional occidental state of mind is flawed. Leaving aside the ambitious generalization, it is Bateson's (1972) thoughts on reactions to this "flaw" that concern us right here. Intoxication offers a correction, albeit problematic, to an alienated state of being. AA offers a way out for the alcoholic by shaping an *epistemology* that overcomes the logic of a self at once cut off from and trying to control the world that contains it. For Bateson (1972), intoxication is a remedy for the radical egocentrism on which the Western worldview rests. It gives the person a short cut to the experience of belonging in the world, of being "part of." It is the sobriety of the alcoholic that is problematic, Bateson (1972) argues, pitting as it does the conscious will against the rest of the personality in a struggle for control and mastery. Intoxication and addiction symptomatically contest the correctness and the adequacy of a view of *human being* based on Cartesian dualism. The point here is not that intoxication is specific to the occident, but that many alcoholics have found an alternative to the prevailing culture. As an alternative to intoxication, AA is not just another modality, *but a culture*, and should be viewed (and studied) as such. Needless to say, this would apply to GA as well. And in either setting, an admission of powerlessness is key. AA's first step—*We admitted that we were powerless over alcohol—that our lives had become unmanageable*—is, in Bateson's (1972) view, not a mere act of surrender, but an epistemological shift in understanding ourselves as human. The style of sobriety, in which an autonomous ego controls its "self" and its behavior, "must have something wrong with it" (Bateson, 1972, p. 310). By recognizing that the self can never be adequate to itself, that it is in fact a part of the full system of life, by accepting its *dependence*, that there is a Power greater than the self—we are, in Bateson's view (1972), moving away from the essential epistemology of the West: "If we deeply and even unconsciously believe that our relation to the largest system which concerns us—the *Power greater than the self*—is symmetrical and emulative, then we are in error" (Bateson, 1972, p. 336).

For Bateson (1972), a society such as AA is in part a response to the Western project of self-mastery and unilateral control. One need not agree with all of Bateson's assumptions (1972) (such as the existence of a distinctive occidental epistemology), or even sympathize with his harsh critique of his own culture, to appreciate some of his suggestions: if pride, drunkenness, willfulness, and hitting bottom are the signs of an anomic subjectivity, then submission, faith, fellowship, prayer, and anonymity are the tools of a redemptive identity.

In his study of AA, *Not God*, Ernest Kurtz (1979, p. 165) offers a formula to help us understand, if not the full span of Western history, then at least the modern age:

$$\text{Enlightenment} = \text{America} = \text{Development} = \text{Modern} \qquad (14.1)$$

The modern (rational) self takes its place under these four signs. While "America" is a questionable equivalent for the three terms, if we let it represent the state, liberalism, democracy, secularization, and republicanism, perhaps it deserves a place in our consideration. To the question, "But what is 'America'?" Kurtz (1979, pp. 164–165) answers: America is "modern," "the first new state," "American development [is] the pattern of the modern."

The Enlightenment project involves the dethroning of absolutes that contest and impede human freedom and the perfectibility of human being. To do this, the logic that describes America as modernity had to institute a new absolute: the Self, understood as the conscious, calculative, rationally focused aspect of the person that is also called the ego. The application and extension of human reason and rationality opens a path to human perfectibility and mastery of nature: in theory, this project knows no limits.

The accomplishments of modernity, driven by this ethic of perfectibility, are magnificent. Yet the problems of modernity work with equal force and an inexhaustible complementarity. Kurtz (1979, pp. 171–172) identifies four paradoxes of modernity in which the logic of the Enlightenment contradicts itself:

1. As rationality and control increasingly encounter their own limits, the identity of modernity is revealed as inherently addictive, the "me" in pursuit of the "more."
2. Identity, the sense of the self as real (the cornerstone of modernity), begins to dissolve; the real self becomes increasingly elusive.

3. Confronted by limitation, and unable to overcome it, the modern self (oriented to growth and progress) becomes confused and demoralized.
4. As universal man divides into diverse communities (as identity gives way to difference, and we are no longer the same), we are less able to relate to one another as equal.

Obviously, societies such as AA and GA do provide a bond based on shared identity: whether alcoholics or compulsive gamblers, members share a common affliction that in many ways can occlude the differences between them. As our discussion of the literature will make clear, studies of GA have tended to follow a similar path: GA is understood as a modality that should be subject to scientific evaluation. While such studies are certainly necessary, and can even be quite sensitive to GA's recovery culture, there has been little accompanying effort to perceive GA as a response to the larger cultural environment from which it hails. Nor has there been much effort to observe GA directly, without judgment pro or con, simply for the sake of understanding. We will now turn to a study of AA that has accomplished both.

Mariana Valverde (1998) has discussed 12-step recovery as a challenge to attitudes one might call bourgeois, liberal, or even masculine. Treating AA practices as a means to governing oneself and others, Valverde (1998) opts to describe rather than evaluate. After all, while AA's unity hinges upon a common alcoholic identity, AA is mainly designed to govern the alcoholic's soul rather than alcohol itself (Valverde, 1998, p. 120). This would be harder to evaluate than abstinence rates. Further, AA initiated a trend (which includes GA) wherein "non-professional forms of expertise" challenge not only the authority of medicine, but also that of science. Valverde's discussion (1998) would suggest that it may be inappropriate to discuss AA from the very perspectives against which it turns: "it could be argued that AA's particular definition of alcoholism as *a non-medical disease*, while at one level amplifying the medical model by labelling the vice of alcoholism as a disease, is nevertheless, at another level, one of the most successful challenges to the authority of medical and psy experts that this century has seen" (Valverde, 1998, pp. 122–123).

Valverde (1998) is, of course, aware that, as expressed in its Big Book (AAWS, 1976), AA has a long tradition of appealing to professional authority and of trying to establish a good rapport with the scientific and professional communities. Nonetheless, AA marginalizes "physicians and other health system workers" who "are not allowed to diagnose alcoholism or to treat anything other than severe physical problems" (Valverde, 1998, p. 123). Alcoholism is not diagnosed by reference to the amount of alcohol consumed or by reference to other clinical criteria. Instead, AA initiates a subjective, experiential journey. Only if a potential member reports loss of control—the inability to stop drinking even when one wants to—is he or she labeled "alcoholic." Since the subject is the only one who knows whether there was (or is) a desire to stop, self-diagnosis is the only acceptable criteria.

It is worth noting that this differs from GA, which employs some objective measures (through its "20 Questions") to establish a compulsive gambler identity. While this also enables GA to marginalize professionals—anyone can ask the necessary questions—it is clear that an understanding of GA practices cannot hinge solely upon "borrowing" ideas from AA studies. Valverde (1998) even notes another AA challenge to psy practices that do not quite apply to GA: AA's refusal to gather information about its members. GA meetings, for example, may keep track of relapses. While this underscores the need to study GA *closely and carefully*, right here we are interested in the ways in which Valverde's analysis (1998) of AA sheds immediate light on GA itself and on how these insights may help to guide further research.

The purpose of AA is more ambitious than getting members to stop drinking. Since AA's gaze is primarily ethical—the target being neither the body (the object in medicine) nor the mind (the object of psy sciences)—Valverde (1998) describes the content of spiritual progress in AA as "vague" (Valverde, 1998, p. 124). Admittedly goals—such as overcoming "egoism, boastfulness, and a misguided feeling of power"—can be identified. Nonetheless, it would be hard to formulate an exhaustive definition of AA's conception of "sobriety" (which involves more than abstinence from drink). This is partly due to the means by which it can be recognized: an introspective gaze that is hybrid (somewhat medical, somewhat religious) in nature. Valverde (1998) points out, for example, that while AA rejects clinical practices, it in fact employs a "manoeuvre used by clinicians against the knowledge of scientific research. Just as GPs sometimes invoke their years of experience to generate a clinical judgement that is at odds with statistical studies or textbook definitions, so too do members of AA often appeal to a quasi-clinical criterion of 'what works' in order to further a rationality of self-governance that is primarily spiritual" (Valverde, 1998, p. 125).

The 12 Steps are, primarily, not something that one believes in (although this can be important), but an activity, something one "works" on. One might ask how best to "study" an object (AA) that consistently defines itself by reference to ethereal postulates, and where even recovery is defined mainly by activities such as "12-stepping" (helping alcoholics who are still drinking) and characteristics that cannot be measured (only the alcoholic can take his or her own "inventory"). Mainly, AA is about what one does more than what one believes (hence the questionable value of attempting to understand AA by pointing out that many of its tenets are inaccurate)."Activity is the key term here: although driven by beliefs and dogmas . . . AA is nevertheless an anti-intellectual, and particularly an anti-scientific, organization. Its knowledge is always justified by reference to the subjective experience of its members, not to either scientific knowledge or factual truths. Stepping is an activity, and the steps are something one works on; the steps as a whole are a programme for governing one's life" (Valverde, 1998, p. 127).

Few critics of AA would disagree with its characterization as "anti-scientific." If we take seriously the notion that an instrument of study should be commensurate with its object, it would follow that scientific instruments could not hold the key to understanding this organization. Valverde's approach (1998) could be described as phenomenological, or empirical—the latter in the old-fashioned sense in that her main "instruments" were her eyes and her ears; and our own experience with AA members suggests quite strongly that most would consider ridiculous any discussion of AA carried on by someone who has never seen a meeting. Valverde (1998) noticed that, despite AA's refusal to proselytize to non-alcoholics, the 12 steps are perceived "more like vitamins than like medicine" in that they would be good for anyone. She also noticed a juxtaposition of a lofty "spiritual awakening" with mundane practices designed to manage day–to-day existence. These two poles are nonetheless mediated by principles such as "powerlessness" and "anonymity."

It is well known that the first and most important step an AA member must take is the admission of powerlessness over alcohol. As opposed to many therapeutic and self-help approaches designed to "empower" the afflicted, AA produces a culture of humility. Further, there is no blaming of one's parents or general upbringing, nor is powerlessness a state to be overcome. A permanent feature of every alcoholic, "powerlessness" entails a never-ending reliance upon "the all-important support of the collective. To this extent, AA indirectly subverts the neoliberal discourse of personal entrepreneurship and perpetual improvement. Members are perpetually in recovery, always working on their souls, but they do not imagine that they will ever re-make themselves from scratch, in contrast to the neoliberal illusion that the poor can become business executives by sheer willpower" (Valverde, 1998, p. 129). American individualism is further taken to task by the conviction that strong beliefs about one's own "power" can simply be a symptom of alcoholism.

The principle of anonymity also serves to instill humility, and again runs counter to the "culture of enterprise." There is far more to it than the right of each member never to be exposed at work or anywhere else by someone he or she had met at a meeting. First, the entire group is thereby protected from "the temptations of money, fame, and power that have crippled other organizations" (Valverde, 1998, p. 129). Valverde (1998) identifies a few facets of "anonymity" as practiced in AA. Members who contribute to official literature can expect neither money nor fame for their efforts. Hence, AA has no "stars." This is also tied to AA's refusal to collect wealth beyond contributions from members for operational requirements. Mentioning AA's refusal to exercise claims to its symbol even as others were using it to make large profits, Valverde (1998) identifies anonymity not as merely a concept that could somehow be pinned down, but as "a panoply of techniques enabling members to maximize the democratic potential of the organization by exercising a certain self-denial—a despotism not so much over one's desires, as in traditional Protestant ethical forms, but over some dominant trends in contemporary culture" (Valverde, 1998, p. 130).

If, for the sake of identification, we would attempt to *think with AA*, we could view AA more as a process than a set of beliefs. Valverde (1998) attempts to do this when defining anonymity as a "panoply of techniques," best understood as a multiplicity of practices with the unifying concept, anonymity, as subsidiary. This on its own is laden with countercultural implications. We in the West tend to perceive ideas as warranting firm definitions, and are often surprised (perhaps pleasantly) when confronted by basic realities such as the need for practice to precede theory in most aspects of education and learning. Persons stemming from cultures influenced by Buddhism, for example, are more likely to take the priority of practice for granted. AA practices confront not only conceptions of rationality we could associate with individualism, free enterprise, or even the Enlightenment. They lead to attitudes that foster interdependence rather than independence, a collective culture of poverty rather than profit-making, and the priority of experiential wisdom over conceptions of rationality hailed by the Enlightenment and today often assuming the shape of positivist scientism. Again, we will point out that science itself dictates that the instrument should be commensurate with the object. Turning briefly to GA, the study of which is still in the formative stages, would it be wise to presume that this "object," GA, is likely to be commensurate with any scientific "tool" currently at our disposal?

Valverde (1998) discusses the many slogans used in AA as exemplary of how this fellowship operates. "One day at a time" applies, first, to the need to focus on the here and now when trying to stop drinking: it is often too hard for an alcoholic to imagine an entire life without drinking, whereas the idea of not drinking "today" is more manageable. The slogan also functions as a way of helping to reintegrate members who have slipped: they are sober "today" and hence welcome. "One day at a time" also serves to equalize all members because even those with years of sobriety tend to accentuate the fact that they are sober "today," and that yesterday is irrelevant and tomorrow could be different just as it could be for the newcomer. This emphasis on a "24-hour cycle" has other applications as well. Persons suffering from the recent loss of a loved one are often advised to deal with it "one day at a time," making it easier to live without a focus of affection—this time a loved one rather than alcohol. This slogan and others—such as "Easy does it" and "Keep it simple"—can in Valverde's view (1998) serve as a lesson for social theorists. The seemingly vacuous slogans—precisely the type of thing many scholars would ignore—are not empty despite a lack of semantic content. Members interpret them at meetings by reference to their own experiences: how they themselves have used a certain slogan in order to get through various difficulties, what that slogan "means to me," etc. It is all in the doing. The real "content" of the slogans, or for that matter most of the AA program, can be found in practices that define the precepts more so than in precepts that determine the practices.

We are, of course, making a case for the ways in which further studies of GA might proceed. While one may question whether the priority of practice over theory just discussed applies to GA as well, our point is precisely that pertaining to GA, such questions have barely been advanced, let alone explored. As the following discussion of the literature reveals, GA is still largely unknown. While some observational work has been done, for the most part GA has been viewed through scientific and clinical lenses without much consideration of whether it is the right kind of "object" for this kind of attention (though it is sometimes mentioned that as an anonymous fellowship GA is not easy to study). At the very least, one should grant that there could be more to GA than such attention could ever reveal.

Yet it is more than likely that some aspects of the above discussion would indeed apply to GA. The goal of the modern self is autonomy and independence, self-sufficiency and self-control. We measure maturity along these vectors, and we determine immaturity by their absence. In AA, the initial and perpetual admission, the fundamental signal of belonging, is, *I am an alcoholic*. In GA, the admission of being a compulsive gambler serves a similar purpose. In a world that prizes self-control and self-mastery, this is a categorical admission of inadequacy. Critics such as Bufe (1991) are surely puzzled. "Why would people do this to themselves?" is a question that one can almost hear between the lines. After the initial acceptance of powerlessness, AA takes the alcoholic even farther away from modern conceptions of individuality and rationality. Steps 2 and 3 speak to alcoholism as a spiritual problem and recovery as a spiritual task: "Came to believe that a Power greater than ourselves could restore us to sanity" and "Made a decision to turn our will and our lives over to the care of God as we understood him." The process of recovery begins with recognition, admission, belief, and surrender. Those events transform the experience of identity. They convert the person, who in an uncanny way is only now an "alcoholic," into someone whose self-understanding and practices become radically different. This is an oft-cited paradox of AA: through admitting their powerlessness, individuals take responsibility for stopping their drinking and changing the way they live (what Bateson [1972] called their "style of sobriety").

Modernism is based on rationality, verifiability, and its complement, falsification. It is an ocean of objective truth fed by many streams of fact determined by many sciences. Yet AA makes few knowledge claims that science would recognize. There is little about AA that conforms to the rules of science. Bill W. did refer to AA as "...a new life and a new science where there was none" (quoted in Kurtz, 1979, p. 57). But this is best read metaphorically. In fact, AA has been the object of suspicious interest by positivist science for some time. Its premise of faith and belief suggest *error*. As already discussed, AA is a pragmatic set of practices for people who feel they have lost control of their lives through an inability to stop drinking. Its knowledge is the knowledge of experience. As such, the "truths" of AA need not be falsifiable.

We would, however, suggest that another reason these mutual aid organizations seem impervious to scrutiny is that science has gotten away from some of its own principles. Science thinks of itself as having two aspects: rational and empirical. Along the way, it has become increasingly rationalistic and less empirical. This is evident in addictions. There is a heavy investment in theory, so that scientific ideas have proliferated. At the same time, empiricism—the precept that something should be accepted as true only if it could be verified by the senses—has gone through a mutation as the senses themselves have been considered more and more fallible and imperfect. As instruments have proven their superior dependability, phenomenological empiricism has been delegitimized. A question arises: is it possible to retrieve the empirical self as a site of knowledge, or will we continue to objectify it and subject it to the gaze of the mind's eye and its instrumental technologies?

Foucault (1975, p. 198) remarks that modernity is the time when "health replaces salvation." The gods recede. It becomes unthinkable that "psychology" might mean the "study of the spirit," or the way of the soul. Yet, as Kurtz (1979) reminds us, this century is the Age of Psychology, but in a way that can mean only the mind, the truer part of the self that has as its external complement the body. Medicine is the science of the body. Its power lies in its ability to objectify the body. Where previously the doctor asked the patient, "what is the matter?" now the doctor asks, "where does it hurt?" (Foucault, 1975). The doctor then identifies the problem by gazing at the body and prescribes the treatment. Medicine works on the basis of the normal. Abnormality is not healthy. Medicine's work is to bring the deviant body toward the norm. Modern medicine approaches alcoholism and addiction along two avenues of logic: bio-logic (in the fabric and tissue of the body of the sufferer) and psycho-logic (an organic or cognitive problem in the mind). Of course, a combination of both logics is possible. It (the complaint) has to have an objective status to be diagnosed.

Although the idea that there is a sociologic to addiction exists at the rhetorical level, the overpowering effect of the bio-psycho gaze of medicine displaces any real consideration of the social domain. The treatment of addictions is given over to dealing with the bodies and minds of addicts. There is a sociopolitical convenience in making the sufferer the locus of the addiction problem, but at what cost to our understanding and the remediation of addiction in our society? The sciences are unlikely to give us a true sociologic of addiction. They pursue remedies based on it as an organic pathology, or one of learning, or skill deficit, or behavioral performance. The rest will have come from communities, a process that has already begun at the level of grassroots harm reduction as well as the rooms of 12-step recovery, in forms of knowledge that science does not at present recognize. While AA has no way of locating alcoholism at a social level—it lacks a sociologic of addiction and makes its appeal to the suffering drinker as a self-contained alcoholic entity— the program takes the alcoholic into an interpersonal world in which a sobriety of interdependence is substituted for a sobriety of independence. The practice of AA becomes a sociologic. Yet if modernity's posture is one of resolute rationality and heroic progress, then AA presents a tragic reading of human being, one based in suffering and disease. This provides the necessary condition for a saving project of recovery. The metaphors of loss-of-control, surrender, faith, recovery, and fellowship have spread far beyond the treatment of extreme alcoholism in this age of mastery, domination, doubt, progress, and self-reliance. GA is one more example. If we wish to understand such a society, how should we proceed?

We have already offered a few suggestions. The following, aside from one last excursion into AA studies, is an account of the ways in which GA has been studied so far. It will be evident that our intention is not to dismiss various scientific approaches, as they have provided a great deal of valuable knowledge. Nor do we suggest that the practitioners of positivist science are blind or one-dimensional. To the contrary, our hope is based on the assumption that these very scientists can appreciate some of the points we have raised and maybe accept that other approaches would also enhance our collective efforts to make sense of organizations—like AA and GA—which to this day leave many in the field a little baffled.

GA as an Unknown Quantity

The rest of this chapter discusses the literature on GA as well as issues that help to contextualize our understanding of this mutual aid association. Despite reflections that may have seemed a little lofty to some readers, at one level our argument can be simplified: as an anonymous, mutual aid organization that seems puzzling to many scientific minds, GA requires more direct observation without interference from a host of scientific filters that, despite adding clarity in some respects, are also designed to ignore whatever they are not designed to "see." Instead of merely talking about GA, there is a need to let GA "speak." Interviews, while important, can miss the point: the target is not just individual GA members, but the fellowship itself, a *culture* that cannot be "described" exhaustively by GA members any more than, for example, Polish culture could be communicated to us by Polish citizens (we would also have to go to Poland).

The following discussion, in the spirit of our critique, is a respectful treatment of some of the work done on GA so far. As the discussion will make clear, overall the scientific literature tends to be critical yet supportive of GA. Some studies have already taken steps in the directions we suggest, but in our view have not gone far enough. In addition, many of the points made about AA as simply inconsistent with much of what contemporary observers take for granted may, or may not, apply to GA. The issue is that we still do not know.

GA's Effectiveness: How It Works

When discussions of GA were in their infancy, endorsements were often less guarded than current assessments (Custer, 1982a; Custer & Milt, 1985; Winston & Harris, 1984), although GA's inability to deal with certain psychiatric issues has long been acknowledged (Custer & Milt, 1985). Since then, more researchers have come to perceive GA as helpful but incomplete, and likely to be more effective in conjunction with other interventions. Such assessments are often based on three considerations:

1. Greater attention to the significance of co-occurring substance addictions (Lesieur & Blume, 1991a)
2. More attention to GA's inability to address other special needs (Rosenthal, 1992)
3. Concerns about the small percentage of gamblers who achieve abstinence after trying GA (Lesieur and Blume, 1991a; Petry, 2002). [Stewart and Brown (1988), for example, found that out of a sample of 232 attendees 8 % had remained completely abstinent and active in the fellowship 1 year after their first meeting, and about 7 % after 2 years.]

There are also questions pertaining to the type of gambler for which GA is effective. For example, both Turner and Saunders (1990) and McCown and Chamberlain (2000) have discussed GA's confrontational approach and how this may alienate some newcomers.

Blaszczynski (2000) has suggested that GA is suitable only for gamblers free of other compounding issues, meaning gamblers who are essentially "normal" save for the gambling problem itself. When Blaszynski (2000) talks about the role of GA in treating gambling problems, he allows that it could be considered as an option for the subgroup he calls as "normal" pathological gamblers who require minimal interventions, but does not acknowledge that it has a role with the two other subgroups he describes—the "emotionally vulnerable" and those with "biological correlates." Yet Blaszczynski (2000) also claims that "normal" gamblers, being relatively well-adjusted, are good candidates for moderation instead of abstinence goals, throwing into question their suitability for a program that insists on abstinence. Brown (1986, 1987a, 1987b) has found that gamblers able to moderate are unlikely to stay for long at GA. Further, Brown has argued that GA may suit only the most severe cases, as GA ideology involves the need to "hit bottom" (in GA this is often called one's "personal low") and insists on abstinence which, as both Brown and Blaszczynski (2000) state, may not be necessary for less troubled gamblers. Brown (1987a, 1987b, 1987c) found that precisely those gamblers who perceived themselves as less troubled were more likely to leave GA. Stirpe (1995) has also argued that GA is appropriate mainly for severe cases. In short, the ideology of "hitting bottom" insists that one must be at the brink—not just financially, but also emotionally—and tends to alienate those who simply cannot relate. Conversely, Blaszcynski's (2000) point is that a compulsive gambler with pressing psychiatric difficulties may require more serious intervention than a nonprofessional society can offer.

This brings to light why, in the literature, the term "effectiveness" often refers to more than just gambling cessation. Browne (1991, 1994) has discussed GA's lesser emphasis on the 12 Steps and spirituality compared to AA, and its more pragmatic focus on gambling itself and issues such as debts. For this reason, Browne considers GA less effective as an overall therapy than AA, which puts more focus on the "whole" self. Browne (1991) has also suggested that the relative absence of spiritual and inner-directed therapies may alienate women and certain minorities. Yet according to Browne (1991) "12-step consciousness" can be found among GA members affiliated with other 12-step fellowships. Lesieur (1990) has made similar observations. This adds weight to suggestions that GA is simply incomplete on its own (Lesieur & Blume, 1991a; Rosenthal, 1992; Petry, 2002) and should be judged on how it can complement other interventions.

As well, many have argued that a program can be "effective" even if it reduces gambling activity without achieving long-term abstinence (Blaszczynski, McConaghy, & Frankonova, 1991), and despite philosophical discrepancies there is no reason to presume that GA could not play a role in such outcomes (McCown & Chamberlain, 2000). It has long been recognized that GA may have a positive effect even on those who attend only once or twice (Allock, 1986).

Yet given the existing state of knowledge, GA's appropriate role is still open to speculation. While most North American gambling treatment programs use GA as an adjunct, a comprehensive understanding of GA's inner workings—its recovery culture and the types of narratives it employs—is lacking. This is due to a dearth of direct, observational accounts of what actually transpires at GA meetings. There is no shortage of attempts to evaluate GA in various ways (Abt & McGurrin, 1991; Allock, 1986; Brown, 1985; Canadian Foundation of Compulsive Gambling, Ontario, 1996; Custer, 1982a; Petry, 2002; Potenza, 2002; Preston & Smith, 1985; Rosenthal, 1992; Steinberg, 1993; Stewart & Brown, 1988; Walker, 1992). Yet Petry (2002) grants that evaluations of GA's efficacy remain tenuous given the current state of knowledge, and argues that large-scale controlled studies of various interventions are necessary for a clearer grasp of what really works for pathological gamblers [though Brown (1985) has discussed some of the difficulties involved in attempting to assess an anonymous fellowship such as GA]. GA members have also been studied outside GA to gauge psychological and other issues (Getty, Watson, &

Frisch, 2000; Kramer, 1988; Lorenz & Yaffe, 1986; Whitman-Raymond, 1988). Yet little descriptive work has been done on the workings of GA itself.

Livingston (1971) provided information that by today's standards would be introductory. Brown (1986, 1987a, 1987b, 1987c) has carried out some of the most useful work on GA, especially regarding the question of why some members drop out. As might be expected, he found that those who left were more likely to consider the talk at meetings to be "meaningless" and were more critical of GA literature than those who remained (Brown, 1987b). Brown (1986) also found that those who were overly elated at their first meeting were more likely to become disenchanted later on than those with a more balanced initial impression. Yet these studies relied on interviews without accompanying observation of GA meetings, so no detailed account is given of what, exactly, some dismiss as meaningless. Further, we are left with speculative evaluation as a solid descriptive base is lacking. For example, Brown (1987a, 1987c) found that only gamblers whose problems had become most severe, or at least those who perceived their problems this way, were likely to remain in GA. Promising explanations for this remain unverified: Brown (1987a) speculates that perhaps some members take pride (possibly competitive pride) in the extreme nature of their gambling careers, with the corollary that many members must either embellish their own stories or be unacknowledged and socially sidelined. Direct observation, accompanied by interviews, would be needed to verify the existence of such a cultural dynamic and then describe its workings.

The study of GA's effectiveness is best understood as a work-in-progress, with important advances identifying better research targets yet still haunted by gaps in available knowledge. When Brown began his studies of GA, little observational work on GA had been done (Cromer, 1978; Livingston, 1971; Scodel, 1964), and both Cromer and Scodel delivered mainly interesting theoretical discussions and only brief empirical accounts of GA's workings. Preston and Smith (1985) claimed that AA is more effective with alcoholics than GA is with gamblers, partly because AA's physical disease conception (of an "allergy" to alcohol) facilitates "relabeling," thereby helping to deflect guilt and shame. While providing valuable insight into the importance of belief systems in mutual aid, Preston and Smith (1985) were nonetheless operating on the premise that the AA and GA programs were virtually identical. Later Browne (1991, 1994) explored the differences between AA and GA. While this does involve some discussion of GA "consciousness" (1991), such as the lesser importance attached to discussing one's feelings than in AA, little attention is paid to how much feelings are actually addressed in GA because Browne's studies are to a large extent comparative. They are also more evaluative than descriptive, containing (beyond criticisms already mentioned) a critical account of GA's version of its own history (Browne, 1994). Browne's work contains some important descriptive material based on direct observation, but does not provide a detailed account of what transpires at a GA meeting.

Similar limits apply to the account given by Turner and Saunders (1990) after a 1-year observational study. Critical of the medical model, these authors discuss the moral and emotional implications of GA narratives. Still, GA narratives are discussed primarily in terms of their negative implications rather than their actual content. Despite some significant descriptive observations, notably concerning the high pressure and confrontational aspects of GA, one is still left mostly in the dark about how GA actually operates. While not nearly as harsh, this account of GA can be compared to Bufe's treatment of AA in that it represents a mindset that we have been questioning from the start. This is not to suggest that Turner and Saunders' (1990) criticisms are without merit (newcomers being tormented and dropouts being made to feel like failures represent serious concerns), but that many criticisms stem from a particular way of viewing humanity, and we believe that other perspectives may be necessary. We will limit ourselves to three examples. "Based upon the solid foundations of the newly constructed GA identity, these individuals are so dependent upon the group for reaffirmation that they become addicted to one another in place of their gambling and all its ramifications" (Turner and Saunders, 1990, p. 75). Here, the suggestion is that dependency, in any form, is negative. Yet maybe GA simply represents one more challenge to this modern perspective. The authors also question the "commitment to a medical model that may not even be accurate" (Turner and Saunders, 1990, p. 76). While certainly not reducing their critique of the medical model to its lack of accuracy, the authors make little attempt to describe it as a myth that has served at least some members very well. The latter is alluded to, but not considered worthy of much discussion, even though this is precisely what a serious *understanding* of GA would require. "Accuracy" may be irrelevant. Our third example involves the authors' account of the "ideal self" to which GA members aspire. The spiritual dimension of this new self is a "mysterious element . . . impossible to define and even harder to attain" (Turner and Saunders, 1990, p. 69). One can appreciate a commentary on the ways in which the medical model alienates those who do not conform, yet still question the validity of a critique that hinges largely on the unattainability of an "ideal self" to which members aspire. The latter, after all, could be said of most spiritual and psycho-emotional endeavors. Further, as Valverde's (1998) discussion of AA demonstrates, beliefs and ideas may have substance despite the absence of solid definitions. While we cannot comment on how difficult GA ideals are to attain, we maintain that the practices by which they are attained require keen elaboration before they can be understood. Only then could a more informed process of evaluation proceed. While we concur with the choice Turner and Saunders (1990) made in opting for qualitative methodology, and have found their study informative, we suggest that these authors have taken one step away from a strictly scientistic mindset and that at least more step would be necessary to take GA studies in a different (and potentially promising) direction.

Nothing we have written should be taken to imply that GA is completely unknown. GA's own literature gives some vindication to Browne's (1991, 1994) contention that "GA consciousness" is pragmatic. The "Pressure Group," for example, sets GA apart from substance-oriented mutual aid societies in that other members take newcomers to task over financial and other issues so they can get honest with their spouses and get their affairs in order (GANSO, 1978). Browne (1991) discusses GA's "Page 17 consciousness," referring to a set of practical (rather than spiritual or psychological) principles found in GA's most important text (GAISO, 1999).

Overall, the available literature does vindicate GA in other, less direct ways. GA's collective wisdom has demonstrated some scientific merit: the "20 Questions" GA poses to help gamblers determine whether they in fact need help has been found to compare favorably to other, professionally developed diagnostic instruments (Ursua & Uribelarrea, 1998). As well, commentators generally appreciate that GA provides social support that professionals could rarely imitate (Rugle & Rosenthal, 1994). Ogborne (1978) has argued that modalities are less important to success than the stability and support (such as family networks) a client brings to treatment, and gamblers with social support have been found to achieve longer-term abstinence than those without it (Stein, 1993). Davison, Pennebacker, and Dickerson (2000) found that AA members lacking outside support adhere more closely to AA's program, and that alienation from one's normal support networks may lead one to mutual aid. In short, mutual aid can alleviate isolation through peer support and encouragement. Walker (1992) claims that GA's main strength lies in its collective belief that compulsive gambling can be beaten.

Yet these endorsements of the mutual aid approach are not specific to GA, and stem from a growing awareness of the importance of social support in general. Involvement in mutual aid has been associated with better results even with biological afflictions such as breast cancer (Davison et al., 2000). Little is known about what, if anything, GA has to offer beyond peer support. Whether GA's recovery program has merit in and of itself, and if so for which type of gambler, remains undetermined.

To complicate matters further, questions concerning "effectiveness" are often laden with assumptions. Answers to whether GA's insistence on abstinence is the best approach, good for some but not for others, or even potentially harmful, will hinge on ideas about the nature of compulsive gambling itself. We now turn to this issue.

The Nature of Problem Gambling

Perceptions of the Problem

Pathological gambling has been called a "pure addiction," given that subjects feel compelled to pursue and continue the activity even when no mind-altering drugs are involved (Rosenthal, 1992). GA uses the disease model, and the way GA is perceived will be greatly affected by the extent to which this model is accepted. In fact, a researcher's position on this issue is a good predictor of whether his or her assessment of GA will be sympathetic. Despite scientific distance from GA, the most prominent view of pathological gambling, at least in North America, is that of GA itself: the standard disease model of addiction, the so-called medical model. Even if DSM IV (1994) calls pathological gambling an impulse control disorder, its description of the problem is quite compatible with (and in places identical to) the disease model.

The disease conception of addiction involves a few major tenets:

1. Addiction is a primary disease, the cause rather than the symptom of other difficulties.
2. Addiction is progressive, meaning that untreated it can only get worse.

3. Addiction is chronic, meaning that it can be arrested but never cured (hence abstinent subjects must forever remain on guard).
4. Abstinence is the only solution (Alcoholics Anonymous World Services, Inc., 1976; GAPC, 1964a; Peele, 1989; World Service Office, Inc., 1982).

Despite the designation "primary disease," medical model proponents in the alcoholism field have pointed out that disease primacy need not involve chronological priority: even if an addiction emerged due to other factors, it can be "primary" once it has taken effect in the sense that alleviating the initial causes would not on its own arrest the addiction (Flavin & Morse, 1991). According to this view, the main consideration is that *active addiction* is not merely a symptom of other difficulties. The medical model (and by implication GA) can, therefore, be compatible with psychodynamic, psychobiological, and other explanations for the problem's onset.

A cursory glance at the literature could easily give the false impression that the medical model is out of favor: it would seem to have more critics than champions. This is mainly a sign of the model's dominance. Its adherents do not necessarily defend it directly, often preferring to vindicate all or most of its tenets either explicitly or implicitly. Critics of this model rarely deny that it dominates, and instead argue that it should not (Abt & McGurrin, 1991; Peele, 1989, 2001; Sartin, 1988; Turner & Saunders, 1990). Also, it is common for researchers critical of one aspect of the disease conception to keep the peace with other tenets and advocate cooperation with GA and its disease orientation. For example, Whitman-Raymond (1988), while at odds with the notion of disease primacy as it downplays the importance of psychoanalytic determinants, also believes that psychoanalysts should collaborate closely with GA. Authors with more sympathy for the medical model of compulsive gambling have even pointed out that newly abstinent gamblers can experience physical withdrawal (Rosenthal & Lesieur, 1992). Blume (1986, 1987) side-steps questions concerning the disease model's scientific validity by simply claiming that it has proven useful for treatment.

Walker (1992) claims that problem gambling research has been marked by an overreliance on data obtained from GA members and other gamblers in treatment who have possibly internalized the medical model and are likely to reconstruct their past experiences in accordance with its tenets. Moreyra, Ibanez, Liebowitz, Saiz-Ruiz, and Blanco (2002) argue that most research suggests that pathological gambling more closely resembles a substance abuse disorder than an obsessive–compulsive disorder, but mention that the addiction and obsession–compulsion models are not mutually exclusive. They also mention that since most research on pathological gambling has come from the substance abuse treatment field, many findings could be biased in that direction. Given that North American substance addiction treatment generally operates along disease model lines, and given the late 20th century trend of perceiving a host of psycho–behavioral ailments in this fashion—often in reference to AA's alcoholism model (Peele, 1989)—it should not be surprising that problem gambling theory and practice have followed suit. This trend has of course been challenged, often because of its propensity to reduce all pathological gambling to one formula (Blaszczynski & McConaghy, 1989).

The existing literature does offer alternatives to the medical model. It has been argued that since problem gamblers score high on both impulsivity and obsessionality, "obsessive–compulsive spectrum disorder" would be a better designation (Blaszczynski, 1999). Some have argued in favor of an overall propensity to addiction, insisting that problem gambling is simply a subset and should not be treated as an independent problem (Jacobs, 1987; Jacobs, Marston, & Singer, 1985), while others have challenged that view (Blaszczynski & McConaghy, 1989; Briggs, Goodin, & Nelson, 1996; Rozin & Stoess, 1993b). Pathological gambling has been associated with risky sexual behavior (Rozin & Stoess, 1993a) and with impulsivity (Blaszczynski, 1999; Castellani & Rugle, 1995), yet the latter view at least has been challenged (Allock & Grace, 1988). Many view compulsive gambling primarily in psycho-emotional terms (Sartin, 1988; Taber, Russo, Adkins, & McCormick, 1986); Brown (1993) has argued that a non-substance addiction such as gambling requires more focus on purely psychological processes, and could possibly steer our grasp of other addictions in similar directions.

Despite the medical model's primacy, there seems to be a trend in the direction of identifying subtypes of problem and compulsive gamblers with the connotation that the medical model—and by implication GA's approach—could not apply to all cases (Blaszczynski 2000; Blaszczynski & Nower, 2002; Peele 2001; Potenza, 2002). The emphasis on typology involves, among other things, the view that two individuals might exhibit similar behaviors for completely different reasons. Blaszczynski (2000) can be taken as exemplary when he divides gamblers into three types: those whose gambling is rooted in genetic difficulties, those with underlying emotional difficulties, and those who are essentially "normal" save for the gambling problem itself. Brown (1986, 1987a, 1987b, 1987c) was already onto the importance of subtypes when attempting to determine what type of gambler is likely to remain in GA. Along these lines, some have argued that the complexities of problem gambling suggest that it is a syndrome rather than a single disorder (Griffiths, Parke, & Wood, 2002; Shaffer & Korn, 2002). Berger (1988) has discussed different personalities attracted to different games of chance whereas Dickerson (1993) has argued that different games produce different types of compulsion.

Perhaps the most controversial implication of one's views on the nature of compulsive gambling is an issue that has haunted other addictions as well: is abstinence the only solution?

Perceived Solutions and the Primacy of the Abstinence Principle

GA emphasizes abstinence, and hence debates over this principle apply directly to evaluations of GA's program of recovery. As well, a researcher's position on this issue is perhaps the best predictor of his or her overall assessment of GA. Arguably the medical model's most important tenet, the abstinence principle, has many critics. Some have argued that the call for abstinence has both positive and negative features (Murray, 2001) while others have been more strongly critical (Peele, 2001; Rosecrance, 1988, 1989; Sartin, 1988). Most common is the claim that abstinence should not be considered the only solution (Blaszczynski, 2000; Blaszczynski et al.,

1991; Blaszczynski & McConaghy, 1989; Peele, 2001; Walker, 1992, 1993), and it has long been argued that GA's call for abstinence can alienate those who do not think that way (Brown, 1987b).

As a subset of the medical model, the abstinence principle may at first glance appear to have more detractors than supporters. Again, this is inaccurate. As abstinence is the dominant solution, many in the field do not defend it explicitly; often success is simply measured, either primarily or exclusively, in terms of abstinence rather than the achievement of less harmful gambling patterns (Johnson & Nora, 1992; Maurer, 1985; Rosenthal & Rugle, 1994). McCown and Chamberlain (2000) provide a more up-to-date defense of abstinence as a goal; they do discuss reduced gambling activity, but primarily with reference to clients who target abstinence.

There is little in the gambling literature on the virtues and drawbacks of abstinence to distinguish it from more thoroughly developed discussions of these ideas among students of substance abuse. Rankin (1982) has argued that since physical dependence is often the criteria for suggesting abstinence in cases of alcoholism, the application of this principle for gamblers is more tenuous. Viets and Miller (1997) have pointed out that even definitions of "abstinence" hinge on definitions of gambling. But for the most part, ideas about abstinence are not specific to gambling, and the gambling literature would probably benefit from greater attention to theoretical discussions of the abstinence principle's role in recovery.

Many perceive the abstinence principle in terms of its ideological function. While critics such as Turner and Saunders (1990) consider GA members' internalization of the medical model to be comparable to collective brainwashing, the designation "ideology" need not be derogatory. Many researchers, rather than attack or defend the belief in abstinence, prefer to study the ways in which the principle can operate. Abstinence, for any addict who accepts it, has been viewed as part of a larger belief system regarding the nature of, and solution to, the ailment in question.

Antze (1979) has discussed the ways in which mutual aid depends on mutual identification and the internalization the group's belief system. Valverde (1998) has claimed that abstinence in AA is not so much a puritanical despotism over desires, but a pragmatic reconstruction of habits rooted in strands of 20th century philosophy as well as ancient, prescientific wisdom. In their study of the 12-Step (AA and NA)–based Minnesota Model, Keene and Rayner (1993) found the approach to favor those with compatible belief systems (e.g., agreement with the medical model, positive attitudes toward spirituality). Keene and Rayner (1993) recommend that clients be served by approaches and theories consistent with their own ways of thinking. There is some evidence for "cognitive profiles" applicable to many AA members (Ogborne & Glaser, 1981), suggesting that similar work could be done on the personality and cognitive profiles of GA members: Are they field dependent? Do they demonstrate authoritarian attitudes and a (often accompanying) need for simple, clear answers (such as abstinence)?

Work already done on AA members could help those of us in the gambling field move ahead more quickly on this score than the AA research pioneers were able to do. On the role of abstinence in AA, Antze (1987) might provide the most thorough account. Antze perceives AA as a "culture"—"in the Geertzean sense, as a coherent web of symbols that directs human conduct." In AA, symbols provide the means by which members reconstruct their experiences "in a standardized way" (Antze, 1987, p. 149), thereby changing their very identities. Obviously, "alcohol" is an important symbol in AA. Yet to appreciate its role, and thereby that of abstinence, we should recall that AA's 12 Steps mention God six times and alcohol only once. Abstinence is not just an end in itself, but a key ingredient to a larger world of recovery. "Where else," Antze (1987, p. 150) quotes from the Big Book (AAWS, 1976), "could you find half a million people dedicated to love, and really loving each other?" Referring to the warmth members show to newcomers, and to the fact that many members tend to "drop nonalcoholic friendships and rebuild their social lives" (Antze, 1987, p. 150) around other recovering alcoholics, Antze points out it is each member's special relationship with alcohol that has made this possible. Hence AA can be described as "totemic": everything about AA is rooted in a substance that members reject; the aversion is not a moral issue, and stems from a perception that members are unique in their vulnerability to the substance. An anthropologist, Antze notes that such totemism is rare in the modern world.

Antze draws a similar analogy with tribal societies, describing AA as a "cult of affliction." Such cults can be based on issues such as "bad luck in hunting, reproductive disorders, and a host of other minor ills . . . they also initiate the victim into a specialized community of former sufferers-turned-healers . . . like AA [they use] mutual confession and the settling of grievances as therapeutic tools." With healing cults involving possession by spirits, "typically, the afflicting spirit is propitiated or 'domesticated' to become a benefactor venerated through cult activity" (Antze, 1987, pp. 151–152). In Antze's view, AA's similarity to these practices can best be understood by reference to the relation AA collectively establishes to the substance its members are instructed to shun, and to the meaning of AA's most important word: "alcoholic"; and the key to grasping the role of abstinence rests in a better grasp of the "alcoholic personhood" espoused by AA (Antze, 1987, p. 153).

For Antze, the fact that medical research has yet to vindicate the disease model of alcoholism, and that some of its tenets are inconsistent with the best research available, suggests that AA's views on this matter should be seen as "elements of a folk system with a logic and coherence of its own" (Antze, 1987, p. 155). To start, AA recognizes no degrees of alcoholism: one either is or is not alcoholic. Alcoholism is said to involve two main problems with respect to alcohol: a physical "allergy" and a mental obsession. The first feature implies that control over intake of alcohol is impossible; to the alcoholic, the substance is poison. "At a metaphorical level in AA's writings, alcohol for the alcoholic becomes the embodiment of death itself" (Antze, 1987, p. 156). For such a person, the need to avoid alcohol is obvious, yet the mental obsession renders the alcoholic incapable of doing that. Though neither of these features could withstand scientific scrutiny, each is close to the experiences of many compulsive drinkers. "But they are also both part of a symbolic scheme that aims to persuade and transform, and their real interest lies at this level" (Antze, 1987, p. 157). Understandably, they can lead to a despair AA describes as "hitting bottom." This is what deflates the alcoholic's sense of self-sufficiency, forcing him or her to accept an absolute dependence on any thing, or being, that could stop the drinking. Only such desperation can, in AA's view, cause an alcoholic to become this "open-minded." The key notion here is "surrender," first the surrender to alcohol which in turn entails a surrender to "God." While alcohol represents death, insanity, or worse, the Higher Power offers "renewed life and strength and companionship." Many AA members will attest to the following: "1) The drinker falls into a serious depression. He may feel himself to be on the verge of dying or may even be close to death for good physical reasons. 2) He sees his condition to be hopeless and/or cries out to God for help. 3) A sudden unexplainable feeling of comfort and release sweeps over him, which he recognizes then or later as the entry of the Higher Power into his life" (Antze, 1987, p. 160).

The abstinence principle, then, is not merely the abnegation of alcohol but also key to what we can safely refer to as a "conversion experience." In AA, the Higher Power is purely benign—forgiving, helpful, ready to provide guidance and support—just like AA itself (and there are members who consider the group to be their "Higher Power"). Of course, alcohol is saddled with the very opposite. AA even manages to supplant alcohol's former role in that it offers many of the things alcohol had promised: strength, courage, companionship. Insofar as AA can exist as a society, a benign order, it must rest upon its rapport with a substance that has essentially been demonized. But it is only a "demon" to alcoholics, and AA does not suggest that nonalcoholics should avoid drinking. AA claims that, beyond the physical allergy (or "sensitivity) to alcohol, alcoholics also suffer from something akin to a spiritual void. This helps to explain the mental obsession to start drinking even before there is any alcohol in the body. Antze discusses two types of abstinence in AA lore: being merely "dry" is a function of willpower, doomed to fail over the long haul and guaranteed to provide misery while practiced; on the other hand there is "sobriety," a state of spiritual fulfillment brought about by working the AA program. Essentially, this new state involves the renunciation of selfishness, self-centeredness, and even willpower. In short, many of the characteristics cherished by entrepreneurial self-starters are anathema. "Empowerment" is supplanted by surrender. The desire to control one's life, along with the behavior of others, is linked inextricably to the obsession to drink. While Antze points out that AA does not explain clearly how this is so, we may note that an idea as simple as "letting go" is sufficient to understand AA's views on this matter (they may be questionable but are not bereft of rationality). The desire for "control," when frustrated, is associated with emotions such as anger, self-pity, and above all resentment—all of which are associated not only with spiritual sickness, but also with drinking.

The function of an act of surrender, abstinence in AA is integral to the overcoming of "pathological selfishness . . . it entails the much broader abdication of ego that comes from putting one's life in God's hands . . . surrender for AA also means the development of a more accepting, less combative approach to the trials of everyday life" (Antze, 1987, p. 166). As AA sees it, its membership is considerably happier than most average (normal) citizens, and Antze refers to an AA official who describes the program as an escape from "enslavement to the false ideals of a materialistic society," who then goes on to critique the very culture out of which AA was born: "millions who are not alcoholics are living today in illusory worlds, nurturing the basic anxieties and insecurities of human existence rather than facing themselves with courage and humility" (Antze, 1987, p. 168). So the AA member is not merely trying to return to predrinking conditions of life and states of mind, but is forging ahead toward something that—as many members will passionately attest—is far better. An AA member who believes in the AA way, and then targets an alternative to abstinence, would be giving up much more than freedom from drink: the very attempt to control one's drinking would amount to the forsaking of a host of ideas, principles, and attitudes upon which a new and purportedly better life is based.

Yet this mode of life is, in one respect, not chosen freely. Since this spiritual state is one's only defense against alcohol, it is the demon itself that ensures ongoing devotion to the program of recovery. "At points in the AA literature, in fact, alcohol emerges as the chief guardian—and a very jealous one—of the moral order the group has constructed." Hence alcohol "stands as a kind of benefactor" (Antze, 1987, pp. 169–170). Persons who once (prior to the onset of alcoholism) were unable to admit to being wrong now do so readily. Persons once unable to acknowledge their own limits, now do so through a culture of humility. Many believe that their alcoholism was part of a Divine plan—without it, they might have remained functional but shallow, free of inebriation but arrogant, resentful, and unfulfilled. Again, AA is a culture that turns against many of the cornerstones of modernity: "Neither self-knowledge nor strength of character can protect him from the impulse to drink, and injunctions to rely of 'willpower' may do more harm than good." Regardless of whether one sympathizes with AA's recovery culture, the parallels with healing cults in different times and places bring home an all important consideration: "we are dealing here with a response to suffering so deeply satisfying that it has emerged in a number of human contexts" (Antze, 1987, pp. 173–174).

There is cause to believe that GA is one more human context where this may apply. But at this point, caution is warranted. GA is also a spiritual organization, but arguably less so than AA. GA is also focused on the cessation of an addictive behavior, but perhaps more directly so than AA. What role, exactly, does the abstinence principle play within the rooms of GA? Work done so far has provided us with some insight, but certainly not with the kind of detail and precision such a topic would warrant. Despite the abstinence principle's popularity, many researchers are coming to the conclusion that while the call for abstinence may be helpful for some gamblers, it might be harmful to others. Given that such questions are nowhere close to settled even in the alcoholism field, we should not expect consensus among gambling researchers anytime soon. Yet the necessary business of client matching would, with respect to GA, be facilitated not only by a better grasp of which clients are best suited to abstinence goals, but also by an appreciation of the "type" of abstinence practiced by GA, and from there the type of gambler best suited to GA's own culture of recovery.

Conclusion

While making a case for direct, observational study, we recognize and expect that there will always be observer bias. Further, if as McCown and Chamberlain (2000) have observed, GA groups tend to be less uniform than their AA counterparts, it will be even more difficult to extrapolate from specific observations to general findings.

From the start, we have recognized that standard scientific instruments have an important role to play. So, is GA a "bad object" for science? Depending on how we define science, it may well be. On the other hand, depending on what we mean science to be, it could be an object of active concern.

As it stands, there is still no consensus on whether GA is suitable for the least, or the most, troubled gamblers. We may yet learn that the extent to which one is troubled may not be the best predictor. An entire culture of recovery is involved, and in order to know it we must get close to it.

Does the scientific gaze construct GA as a cult and something that occurs outside the realm of normal practices and knowledge? Is there something to be learned about it as a cult of affliction? Modern medicine is an expert domain. The tracing and topologizing of the regions of health and disease are the provinces of specialists. Yet we have tried to identify the mutual aid group as a culture, a society in itself. The map is not the territory, we must remember. The templates of science have not served us well in the social sphere. Perhaps we can no longer approach from the outside the suffering that in this age gives rise to addiction. Griffith Edwards (1990) cites a case, the study of withdrawal symptoms, in which for a full century, science, for all its powers of understanding, became so absorbed in the abstract world of scientific hypotheses that it forgot that what it was looking for had been in front of it all the time, and had been documented by clinicians years earlier: ". . . over a period of time [the last 100 years] the best scientific minds were able to dismiss from their field of vision the facts that any shaking patient would have demonstrated or reported to them at any time." He asks how scientists could ". . . fail to test our received scientific wisdom against what our patients can tell us if only we will listen" (Edwards, 1992, p. 46). Too often, science has stopped listening to the sufferer, for whom it has little use beyond fitting him or her into its designs. Edwards calls for a redirection away from a rarefied rationality and toward the phenomenological self of the drinker, the drug user, the addict. He speaks out for ". . . a type of research that has no precise designation but which for shorthand one might call "listening and looking." The research community needs to set about the task of strengthening an investigative tradition that is rooted in listening to what patients have to tell us and observing what they have to show" (Edwards, 1992, p. 59).

It is toward this possibility, so unacknowledged by a science dominated by instrumental technologies, that a more authentic study of addiction needs to turn. Edwards cautions that it would be wrong to dismiss such an approach as "soft." There is need to turn toward a "science" of experience, to the raw empiricism of the lived world. It is there that we will find GA and its kind, doing their work, one day at a time.

Acknowledgments The authors acknowledge with gratitude the Ontario Problem Gambling Research Centre for their support of this research initiative. We also want to acknowledge and thank the Journal of Gambling Issues; this report draws heavily on material originally presented there. The opinions expressed are those of the authors and not necessarily those of the Centre for Addiction and Mental Health.

Chapter 15
Problem Gambling and Anger: Integrated Assessment and Treatment

Lorne M. Korman, Emily Cripps, and Tony Toneatto

Recently there has been increasing awareness of the role of dysregulated emotions among individuals with gambling problems. Problems of anger and intimate partner violence appear to be particularly prevalent among gamblers. In this chapter, we discuss the available research on comorbid gambling and anger, and discuss issues in the assessment of these problems. We then describe an integrated emotion and behavior regulation treatment for comorbid gambling and anger problems. In this chapter, we use the diagnostic term "pathological gambler" to describe an individual who meets at least at least five of the ten criteria in the Diagnostic and Statistical Manual (DSM-IV) of the American Psychiatric Association (1994). The term "problem gambler" (Lesieur & Rosenthal, 1991) is used to describe individuals who have gambling problems but who may not meet full DSM-IV criteria for pathological gambling.

The Role of Emotion in Problem Gambling

Research on the etiology and treatment of problem gambling generally has focused on the role of cognitive errors and distortions that are frequently observed in this population. In 1999, Toneatto summarized the extensive research literature regarding the cognitive distortions observed in problem gamblers. Toneatto highlighted several cognitive distortions believed to play a role in problem gambling, such as the magnification of one's own gambling skills, the minimization of the skills of other gamblers, superstitious beliefs, interpretive biases, selective memory, illusion of control over luck, predictive skill, illusory correlation, and several self-relevant beliefs (e.g., entitlement, magical thinking). Since the publication of Toneatto's review, both research (e.g., Hodgins & el-Guebaly, 2004) and theory (e.g., Delfabbro, 2005) have tended to continue to focus on the role of cognitive factors in the etiology, maintenance, and treatment of problem gambling.

Lorne M. Korman
British Columbia Children's Hospital, The Provincial Health Services Authority of British Columbia, and the University of British Columbia, Canada

M. Zangeneh, A. Blaszczynski, N. Turner (eds.), *In the Pursuit of Winning.*
© Springer 2008

Recently, however, there has been growing awareness of the possible role of dysregulated emotions in problem gambling. For example, Blaszczynski and Nower (2002) theorized that "emotionally vulnerable" problem gamblers constitute one of three subgroups in problem gambling. They describe the gambling behavior of these individuals as motivated by a desire to regulate emotional states, in particular to provide escape from aversive feelings like anxiety or depression or to increase arousal. Blaszczynski and Nower point to the factor analytic studies of Gonzalez-Ibanez et al. (1999) and Steel and Blaszczynski (1996) as evidence in favor of the existence of this subgroup. This view is also supported by studies finding high rates of depression (Bland, Newman, Orn, & Stebelsky, 1993; Ramirez, McCormick, Russo, & Taber, 1983; McCormick, Russo, Ramirez, & Taber, 1984) and anxiety disorders (Specker, Carlson, Edmonson, Johnson, & Marcotte, 1996) among pathological gamblers. Other theorists have also discussed the role of emotion regulation in problem gambling (e.g., Jacobs, 1986), and several of these discussions (e.g., Diskin & Hodgins, 2001; Mark & Lesieur, 1992) include the opinion that female problem gamblers may be more likely than male problem gamblers to have emotion regulation motivations.

Studies have also found high rates of Axis II comorbidity among pathological gamblers (Black & Moyer, 1998; Blaszczynski and Steel, 1998; Fernandez-Montalvo & Echeburua, 2004; Lesieur & Blume, 1990). Personality disorders characterized by emotional lability and/or problems with anger have tended to be most prevalent. Blaszczynski and Steel (1998), for example, found that 92 % of a sample of 82 treatment-seeking problem gamblers met criteria for at least one personality disorder. The majority of participants met criteria for more than one personality disorder. Cluster B DSM-IV personality disorders were by far the most prevalent, with between 57.3 % and 69.5 % of pathological gamblers meeting criteria for borderline, histrionic, and/or narcissistic personality disorders. Borderline and histrionic personality disorders were characterized by both high anxiety and depression scores, while narcissistic personality disorder was characterized by high anxiety.

Several researchers have more directly examined the role of emotions in problem gambling. For example, Beaudoin and Cox (1999) found that more than 80 % of their sample of treatment-seeking problem gamblers reported gambling in order to relieve dysphoria or to escape from life stressors. Similarly, Griffiths (1995) observed that both problem and non-problem gamblers reported experiencing depressive moods prior to gambling behaviors.

Ricketts and Macaskill (2003) conducted two studies aimed at examining the role of emotion in gambling. In their 2003 study, they analyzed themes from interviews, therapy sessions, and open-ended questionnaires with 14 treatment-seeking individuals who met criteria for pathological gambling. They concluded that these individuals gambled purposefully to manage unpleasant emotional states and described three particular emotion-altering effects (experiencing positive emotions and arousal, suppressing unpleasant emotions or worries, and feeling a sense of achievement).

Ricketts and Macaskill followed the same procedure in their 2004 study with a sample of frequent gamblers who did not report experiencing associated problems or feeling a lack of control over gambling. Most of these nonpathological gamblers did not report using gambling to deal with negative emotions. The authors also noted that those nonpathological gamblers who did manage emotional states through gambling also employed a range of other emotion management strategies; they contrasted this finding to their 2003 sample of pathological gamblers who tended to use gambling as their primary emotion regulation strategy. Based on these two studies, Ricketts and Macaskill concluded that it is the use of gambling to manage negative emotions that differentiates normal from problem gambling.

In their retrospective and prospective study of gambling relapse, Hodgins and el-Guebaly (2004) included an examination of the role of emotions. While they found that the most commonly identified predictors were cognitive (e.g., optimism about winning) and financial (e.g., needing money), they also observed that dealing with negative situations or emotions accounted for approximately 11 % of relapses. Further, Hodgins and el-Guebaly stated that female participants reported gambling to regulate emotions more than their male participants, a finding that they noted to be consistent with the theories of Diskin and Hodgins (2001) and Marks and Lesieur (1992).

Overall, despite the emphasis on cognitive factors, the gambling literature is beginning to provide support for a role of emotion regulation in understanding problem gambling. Further research exploring the role of emotion regulation in gambling behavior is important in understanding the etiology of, and designing appropriate interventions for, this problem. At the present time, research and theorizing in this area have primarily considered the emotions of depression and stress; the possible role of anger regulation in problem gambling has so far received little attention.

Gambling and Anger

Until recently, little attention has been given to the role of anger in problem gambling. We had already observed anecdotally that high proportions of individuals seeking treatment for substance use also reported problems with anger and violence, leading to the establishment of a specialized clinic for the integrated treatment of comorbid anger and addictions. Our interest in comorbid gambling and anger problems was in part kindled by our anecdotal observation that a high proportion of problem gamblers presenting for treatment in our hospital also self-reported comorbid anger problems.

A recent study reported that treatment-seeking substance use clients were significantly more likely have anger problems if they also had gambling problems. Collins, Skinner, and Toneatto (2005) compiled a comprehensive clinical database of 4985 clients seeking substance abuse treatment between December 1996 and March 1999 at the Addictions Program of the Centre for Addiction and Mental Health. In this large outpatient sample, 5.6 % (277) clients reported problem gambling. When problem gambling and nonproblem gambling substance users were compared, there was a significantly higher incidence of reported anger problems among patholog- ical gamblers (60 %) than among nonproblem gamblers (41 %). In addition, there also were more self-reports of verbal and physical abuse in the 90 days leading up to treatment among problem gambling substance users (25.2 % verbally abusive, 9.6 % physically abusive) than among nonproblem gambling substance users (9.4 % verbally abusive, 3.9 % physically abusive). These data cohere with the findings of another large cohort of treatment-seeking substance users indicating that the severity of gambling problems was also associated with greater hostility and negative affect (McCormick, 1993).

Research on Gambling and Intimate Partner Violence

Though the research on gambling and intimate partner violence is limited, the available empirical data suggests that an association exists between gambling and domestic violence. Lorenz and Shuttlesworth (1983), for example, surveyed 144 spouses of compulsive gamblers, and found that 50 % were physically and verbally abused by their partners. In interviews with pathological gamblers, 23 % reported having hit or thrown things at their partners on more than one occasion (Bland et al., 1993). There is also some survey data suggesting a rise in intimate partner violence associated with the establishment of new casinos in local communities (National Opinion Research Center, 1999). Finally, a recent study of 300 women attending an emergency room in Nebraska found that women who reported their partners had gambling problems were significantly more likely to have been the victims of domestic violence (Muellerman, DenOtter, Wadman, Tran, & Anderson, 2002). Of women who reported experiencing domestic violence, 64 % believed there was a relationship between their partners' gambling and violence. In addition, the preva- lence of domestic violence was higher among women who reported their partners had a drinking problem.

In a recently completed randomized control study of problem gamblers with comorbid anger problems (Korman (2005); Collins, McMain, & Skinner, (2006)), 74 % reported being verbally abusive and 25 % reported committing acts of physical violence against others in the 3 months prior to treatment. While this study did not specifically examine intimate partner violence, the findings suggest a high degree of self-reported violence and abusive behaviors among angry problem gamblers.

The study of Korman et al. also found gambling and anger outcomes were sig- nificantly better when both gambling and anger issues were addressed in treatment, compared to a specialized treatment exclusively addressing gambling problems. This finding likely underscores the importance of assessing problem gamblers for comorbid anger problems, and treating comorbid gambling and anger problems in an integrated fashion when both are present. In the balance of this chapter, we describe our assessment procedure and treatment for comorbid gambling and anger problems.

Assessment and Treatment

Assessment of Gambling and Anger

The assessment process in this treatment involves several questionnaires and structured interviews used to gather information about gambling, anger, and substance use for use in planning and implementing the treatment protocol.

Gambling

The primary measure of gambling used in our treatment is the Canadian Problem Gambling Index (CPGI; Ferris & Wynne, 2001). The CPGI is a 31-item self-report measure, that, using nine of the items produces scores that lead to a categorization of non-gambling, non-problem gambling, low risk gambling, moderate risk gambling, or problem gambling. The authors designed the CPGI to be consistent with the DSM-IV criteria for Pathological Gambling and have demonstrated acceptable reliability (i.e., internal consistency and test–retest reliability estimates greater than .78), validity (i.e., high correlation between CPGI classification and DSM-IV diagnosis), and classification accuracy (i.e., correctly identifying individuals as having a problem with gambling). The CPGI categorization score is helpful because it provides a sense of the clinical severity of the client's gambling problems. For example, information regarding level of problem awareness and negative consequences associated with gambling are helpful in addressing commitment to treatment and can help direct a clinician with regard to the use of commitment strategies. Further, the CPGI items not used to create the categorization score provide useful clinical information about components and correlates of problem gambling, such as type of gambling, loss of control, problem recognition, and adverse consequences.

Substance Use

Information about substance use was gathered through the Drug Use History Questionnaire (Sobell, Kwan, & Sobell, 1995). This self-report questionnaire has been in use at the Centre for Addiction and Mental Health since 1997 and is currently part of the Ontario Substance Abuse Bureau's required assessment instruments. The measure provides detailed information about type, frequency, and amount of substances used in the past 3 months. This information, coupled with the information from the VAHI regarding the links between substance use, gambling, and anger, can aid the clinician in guiding the direction of treatment.

Anger

Clinical information about anger was gathered through a self-report questionnaire and a structured interview. The State-Trait Anger Expression Inventory (STAXI;

Spielberger, 1988) is a self-report questionnaire that provides quantitative measures of different components of anger. The STAXI has been demonstrated to be a reliable and valid measure of anger, and contains norms for a range of different populations (e.g., outpatients, prison inmates). The STAXI has been recently updated in the STAXI-2 (Spielberger, 1999) and it is this updated version that continues to be used in the Anger and Addiction Clinic.

The STAXI-2 contains six scales, five subscales, and an overall Anger Expression Index. The first scale, State Anger, measures the intensity of angry feelings and the extent to which a person feels like expressing anger at the time of completing the questionnaire. The State Anger scale contains three subscales: Feeling Angry (the intensity of angry feelings currently being experienced), Feel Like Expressing Anger Verbally (the intensity of current feelings related to the verbal expression of anger), and Feel Like Expressing Anger Physically (the intensity of current feelings related to the physical expression of anger). The second STAXI-2 scale is Trait Anger, which measures how often angry feelings are experienced over time. The Trait Anger scale contains two subscales: Angry Temperament (the disposition to experience anger without specific provocation) and Angry Reaction (the frequency that angry feelings are experienced in situations that involve frustration and/or negative evaluations). The third STAXI-2 scale is Anger Expression—Out, which measures how often angry feelings are expressed through verbal or physical aggression. The fourth scale, Anger Expression—In, measures how often angry feelings are experienced but not expressed (i.e., are suppressed). The fifth STAXI-2 scale is Anger Control—Out, which measures how often a person controls the outward expression of angry feelings, and the final scale, Anger Control—In, measures how often a person attempts to control angry feelings by calming down. The Anger Expression Index of the STAXI-2 provides an overall measure of the expression and control of anger based on the responses to the Anger Expression and Anger Control scales.

The information gathered from the STAXI is helpful because an individual client's scores are compared to the measure's standardization sample and can be expressed in terms of percentile ranks. The ability to compare a client's scores to those of other relevant individuals (in this case, people seeking outpatient treatment) can help the clinician determine the clinical relevance of the various STAXI subscale scores. Scores equal or above the 75th percentile (or below the 25th percentile on Anger Control) are considered to fall in the clinical range.

Structured Violence and Anger History Interview

Another part of the assessment involves a more detailed behavioral examination of client's angry and violent behaviors, as well as an assessment of the idiopathic relationship between an individual's anger and addictive behaviors. For this purpose, we use the Violence and Anger History Interview (VAHI; Korman & Collins, 2005), a structured interview that was designed in part to assess the relationship between an individual's angry and addictive behaviors (such as gambling and substance use). The first section of the VAHI provides an overview of an individual's history of angry and violent behaviors. Next, salient anger and violent episodes are selected for more detailed analysis using methods adapted from behavioral assessment and theory. Angry and violent episodes with the most serious consequences to self (e.g., being fired or arrested, spouse leaving) and others (e.g., violence and physical harm), and more recent episodes, generally are selected for analysis.

The VAHI assesses variables such as the emotions, cognitions, actions, and situational/environmental events that have occurred before, during and after salient episodes of anger and violence. The VAHI also helps identify the links between prompting events, situational factors (including substance use and gambling), actions, and consequences associated with angry and violent behaviors. Particular emphasis is placed on identifying addiction behaviors that may have served as prompting events (e.g., gambling losses, gambling-related spousal conflict) or vulnerability factors (e.g., alcohol intoxication or withdrawal) for angry behaviors, or that were consequences of angry and violent behaviors (e.g., gambling or drinking alcohol to modulate angry affect). The information gathered regarding prompting events and the links between anger and other behaviors such as substance us and gambling is essential in aiding the clinician in organizing and directing treatment. In addition, similar to the gambling measures, the VAHI information regarding consequences of angry and violent behaviors can also aid clinicians in using commitment strategies to increase clients' dedication to treatment.

Assessing Functional Relationships Between Anger and Gambling

An integral component in the assessment of individuals with concurrent anger, gambling, and other addiction problems is the evaluation of functional relationships between angry and addictive behaviors. In the general field of concurrent disorders, a number of models of possible relationships between addiction and mental health problems have been identified (Flett & Hewitt, 2002; Skinner, 2003). These have been applied to concurrent anger and addictions and are summarized briefly below.

Anger and Gambling Problems Are Independent

When anger and addiction behaviors are not functionally related, they are deemed to be independent. An example of this is an individual with a history of perpetrating domestic violence but who has no history of addictive behaviors. However, after being laid off in a company "downsizing," the individual subsequently develops a gambling problem.

Key Assessment Data

When anger and addiction problems are independent, the onset of symptoms is not contingent upon one another. Changes in the intensity and/or frequency of one type of behavior are unlikely to affect the other behavior.

Gambling or Substance-Engendered Anger

Anger is considered addiction-engendered when angry behaviors are related principally to the consequences of chronic, excessive, or acute gambling or substance use, or from withdrawal from that behavior. For example, an individual with no history of problematic angry or belligerent behaviors may become angry and hostile following a gambling binge and/or when challenged with the consequences of her gambling addiction. Similarly, the disinhibitory effects of acute alcohol intoxication may contribute to anger and aggression.

Key Assessment Data

When anger is engendered by addictive behaviors, there typically is minimal history of maladaptive aggression until the initiation or cessation of gambling or substance use behaviors.

Gambling or Substance Use as Anger Regulation

Gambling and substance use both can serve to modulate dysregulated emotions, including anger. In the area of substance use, Khantzian (1985) has referred to this as the self-medication hypothesis. Gambling may be particularly well suited to modulate dysregulated anger because the attentional demands associated with gambling make it likely that attention will be reallocated away from the object of perceived violation. The intensity of anger is likely to be reduced, as a result.

In a recent study (Brunelle, Korman, Collins, & Cripps, 2005), angry, problem gamblers underwent structured interviews about salient episodes of their anger and violence resulting in serious consequences to themselves or others. In anger episodes involving serious consequences to self, 45.2 % of respondents reported they had gambled after their anger episodes, and of these, 60.7 % reported their anger decreased while gambling. Among anger episodes with serious consequences to others, 30.6 of respondents reported they had gambled after their anger episodes, and of these 68.4 % reported their anger decreased while gambling. These findings lend support to the notion that gambling may function to modulate dysregulated anger in some individuals. Interestingly, among participants who both gambled and drank, gambling was reported to be more effective at reducing angry feelings than alcohol.

Key Assessment Data

Minimal or nonproblematic gambling or substance use until the life event associated with violation. It is important to note that deficits in anger regulation can involve not only the inability to tolerate intense emotions but also the inability to symbolize anger and the experience of other emotions (Korman, 2005). Thus, when assessing for the presence of anger immediately prior to gambling behaviors, it may be important to also assess for the presence of perceived violations and relationship difficulty, as individuals may be unaware that they have been angry. This may be particularly important for individuals who are overregulated in their expression of anger.

Personality/Trait Mediational Risk Factor

In some circumstances, an individual's problem anger and addiction behaviors may be both mediated by a third factor. The third factor may be either a personality trait or a constellation of traits as seen in personality disorders. Blaszczynski and Steel (1998) found very high rates of personality disorders among pathological gamblers. Borderline personality disorder, for example, can be characterized by intense anger, and by impulsive, self-destructive behaviors, like gambling and substance use.

Key Assessment Data

Pervasive deficits in functioning in relationships, work, and self-care. Chaotic lifestyle. The presence of a personality disorder or personality disorder traits.

Treatment

Inclusion and Exclusion Criteria

There a number of inclusion and exclusion criteria for participation in our integrated treatment. Many of our clients have had legal problems, and we accept clients who are mandated by courts to engage in treatment. However, in order to maintain continuity of care, individuals with outstanding legal charges are excluded from treatment until their charges are resolved. Clients who are under probation or parole must provide their probation or parole reports to our clinic, permit ongoing two-way communication between our treatment team and probation and parole services. Clients with thought disorders and/or with severe paranoid features and those with intellectual disabilities are excluded because they are unlikely to benefit from this treatment. Finally, we would note that many of our clients meet criteria for diagnoses of personality disorders and/or have histories of suicidal and violent behaviors; these clients are welcomed into our treatment

Orientation Phase

After being assessed, prospective clients enter an orientation phase. Entry into the treatment program is contingent on successful resolution of the orientation phase. The orientation phase is based in part on Motivational Interviewing (Miller &

Rollnick, 1991), and on orientation and commitment principles from Dialectical Behavior Therapy (DBT) for borderline personality disorder (Linehan, 1993a).

Orientation includes the following:

- Exploring clients' reasons for seeking treatment. To proceed into treatment, prospective clients must express some interest in addressing their gambling, substance use, anger, and/or violent behaviors.
- Exploring the consequences of gambling and angry and violent behaviors.
- Psychoeducation about gambling, substance use, and anger, and a brief review of the empirical evidence supporting the efficacy of this treatment for concurrent gambling and anger problems.
- The use of motivational interviewing (Miller & Rollnick, 1991) and DBT commitment strategies to establish and strengthen clients' motivation to reduce gambling, substance, and problem anger behaviors and to engage in this treatment.
- Reviewing behavioral expectations of clients (e.g., attending all sessions, completing diary card on a daily basis, completing homework assignments).
- Establishing concrete and realistic treatment goals.
- Introducing and establishing agreement about the hierarchy of targets to be addressed in this treatment. This is discussed in more detail in the next section of this chapter.
- Teaching prospective clients about learning theory: Clients are informed about operant and respondent conditioning. The aim is to teach clients how their gambling and angry behaviors may be controlled, and orienting them to how treatment will seek to identify factors controlling their behaviors.
- Briefly orienting clients to behavioral analysis.
- Briefly orienting clients to exposure, response prevention, and skills rehearsal and acquisition/generalization.
- Briefly orienting clients to the various skills taught in this treatment.
- Introducing the diary card.
- Reviewing clients' beliefs about how treatment works, and as appropriate, addressing misconceptions.

Orienting Clients to Angry Behaviors

Like gambling and substance use behaviors, many of the problem anger behaviors with which clients present in therapy, like physical violence and yelling, are overt. Such behaviors are relatively easy to define. However, many other problem anger behaviors and their behavioral antecedents are covert. For example, angry clients often ruminate about perceived violations and the objects of their anger (typically the perceived "instigator" of the violation). Like other covert angry behaviors, ruminating about the object of a grievance often increases anger and general arousal, and also serves frequently as an antecedent for overt angry actions. For example, after his wife arrived 15 minutes late for a movie date, one client reported "winding himself up" during the entire duration of the movie by ruminating about his wife's tardiness.

He subsequently yelled at her, accusing her of being inconsiderate and destroying his enjoyment of the movie, and then abandoned her at the cinema.

Because many angry behaviors are not obvious, overt, or necessarily recognized by individuals as problematic, an important part of pretreatment involves educating prospective clients about angry behaviors so that clients (1) fully understand anger-related treatment targets; (2) are able to provide informed consent and commitment to engage in all aspects of the treatment; (3) can identify their own angry behaviors; and (4) can target these behaviors with their therapists. Various types of angry actions and cognitions have been described elsewhere (Deffenbacher & McKay, 2000; Korman, 2005). We divide them into covert and overt behaviors.

Covert angry behaviors include the following:

- "Injustice collecting," which involves remembering multiple perceived injustices one believes one has experienced, or mentally listing grievances one has
- Scanning for violation, or actively looking for grievances in the environment, or looking for a fight
- Hostile attributions that involve imputing motives of deliberate malice to others
- Blaming thoughts
- Judging thoughts
- Ruminating/obsessing
- Revenge fantasies

In addition to more overt problem anger behaviors such as physical violence and yelling, clients are also oriented to overt angry acts like sarcasm, spite, abandoning others, judging, blaming, commanding, demanding, threatening, acting punitively, and "giving others the silent treatment." To proceed into the treatment phase, clients must acknowledge they have a problem with anger, express an interest in and commitment to work toward reducing their angry behaviors.

Therapy Phase

Treatment is offered on an outpatient basis via once-weekly, one-hour individual sessions. The therapy is largely behavioral, and adapts many structural strategies, principles, and skills from DBT (Linehan, 1993a); structured relapse prevention (Annis, Herie, & Watkin-Merek, 1996); and other behavioral treatments.

Diary Card

Clients complete a weekly log of relevant behaviors and emotions. The card is completed by clients on a daily basis, and is brought to each individual session. The gambling and anger diary card is presented in Fig. 15.1. The card was adapted from logs used by Linehan (1993a) and other behavioral therapies. On the card, clients monitor daily gambling behaviors, urges to gamble, and any amounts of money they have may have wagered. Clients also identify and log any overt or covert angry or violent behaviors they have engaged in, as well as any substance use and urges to use substances. They also monitor the intensity of any emotions they have experienced, urges to harm themselves and/or others, coping skills they used, and the effectiveness of these skills. In addition, at the beginning and end of each session, clients are asked to rate the intensity of any urges to harm themselves or others, and their urges to gamble, use substances, or quit treatment. At the beginning of each therapy session, the agenda for that session is established primarily through an examination of the card by client and clinician for the presence (or absence) of treatment target behaviors. When clients have not completed their diary cards for the previous week, they are asked to complete the card at the beginning of the session before the session proceeds.

Target Priorities for Individual Sessions

Targets to be addressed in individual therapy sessions are determined by a target hierarchy system adapted from Linehan's DBT (1993a). The hierarchy of targets for individual sessions is as follows:

1. Life-threatening behaviors (e.g., physical violence, child abuse or neglect, suicide or other intentional self-harm)
2. Treatment-interfering behaviors (e.g., missing previous sessions, not completing behavioral assignments, poor motivation to engage in treatment)
3. Gambling, anger, and substance use behaviors
4. Other quality-of-life behaviors (e.g., depression, anxiety, vocational, financial, or relationship problems)

Structure of Sessions

Clients and therapists begin sessions by reviewing the diary card from the previous week. Using the target hierarchy discussed earlier, one or two discrete behaviors (e.g., an episode of gambling or attacking someone) are then selected for detailed analysis. Functional analyses are used to identify the prompting event, dysfunctional links that may have preceded the target behavior, and any consequences following the target behavior. General behavior therapy principles are used in examining if targeted behaviors are under the control of respondent and/or instrumental factors, if they are related to specific skills deficits and/or cognitive dysfunction. Particular emphasis is placed on identifying deficits in the ability to recognize, symbolize, and regulate anger and other emotional experience.

Depending on the type of problem discovered in the behavioral analysis, the last segment (usually 20 to 30 minutes) of individual sessions is dedicated to the following: exposure and response prevention for problem behaviors under the control of a stimulus or cue (i.e., respondent behaviors; e.g., intense sensitivity to cues of criticism resulting in angry, hostile behaviors); contingency management for behaviors under the control of consequences (i.e., instrumental behaviors; e.g.

gambling results in attenuation of aversive affect), skills training and rehearsal for skills deficits (e.g., inability to tolerate gambling urges or inability to express anger in a nonabusive manner); and establishing homework assignments.

Skills Training

Skills are derived from three major sources. Structure relapse prevention strategies are used primarily to identify high-risk situations and to develop strategies to manage intense urges to gamble or abuse substances. These have been adapted from strategies described in detail by Annis et al. (1996). Mindfulness, interpersonal effectiveness, emotion regulation, and distress tolerance strategies from DBT (Linehan, 1993b) are used to help clients identify, tolerate, and understand their emotional experience, tolerate painful affect, and assert themselves adaptively.

Clients are instructed that in relation to anger, the goal of treatment is not to give up anger but rather to increase mindfulness of anger and control over emotion intensity and action. With this aim in mind, a set of "anger awareness" skills has been developed to help clients identify and regulate their anger (Korman, 2005). These skills were created by modifying salient interventions from a number of different treatment approaches and by consulting theories of human functioning, and are described in the following paragraphs.

Primary Emotion Check

The skill termed "primary emotion check" derives from emotion theory (e.g., Frijda, 1986) and emotion-oriented therapy approaches (e.g., Greenberg & Safran; Korman & Greenberg, 1996). Primary emotions are initial adaptive responses to situations that serve to orient the individual, provide information about the personal significance of situations in relation to the individual's well-being, and ready the person for adaptive action. Secondary emotional expressions, on the other hand, are considered learned reactions to primary emotions, (e.g., secondary anger to primary feelings of fear), and are often associated with problematic expressions of anger. Dutton and Golant (1986), for example, have argued that many instances of domestic violence are preceded by primary emotions of shame or fear.

To help clients recognize primary emotions, clients are taught about core relational themes (Lazarus, 1991). These are generic categories of emotion-related themes or interpretations (e.g., loss) that provide information about attendant, basic, adaptive emotions (e.g., sadness). The aim of the primary emotion check skill is to identify and symbolize primary emotions, which are most likely to yield adaptive information and motivate adaptive behavior. For example, primary feelings of sadness associated with interpersonal loss are adaptive because they organize the individual for healing, and engender compassion and assistance from others. On the other hand, the expression of secondary emotion is discouraged, as they typically are incongruent with the individual's goals. In the example above, anger is likely to interrupt resolution of loss-related healing and alienate others.

Anger Interpretation Check

"Anger interpretation check" is a skill adapted from Beck's cognitive approaches to emotions (Beck, 1976; Beck, Rush, Shaw, & Emery, 1979) and from cognitive approaches to the treatment of problem anger (Novaco, 1975, 1976). This skill involves first identifying the often tacit interpretation or appraisal associated with the generation of anger. Once identified, the individual evaluates the accuracy of the interpretation. In conjunction with this skill, as appropriate, clients are also taught to identify their own particular types of cognitive distortions (Deffenbacher & McKay, 2000) and irrational beliefs (Ellis & Tafrate, 1999) associated with their problem anger, as well as fundamental attribution errors they may be making (Ross, 1977).

Humor

Humor is a skill adapted from CBT approaches to problem anger (Deffenbacher, 1995). This skill uses an acronym (humorous ANGLE) to prompt clients to use silly, gentle, and nondeprecating humor to attenuate intense, unwanted anger. This is often a difficult skill for clients to master, with initial attempts often descending to belittling sarcasm. Clients are prompted to look for what is cosmically absurd when they are angry, often by using concrete imagery to exaggerate a problem until it seems silly and funny. For example, a client who frequently became enraged on the roadway when he perceived being cut off by other motorists imagined following a bus that had cut him off across the country, passing howling coyotes under a crescent moon.

Actual Damage Evaluation

"Actual damage evaluation" is a skill adapted from rational–emotive–behavior therapy (Dryden & Ellis, 1988; Ellis & Tafrate, 1999). The skill involves having clients systematically evaluate the actual short- and long-term damage to their welfare caused by perceived violations. Clients then evaluate the intensity of their anger in relation to the actual damage they have experienced. If the intensity of their anger is disproportionate to the actual damage they have experienced (e.g., intense anger and verbal abuse of a partner who provided critical feedback), clients are asked to use DBT skills to (1) assess the pros and cons of expressing the emotion; (2) consider using distress tolerance to tolerate the intensity of the emotion without acting on it; and (3) using change-focused strategies such as acting-opposite-to-anger to reduce the intensity of anger and maintain important relationships.

Cue-Focused Strategies

A number of skills focus primarily on either withdrawing from or managing in the face of cues or situations engendering anger. Adapted from many approaches to problem anger, taking a "time out" is a skill involving a gentle, structured withdrawal (physical and attentional) from anger-prompting situations. This skill is emphasized when clients are unable to use skills effectively to attenuate their anger *in situ*. Similar to time outs, stimulus control involves avoiding situations likely to engender anger. Both of these skills are taught earlier in treatment, when clients have not yet acquired sufficient skills to regulate their anger in the face of the prompting cue. Toward the end of treatment, stress inoculation training (Meichenbaum, 1985; Novaco, 1975, 1976) is emphasized to ensure that clients are able to use a wider array of skills effectively while in the presence of anger-prompting cues.

Case Examples

Peter

Peter is a 45-year-old divorced skilled tradesman who presented in treatment for concurrent gambling and anger problems. He presented as friendly though lonely and somewhat irritable. Peter gambled on average two or three times per month, playing card games at casinos, and typically lost $300 to $500 per occasion. On the Violence and Anger History Interview, he reported having had sporadic angry verbal outbursts against contractors for whom he conducted work contracts. These outbursts typically were preceded by him feeling exploited by contractors and by Peter responding passively and unassertively. Eventually, he would respond with verbal abuse, leading to the loss of work job contracts on a number of occasions. As a result, he was essentially a "journeyman" tradesman, searching for new contractors to work for despite his considerable expertise. He also reported that he sometimes gambled following his "blowups." He also reported frequently feeling irritated by everyday situations such as waiting in lines or driving in traffic, and consequently feeling drained and sour.

Together with his gambling, Peter's work problems resulted in him having little money in his pocket, although he was for the most part able to pay his bills and reported minimal debt. He also reported longstanding feelings of frustration with his ex-wife, with whom he maintained occasional contact. He reported drinking about four to six beers about three or four times per week. Peter's goals were to stop gambling, get control of his temper, and reduce his alcohol consumption.

Behavioral analyses of Peter's drinking revealed that his alcohol consumption was typically prompted by feelings of loneliness, which he had difficulty symbolizing. His drinking was reinforced by reductions in the intensity of his loneliness associated with intoxication (when he drank alone) and by affiliation with others when he drank at bars. Through the use of relapse prevention strategies, Peter was largely successful on his own in reducing his alcohol consumption. For example, he avoided bars, and kept only one or two beers in his home at any time. There was no indication that Peter's gambling was associated with his alcohol use.

During the sixth session, Peter reported that he had, despite considerable effort, relapsed the previous weekend, losing $400 at a casino. Initially he remembered little of the episode or of what preceded it. Behavioral analysis of the episode revealed that he had met with his ex-wife earlier in the day to discuss financial issues. He reported that they had argued, and he remembered only that while leaving he felt "bad." He next recollection was of being in his car driving to a casino. On more detailed analysis, it became apparent that he had felt ashamed while discussing his gambling problem with his ex-wife, and that he then became argumentative with her. He was unable, at the time, to symbolize his feelings of shame or anger. Initially, he remembered little until he was well on his way to the casino, recalling only that he felt "bad." On analysis, he reported that his anger attenuated as he approached the casino, replaced by feelings of excitement as he anticipated gambling.

Peter's therapy initially focused on him learning to recognize emotions such as anger, shame, and sadness (including loneliness). This involved teaching him to attend to and symbolize the bodily referents associated with basic emotions as well as the core relational themes associated with them. Therapy then focused on helping Peter to distinguish primary from secondary emotions; to this end, Peter used the skill of primary emotion check to identify his primary emotions. DBT distress tolerance skills were used to withstand intense primary affect without acting in self-defeating ways, and to manage urges to gamble. In behavioral analysis, considerable emphasis was placed on increasing his insight into how his gambling served to modulate his dysregulated anger and other emotions. DBT interpersonal effectiveness skills were also taught, rehearsed in therapy (earlier in treatment), and practiced outside treatment (later in treatment), in order to increase Peter's capacity to act assertively with his employers and with his wife. In role-playing these scenarios in sessions, the therapist also challenged Peter to use skills like actual damage evaluation and humor in responding to challenging conflicts with his employer and ex-wife.

Sylvia

Sylvia is a 28-year-old single woman who presented for treatment to address gambling problems and general feelings of unhappiness. Sylvia is single, unemployed, and has been receiving social assistance. She recounted an unhappy childhood, with an absent father and an alcoholic, neglectful, and sometimes punitive mother. Sylvia presented with a number of symptoms of borderline personality disorder, including pervasive feelings of boredom and emptiness, and intense anger, though she did not meet full criteria for the disorder.

Sylvia reported gambling four to five times per week, purchasing instant lottery tickets from convenience stores and attending bingo halls in her neighborhood. She estimated that she spent about $25 a week on gambling activities, which represented about 20 % of the income she received from social assistance payments. She also reported smoking about two or three cannabis cigarettes per month. Sylvia's meagre social assistance payments, coupled with her gambling and her occasional cannabis use, left her with insufficient money to pay for her rent and food, and she occasionally exchanged sex for money or cannabis with two male acquaintances.

Sylvia reported considerable conflict with many individuals in her life.

On the Violence and Anger History Interview, Sylvia reported frequent angry, verbally abusive episodes, during which she typically yelled at others like her mother, her social assistance worker, care providers, and bingo hall acquaintances. Behavioral analyses of these anger episodes indicated that many of such anger episodes were secondary reactions to primary feelings of intense shame, prompted by ultrasensitivity to perceived criticism and the demands of others. For example, Sylvia swore at a community mental health counselor and stormed out of an important meeting when the counselor suggested she address her gambling behaviors. On exploration, Sylvia had interpreted the counselors' communication as a vicious attack on what she perceived as an unforgivable weakness in her character. Sylvia also reported that she had on a number of occasions punched, scratched, or kicked intimate partners, typically when she felt ashamed or disappointed. She denied ever having been arrested.

Behavioral analyses of Sylvia's gambling and cannabis use indicated that these behaviors typically were precipitated by feelings of boredom and emptiness. She reported feeling excited by the anticipation of playing scratch-and-win lottery tickets, which served to relieve her feelings of boredom and emptiness. This excitement typically was short lived, and was followed by irritation and anger prompted by losing. Sylvia reported that her cannabis use also salved her feelings of boredom, as well as her feelings of discomfort associated with selling sex. She reported that playing bingo also attenuated her boredom, as well as giving her something to do with her time. Finally, despite Sylvia's irritation with others, she reported that attending bingo halls reduced her sense of isolation.

Sylvia's therapy initially focused on establishing clear treatment targets based on the client's goals (e.g., abstinence from lottery gambling, reducing her yelling, eliminating violence, stopping her prostitution, finding a job). Motivational Interviewing principles (Miller & Rollnick, 1991) and commitment strategies from DBT (Linehan, 1993) were used to enhance Sylvia's commitment to work on therapy targets and to engage fully in therapeutic tasks pin all aspects of the treatment. The client did not want to work to reduce her bingo playing or cannabis use, and it was agreed that these would be tabled later in therapy should they be found to interfere with progress on other treatment goals.

Sylvia's intense, angry reactions posed an immediate obstacle to treatment, as many of the therapist's communications and probing about the client's problematic behaviors typically prompted reactions such as yelling, attacking, and withdrawing from the client. Thus, considerable emphasis was placed on establishing clear agreements with the client about addressing her problem anger behaviors. Sylvia agreed that her angry reactions often damaged important relationships and otherwise disadvantaged her. In the context of warm, validating responses from her therapist, Sylvia also agreed that it would be hard to address her addictive behaviors because of her tendency to feel defensive and get angry. Her therapist then informed Sylvia about learning theory and how angry behaviors are learned and maintained, and about exposure and extinction as means to reducing these reactions. Sylvia then consented to be exposed to anger-prompting cues like respectful feedback about her behaviors as a means of extinguishing her raging responses to criticism.

Many of Sylvia's early sessions were devoted to deliberate, increasingly longer exposures to critical feedback about her gambling and angry behaviors. These were paired with teaching Sylvia mindfulness strategies from DBT to help her attend to cognitions and the bodily referents (e.g., feeling hot), and to the feelings of shame and disappointment that often precipitated her angry reactions. Relaxation strategies were used to reduce the intensity of her emotional arousal. The therapist used praise to reinforce and shape any of Sylvia's non-attacking behaviors in the face exposure to the therapist's demands and critical feedback. The client's angry reactions were ignored by the therapist. To teach the client incongruent, adaptive behaviors, and a means of emotion regulation, Sylvia was also taught the "opposite-to-emotion-action" strategies from DBT: In the midst of her angry feelings, this skill involved Sylvia smiling and thanking the therapist for taking the trouble to raise Sylvia's gambling and anger problems. Sylvia was also coached to praise herself for responding in a gentle manner when she felt angry. Finally, the client was also taught "anger interpretation check" as a means of reexamining the accuracy of her emotional appraisals that were associated with her angry responses. For example, Sylvia often explicitly reexamined her implicit assumption that the therapist's questions about her gambling constituted an attack on her character.

Because Sylvia's urges to gamble were often precipitated by feelings of loneliness and emptiness, Sylvia was taught DBT distress tolerance skills in order to tolerate these painful feelings without resorting to gambling. These skills involved strategies like deliberately directing her attention away from painful feelings and urges to gamble, towards soothing sensory stimuli like pleasant smells, hot and cold sensations, and physical activities. The therapist paid particular attention to ensuring that the client practiced and mastered these skills under situations of both low and high stress, so that Sylvia both acquired these skills, and mastered them for use when she felt high distress and strong urges to gamble. Initially, Sylvia also indicated that entering convenience stores prompted urges to gamble she had difficulty resisting, and so a temporary plan was made for Sylvia to avoid convenience stores. As Sylvia's skills and confidence increased, a plan was made for Sylvia to gradually expose herself to the cues associated with convenience stores in order to extinguish her urges to gamble.

Sylvia had numerous serious problems other than anger and gambling, including general feelings of unhappiness, a lack of meaningful and healthy relationships, the lack of work, and painful memories from childhood. Though substantial problems, these issues were easier to address later in treatment once Sylvia was able to bring her anger and gambling problems under control.

Conclusion

Research on the etiology of problem gambling generally has focused on the cognitive distortions associated with problem gambling. Correspondingly, treatments for gambling problems have focused largely on identifying and correcting these errors. However, recently there has been increasing recognition of the role of emotions in problem gambling.

Table 15.1

Day	Harm Urges: Self (rate intensity 0-5)	Harm Urges: Other	Harm Acts: Self Harm (Y/N)	Angry acts (See code list below)	Emotions: Anger	Emotions: Fear	Emotions: Guilt/Shame	Emotions: Sad/Hurt	Emotions: Joy/Love	Gambling Urges (0-5)	Gambling Acts (See code list below)	Time Spent	Alcohol/Drug Urge to use (Rate intensity 0-5)	Alcohol	Prescription drugs	Over-the-counter drugs	Illicit drugs	Did you use Skills? (See code list below)
					rate intensity of emotion (0-5)						*Enter $ spent gambling (not including winnings)*		*What did you use? Amount used?*					
Mon																		
Tues																		
Wed																		
Thur																		
Fri																		
Sat																		
Sun																		

Angry Acts: Code List

A = Abandon Other   R = Ruminate/Obsess
B = Blame
C = Command/Demand   S = Scan for Violation
F = Fantasize Revenge   T = Threaten
H = Huff/puff, Silent Tx   V = Violence

Gambling Acts: Code List

L = Lotto
HR = Horse Racing
IS = Instant win/Scratch

Rate yourself before & after Session:	Before (0-5)	After (0-5)
Urge to gamble		
Anger		
Urge to use		
Urge to quit therapy		
Urge to harm yourself		
Urge to harm other(s)		

New research suggests that anger problems may frequently be present among problem gamblers, and that an integrated treatment addressing both gambling and anger issues may result in better outcomes than traditional treatment focusing on gambling alone.

We have outlined an integrated assessment and treatment model for comorbid gambling and anger. We have argued that clinicians who treat individuals with comorbid gambling and anger problems need to assess the idiopathic relationships between clients' problem gambling and anger behaviors. Once these relationships are understood, clinicians need to ensure that clients with comorbid gambling and anger problems acquire and master the skills necessary to help control their dysregulated emotions and actions.

Chapter 16
A Treatment Approach for Adolescents with Gambling Problems

Rina Gupta and Jeffrey Derevensky

It is not uncommon for an adolescent to be participating in one form of gambling or another, be it the lottery, card playing for money, sports wagering, or gambling on electronic gambling devices. The results of the National Research Council's (NRC) (1999) review of empirical studies suggest that 85% of adolescents (the median of all studies) report having gambled during their lifetime, with 73% of adolescents (median value) reporting gambling in the past year. This raises serious mental health and public policy concerns (Derevensky, Gupta, Messerlian, & Gillespie, this volume; NRC, 1999).

Meta-analyses (Shaffer & Hall, 1996) and a review of more recent studies (see Jacobs, this volume) confirm that between 4% and 8% of youth experience very serious gambling-related problems, with another 10% to 15% at-risk for the development of a gambling dependency. More recent debates have raised the question as to the accuracy of prevalence rates of problem gambling among youth. Some have recently argued that our current instruments and screens are not accurately assessing pathological gambling among adolescents but are overestimating the prevalence rates (i.e, Jacques & Ladouceur, 2003; Ladouceur et al., 2000). Yet, in a comprehensive discussion of the arguments, Derevensky, Gupta, and Winters (2003) and Derevensky and Gupta (this volume) suggest that many of the assertions raised have little merit. Nevertheless, while this debate plays itself out in the research community and the search for the gold standard instrument continues, it remains clear that a small but identifiable number of youth actually develop serious gambling-related problems. While the need for treatment of youth who gamble problematically is evident, little progress has been made in understanding the treatment needs of this population, a conclusion also reached by the NRC (1999) review. Treatment studies reported in the literature have generally been case studies with small sample sizes (Knapp & Lech, 1987; Murray, 1993; Wildman, 1997) and have been criticized for not being subjected to rigorous scientific standards (Blaszczynski & Silove, 1995; Nathan, 2001; National Gambling Impact Study Commission, 1999; NRC, 1999).

A critical review of treatment issues pertaining to pathological gambling highlights the stringent and rigorous criteria that treatment outcome studies must meet

Rina Gupta
McGill University, Canada

M. Zangeneh, A. Blaszczynski, N. Turner (eds.), *In the Pursuit of Winning.*
© Springer 2008

to be considered an Empirically Validated Treatment (EVT) approach (Toneatto & Ladouceur, 2003) or falling within the parameters of Best Practices. Both models base their criteria on recommendations put forward by the American Psychological Association (Kazdin, 2001) and Substance Abuse and Mental Health Services Administration (SAMSHA) and Centre for Substance Abuse Treatment (CSAT). Along with replicability of findings, randomization of patients to an experimental group, the inclusion of a matched control group, and the use of sufficiently large enough samples are viewed as the minimum requirements necessary to validate effective treatment paradigms. Unfortunately, the treatment of adolescent pathological gamblers has not yet evolved to the point that treatment evaluation studies have met the criteria for EVT or Best Practices.

There are several reasons to explain why more stringent criteria, scientifically validated methodological procedures, and experimental analyses concerning the efficacy of treatment programs for youth have not been implemented. Primarily, these reasons include the fact that there exist very few treatment programs prepared to include young gamblers among their clientele and few underage problem gamblers actually present themselves for treatment in centers with trained personnel. This small number of young people seeking treatment in any given center results in the difficulty of obtaining matched control groups. Matched controls are even more difficult to obtain when considering that young gamblers often present with a significant number and variety of secondary psychological disorders. Another obstacle to treatment program evaluation is that treatment approaches may vary within a center and may be dependent upon the gamblers specific profile, developmental level, or therapist's training orientation. Given the lack of empirically based treatment in the field of pathological gambling, this therapy issue is relatively new compared to existing treatment models for youth with other addictions and mental health disorders. There nevertheless remains a growing interest in identifying effective treatment strategies to help minimize youth gambling problems.

Existing Treatment Approaches

Treatment paradigms used for adults have in general been based on a number of theoretical approaches. These paradigms fundamentally include one or more of the following orientations: psychoanalytic or psychodynamic (Bergler, 1957; Miller, 1986; Rosenthal, 1987; Rugle & Rosenthal, 1994), behavioral (Blaszczynski & McConaghy, 1993; Walker, 1993), cognitive and cognitive–behavioral (Bujold, Ladouceur, Sylvain, & Boisvert, 1994; Ladouceur & Walker, 1998; Toneatto & Sobell, 1990; Walker, 1993), pharmacological (Grant, Chambers, & Potenza, this volume; Grant, Kim, & Potenza, 2003; Haller & Hinterhuber, 1994; Hollander, Frenkel, DeCaria, Trungold, & Stein, 1992; Hollander & Wong, 1995), physiological (Blaszczynski, McConaghy, & Winters, 1986; Carlton & Goldstein, 1987), biological/genetic (Comings, 1998; DeCaria, Hollander, & Wong, 1997; Hollander et al., 1992; Saiz, 1992), addiction-based models (Lesieur & Blume, 1991a;

McCormick & Taber, 1988), or self-help (Brown, 1986, 1987b; Lesieur, 1990) (For a more comprehensive overview of these models the reader is referred to the reviews by Griffiths, 1995b; Lesieur, 1998; NRC, 1999; Rugle, Derevensky, Gupta, Winters, & Stinchfield, 2001.)

The resulting treatment paradigms have in general incorporated a rather restrictive and narrow focus depending on one's theoretical orientation of treatment (see Blaszczynski & Silove, 1995 for their analyses of the limitations of each approach). The application of theory and research findings to clinical practice has been similarly limited. Ladouceur and his colleagues have long argued for a cognitive–behavioral approach to treating both adults and youth with gambling problems (Bujold et al., 1994; Ladouceur, Boisvert & Dumont, 1994; Ladouceur, Sylvain, Letarte, Giroux, & Jacques, 1998; Ladouceur & Walker, 1996, 1998). The central assumption underlying the cognitive–behavioral approach is that pathological gamblers will continue to gamble in spite of repeated losses given they maintain an unrealistic belief that losses can be recovered. As such, this perspective assumes that a number of erroneous beliefs (including a lack of understanding of independence of events, perceived level of skill in successfully predicting the outcome of chance events, and illusions of control) result in their persistent gambling behavior (Ladouceur & Walker, 1998).

In one of the few empirically based treatment studies with adolescents, Ladouceur et al. (1994), using four adolescent male pathological gamblers, implemented a cognitive–behavioral therapy program. Within their treatment program, five components were included: information about gambling, cognitive interventions, problem-solving training, relapse prevention, and social skills training. Cognitive therapy was provided individually for approximately 3 months (mean of 17 sessions). Ladouceur and his colleagues reported clinically significant gains resulting from treatment, with three of the four adolescents remaining abstinent 3 and 6 months after treatment. They further concluded that the treatment duration necessary for adolescents with severe gambling problems was relatively short compared to that required for adults, and that cognitive therapy represents a promising new avenue for treatment for adolescent pathological gamblers. This therapeutic approach is predicated on the belief that (1) adolescents persist in their gambling behavior in spite of repeated losses primarily as a result of their erroneous beliefs and perceptions and (2) winning money is central to their continued efforts. However, their limited sample (four adolescents), while somewhat informative, is not sufficiently representative to depict a complete picture.

Research with adolescents suggests that the clinical portrait of adolescent problematic gamblers is much more complex than merely that of erroneous beliefs and the desire to acquire money. Our earlier research demonstrates strong empirical support for Jacobs' *General Theory of Addictions* for adolescent problem gamblers (Gupta & Derevensky, 1998a). Adolescent problem and pathological gamblers were found to have exhibited abnormal physiological resting states (resulting in a tendency toward risk-taking), greater emotional distress in general (i.e., depression and anxiety), reported significantly higher levels of dissociation when gambling, and had higher rates of comorbidity with other addictive behaviors.

More recently, a series of studies have uncovered that adolescent problem and pathological gamblers differ in their ability to cope successfully with daily events, adversity, and situational problems (Gupta & Derevensky, 2001; Gupta, Derevensky, & Marget, stay as in press; Hardoon, Gupta, & Derevensky, stay as in press). The empirical knowledge of the correlates and risk factors associated with adolescent problem gambling has been described in more detail elsewhere (Derevensky & Gupta, 2004; Griffiths & Wood, 2000; Hardoon & Derevensky, 2002; Stinchfield, this volume). Further, contrary to common beliefs and the tenets of the cognitive–behavioral approach, our research and clinical work suggests money is not the predominant reason why adolescents with gambling problems engage in these behaviors (see Gupta & Derevensky, 1998b). Rather, it appears that money is often perceived as a means to enable these youth to continue gambling.

Blaszczynski and Silove (1995) further suggest that there is ample empirical support that gambling involves a complex and dynamic interaction between ecological, psychophysiological, developmental, cognitive, and behavioral components. Given this complexity, each of these components needs to be adequately incorporated into a successful treatment paradigm (to achieve abstinence and minimize relapse). While Blaszczynski and Silove addressed their concerns with respect to adult problem gamblers, a similar multidimensional approach appears to be necessary to successfully address the multitude of problems facing adolescent problem gamblers.

This chapter serves to add to the growing body of literature focused on youth gambling problems. In particular, we seek to provide an example of our treatment approach, which is conceptually linked to, based on, and derived from existing empirical research. Nonetheless, it is important to note that we have not empirically tested our approach to the standards set forth by SAMSHA or American Psychiatric Association (APA) owing to the lack of a sufficiently large control group. It is our contention that placing youth requesting treatment on a waiting list for an extended period of time is problematic because of the high level of distress evidenced by these youth, the belief that if they remain in a control group their problems will escalate, and the concern that they will no longer seek treatment after waiting in a control group. As such, to date, we have elected to provide immediate treatment to all youth requesting services.

Finding a Treatment Population

Adolescents with gambling problems in general tend not to present themselves for treatment. There are likely many reasons that they fail to seek treatment, including (1) fear of being identified, (2) the belief that they can control their behavior, (3) adolescent self-perceptions of invincibility and invulnerability, (4) the negative perceptions associated with therapy by adolescents, (5) guilt associated with their gambling problems, (6) a lack of recognition and acceptance that they have a gambling problem despite scoring high on gambling severity screens, and (7) their inherent belief in natural recovery and self-control (for a more detailed explanation see Derevensky et al., 2003; Derevensky & Gupta, 2004).

Referrals from parents, friends, teachers, the court system, and the local help/referral line are the primary sources through which we acquire our treatment population. As part of an effective outreach program, posters and brochures are distributed to schools; media exposure and media campaigns are frequent; and workshops are provided for school psychologists, guidance counselors, social workers, teachers, and directly to children and adolescents. As a result of this outreach program, we receive a number of calls from adolescents directly requesting treatment. Interestingly, our Internet site has generated several inquiries for online help and assistance.

Research and our clinical experience suggest that adolescent problem gamblers develop a social network consisting of other peers with gambling problems (Wynne, Smith, & Jacobs, 1996). This results in clients recommending their friends for treatment. Once adolescents accept and realize that they have a serious gambling problem, they become astutely aware of gambling problems among their friends. Eventually, some successfully convince their peers to seek help as well.

Since adolescents with gambling problems have little access to discretionary funds and many initially seek treatment without parental knowledge, treatment is provided without cost. While this is not practical for treatment providers in independent practice, state or provincial funding (or support by insurance providers when available) appears to be fundamental when treating these adolescents.

The location of the treatment facility plays an important role in successfully working with youth. Concerns about being seen entering an addiction center, mental health facility, or hospital may discourage some youth from seeking treatment. Accessibility by public transportation is essential since most young clients do not own cars or have money for taxi fare. Although our clinic is adjacent to a University counseling centre, it operates as a self-contained facility exclusively for work with youth experiencing gambling problems.

The McGill Treatment Paradigm

The McGill treatment approach has been refined through our continued work over a 7-year period with more than 50 young problem gamblers, ranging in age from 14 to 21 years. While not a sufficiently large number of clients on which to draw firm conclusions, it nevertheless has provided us with sufficient diversity of experience to appreciate the broad applicability of our approach considering the variability of the age range of clients and the concomitant co-occurring problems often accompanying their gambling problems. Based on empirical findings and our clinical observations with these individuals, their reported success in remaining abstinent, and their improvement in their overall psychological well-being, the approach adopted in our clinic is generally successful in assisting youth to resume a healthy lifestyle.

The criterion by which to evaluate success differs from one treatment facility and approach to the next. In a recent review of treatment literature, Toneatto and Ladouceur (2003) suggested that several different outcome measures have traditionally been used when assessing treatment effectiveness; these being personal ratings of urges, reduction of gambling involvement, and gambling cessation. Our treatment philosophy is predicated on the assumption that sustained abstinence is necessary for these youth to recover from their gambling problem and that their general overall psychological well-being and mental health must be improved (this also includes improvement in their coping skills and adaptive behaviors). During the past 7 years, we have observed a large percentage of youth in treatment who initially had as their primary goal controlled gambling. Our clinical work suggests that while controlled gambling (ability to respect self-imposed limits) can be an interim goal, abstinence is eventually necessary. Attempts are made to closely monitor these youth for at least 1-year posttreatment; however, it becomes difficult to maintain contact with many of these youth after this point in time. Several youth call periodically beyond the 1-year follow-up period to report their progress, but we remain acutely aware that youth who may have relapsed may be unwilling to contact the treatment centre unless they are prepared to reenter treatment. There is also some recent evidence with adults that pathological gamblers who have successfully completed treatment and who have relapsed often fail to return to the same treatment center for assistance but are more likely to seek treatment elsewhere (Chevalier, Geoffrion, Audet, Papineau, & Kimpton, 2003).

For the most part, our treatment philosophy is predicated upon the work of Jacobs' General Theory of Addictions and the work of Blaszczynski and his colleagues' Pathways Model (see Nower & Blaszczynski, this volume, for a comprehensive discussion of the model and an adaptation of the Pathways Model for youth problem gambling). This model presupposes that there are three different subtypes of pathological gamblers, with each subtype having a different etiology and different accompanying pathologies. It is further assumed that these different subtype pathological gamblers would by necessity require different types of intervention (with different emphases) and that the duration for treatment will likely differ. While there is some overlap between the two models, with both describing the etiology, trajectory, and psychology of the addicted gambler, Jacobs' model primarily describes the Pathway 3 gambler articulated by Nower and Blaszczynski. The commonalities lie in the belief that these youth have a combination of emotional and/or psychological distress coupled with a physiological predisposition toward impulsively seeking excitement. This subset of problem gamblers represents our most typical young clients who seek therapy: those tending to gamble impulsively primarily for purposes of escape and as a way of coping with their stress, depression, and/or daily problems. Longitudinal data recently published following young boys 11 to 16 years of age suggests that early indicators of gambling problems include indices of anxiety and impulsivity (Vitaro, Wanner, Ladouceur, Brendgen, & Tremblay, 2004). Recent research has also replicated earlier findings that adolescent problem gamblers are more likely to be exposed to peer and parent gambling, are more susceptible to peer pressure, are more likely to exhibit conduct problems and antisocial behaviors, engage in substance use, and have suicide ideation and indicate more suicide attempts (Langhinrichsen-Rohling, Rhode, Seeley, & Rohling, 2004). Such a constellation of correlates and risk factors is sure to result in different profiles of young problem gamblers.

A General Profile of Youth Seeking Treatment

It has been suggested that individuals who present themselves for treatment are distinct, representing a minority of young pathological gamblers. It is important to note that while our clients voluntarily come for treatment a number may be less than motivated to participate at first. A considerable number attend because of parental pressure, mandatory referrals from the judicial system, or are strongly encouraged by significant others (i.e., boyfriends, girlfriends) and comply for fear of losing relationships.

The youth who do present for treatment tend to share a similar constellation of behaviors. Other than the psychological variables of depression, anxiety, impulsivity, and poor coping abilities previously mentioned, it is not uncommon to see youth who have a history of academic difficulties (usually owing to a learning disability and further compounded by their gambling preoccupation and gambling behavior), stressed interpersonal relationships with family members and old friends, involvement with unhealthy peer groups, and a history of delinquent criminal behaviors to support their gambling (e.g., shoplifting, check forgery, credit card scams). Despite these commonalities, individual differences exist that result in three distinct profiles.

The following represents a brief synopsis profile of the three predominant types of young gamblers we have treated in our practice, with those fitting in Nower and Blaszczynski's Pathway 3 being most representative of the majority of youth with whom we have worked.

Pathway 1: Behaviorally Conditioned Problem Gamblers

Seventeen-year-old Joe is primarily a blackjack casino player (in spite of legal prohibitions). On one of his early visits to the casino, Joe reportedly won more than $200, leading him to believe that gambling could provide a good and easy source of revenue. Personal accounts suggest he played, on average, between $300 and $500 per week before seeking treatment. Joe also revealed that he had lost up to $2000 on several visits to the local casino. He attends a postsecondary business school, but was failing because of his problem gambling and preoccupation with gambling debts. He presents with occasional drug use and antisocial behaviors related to his gambling behaviors.

Motivation for Gambling

Joe reports that gambling is very rewarding, as it makes him feel exceptionally good. He revealed that gambling is highly exciting and he perceives it to be the ultimate challenge to outsmart the casino, recoup his losses, and to win large amounts of money.

Financial Resources

Joe works part-time in father's company while attending school. He takes money from the company coffers, steals money from family members, and has even stolen and cashed alimony checks sent to his mother to enable him to gamble. He reportedly has borrowed money from friends, and while he does his best to repay them he remains in constant debt.

Therapeutic Objectives

Joe entered treatment reporting that he could stop gambling by himself but likes the support and supervision therapy provides. He acknowledged his need for an outlet to deal with the frustration and agitation resulting from his gambling withdrawal. The primary therapeutic objectives were to help him reduce his gambling participation gradually by setting frequency, time, and money limits on his activities while simultaneously addressing his erroneous beliefs about wagering and winning. Restructuring his time was essential to ensure he had minimal free time to think about gambling. This included helping him prioritize school work, seeking and developing healthy peer relationships, and minimizing his use of drugs.

Pathway 2: Emotionally Vulnerable Problem Gamblers

Seventeen-year-old Candice primarily wagers on sports and casino playing (blackjack was her preferred game of choice). She reported wagering on average between $500 and $1500 per week. She generally plays until all her funds are depleted. She readily understood that the gambling cycle involves wins and losses, with the casino holding the edge over the player. On entry into treatment she was enrolled in the first year of CEGEP (Junior College), but rarely attended, as she spent much of her time at the casino. She also held a part-time job that she approached in a responsible manner.

Motivation for Gambling

Candice reports gambling primarily to make herself feel special; impress friends; become closer to her father (also a pathological gambler); and as a way of dealing with depression, low self-esteem, agitation, and anxiety. She indicates that she had always experienced academic difficulties and preferred to spend time at the casino versus attending class and completing assignments.

Financial Resources

Since all of her expenses were paid by her family (pocket money, car expenses, clothing, cell phone), the money Candice earned from her job was used almost exclusively for gambling. In addition, she would regularly take cash advances on her credit card (approximately $300 per week), which was readily paid by her father.

Therapeutic Objectives

The primary goals established for Candice focused on the identification of her underlying stressors and unresolved issues, addressing the underlying depression and anxiety, and improving her coping skills and adaptive behavior. There was also a need to directly address her gambling behavior and determine her willingness to abstain from gambling. This was accomplished through the gradual introduction of limit setting (money spent, frequency, and time spent at the casino).

Pathway 3: Antisocial Impulsivist Problem Gamblers

Eighteen-year-old Sonny is primarily a casino card player. He reports playing on average between $300 and $600 per week depending on his success at the casino. He acknowledges being a thrill-seeker and was diagnosed with attention deficit/hyperactivity disorder (ADHD) at the age of 12. He frequently engages in drug use, primarily cannabis, to "take off the edge." Sonny has a family history of depression, meets the criteria for a mild chronic depression (dysthymia), and reports having repeated suicidal ideations.

Motivation for Gambling

Sonny reports that while he is unhappy about his inability to control his gambling it provides him with such a thrill and escape that he cannot stop. He has also calculated that the casino "owes" him $7000, and that it would be easier to stop once he wins back that money (a frequent form of logic seen with our clients). When explained that he would be unlikely to recoup the money lost, he acknowledged that most people lose money over time when gambling but that he is the exception to the rule. His erroneous belief system about his ability to control the outcomes of random events was pervasive. Sonny gambled primarily for escape, excitement, and to recoup lost money.

Financial Resources

Sonny has little access to gambling funds as he was attending school and only holds a small part-time job. His parents are divorced and he works in his father's company on the weekend. His psychological profile indicates antisocial tendencies, often stealing money from his father's company. He also reports repeatedly lying to and manipulating his mother and friends to obtain money to gamble.

Therapeutic Objectives

Sonny's impulsivity was underlying his inability to control his gambling. Thus, controlling impulsive tendencies (ADHD) and finding more appropriate ways to channel them were primary 1objectives. Sonny also met the criteria for a mild depression that required treatment and monitoring. His lying, stealing, and manipulation of his family and friends were without remorse, representing an important treatment goal. Sonny's peers were perceived to be a negative influence and as such fostering a healthier choice of peers was important. The treatment plan also included a gradual reduction of his gambling participation and modifying erroneous cognitions.

The Treatment Procedure

Intake Assessment

The intake procedure includes a semistructured interview using the DSM-IV criteria for pathological gambling as well as other pertinent gambling behaviors (e.g., preferred activities, frequency, wagering patterns, accumulated losses, etc.). Current familial situation and relationships, academic and/or work status, and social functioning are ascertained. Information concerning alcohol or drug use, the presence of other risk-taking behaviors, self-concept, coping skills, and selected personality traits are ascertained through a variety of instruments and clinical interviews. An evaluation for clinical depression as well as a history of suicidal ideation and attempts is included.

An explanation of our procedures, requirements, and goals are provided to each client to avoid any misconceptions. Client expectations and personal goals are also ascertained. Many youth report that they desperately want their unbearable situation to improve. However, approximately 60% of clients are initially ambivalent about abstinence.

Tenets of Therapy

A staff psychologist provides all therapy individually. Initially, therapy is provided weekly; however, if the therapist deems more frequent sessions are required, appropriate accommodations are made. All clients are provided with a pager or cell phone number for emergency contacts. The number of sessions varies significantly with the motivation and degree of gambling severity of the client and the concomitant disorders. The number of therapy sessions generally range between 20 and 50 sessions. The following paragraphs describe the basic therapeutic process.

Establishing Mutual Trust and Respect

Mutual trust and respect are fundamental to the therapeutic relationship. Total honesty is emphasized and a nonjudgmental therapeutic relationship is provided. This results in the adolescent not fearing reactions of disappointment if weekly personal goals are not achieved. However, since treatment is provided without cost, clients are required to respect the therapist's time. This involves calling ahead to cancel and reschedule appointments, punctual attendance of sessions, and a commitment to complete "homework" assignments.

Assessment and Setting of Goals

Since the emphasis of different therapeutic objectives is tailored to the individual, a more detailed profile of the client is required. This is accomplished through comprehensive clinical interviews (beyond intake assessment), usually taking place over the first three sessions. The initial interview consists of the completion of several instruments primarily designed to screen for gambling severity, impulsivity, conduct problems, depression, antisocial behaviors, and suicide ideation and attempts. Their responses to these measures are followed up through more in-depth diagnostic interviews over the next few sessions and more details about the consequences associated with their gambling (i.e., academic and/or occupational status, peer and familial relationships, romantic and interpersonal relationships, legal problems, etc.) are obtained.

This comprehensive evaluation allows for the therapeutic goals to be established. For example, an adolescent who presents with serious depression will not be approached in the same manner as one who does not evidence depressive symptomatology. If a client presents with a severe depression, this becomes the initial therapeutic objective while the gambling problem becomes a secondary objective. Interestingly, for many youth, once gambling has stopped, depressive symptomatology actually increases as youth report that their primary source of pleasure, excitement, and enjoyment has been eliminated. It is therefore important to screen periodically for depressive symptomatology throughout the therapeutic process.

Assessment of Readiness to Change

An important factor influencing the therapeutic approach relates to the client's current willingness to make significant changes in their life. Our experience suggests that most adolescents experiencing serious gambling-related problems are reluctant and are not convinced that they really want to stop gambling completely. Rather, most state that they believe in *controlled gambling* and hold onto this belief for some time in spite of our reluctance. Some individuals seek basic information but remain open to the idea of making more permanent changes. Others have decided that they really must stop gambling but are unable to do so without therapeutic assistance and support. Finally, some adolescents have made the decision to stop gambling and do so before their first session but require support in maintaining abstinence. These three examples depict adolescents in different stages of the process of change (see the chapter by DiClemente, Delahanty & Schlundt, this volume, for a comprehensive discussion of the Stages of Change Model).

While there are a multiplicity of approaches taken depending upon one's severity of gambling problems, underlying psychological disorders or problems, age, and risk factors, the overall therapeutic philosophy remains similar, with different weightings of therapeutic goals placed where most needed.

Goals of Therapy

DiClemente, Story, and Murray (2000) initially proposed a *Transtheoretical Model of Intentional Behavior Change* for adolescent gambling problems whereby they contend that paths leading from addiction to recovery involve interactions between biological, psychological, sociological, and behavioral elements in a person's life (see also the chapter by DiClemente, Delahanty & Schlundt, this volume). As such, a multimodal, multigoaled therapeutic approach is necessary. Within our treatment philosophy, the overall framework is to address multiple therapeutic goals simultaneously over time, tailoring the time allocated to each goal to the client. Some will require more emphasis on psychological issues, others on their physiological impulses, others on environmental /social factors, while others will require examining their motivations to change. Nevertheless, each client receives individualized therapeutic attention in all areas to ensure he or she is achieving a balanced lifestyle. The goals of therapy can be conceptualized as described in the following paragraphs.

Understanding the Motivations for Gambling

Adolescents experiencing serious gambling problems continue gambling in the face of repeated losses and serious negative consequences as result of their need to dissociate and escape from daily stressors. Without exception, youth with gambling problems report that when gambling they enter a "different world," a world without problems and stresses. They report that while gambling, they feel invigorated and alive;they are admired and respected; that time passes quickly; and all their problems are forgotten, be they psychological, financial, social, familial, academic, work-related, or legal. As such, gambling becomes the ultimate escape.

Adolescents are required to write a short essay on why it is they feel they gamble, entitled, "What gambling does for me." We contend that the youth must be benefiting in some way from their gambling experiences, albeit temporarily, to continue playing despite serious negative consequences. This exercise is important for two reasons. First, it enables us, in a general way, to understand the individual's perceptions of the reasons underlying why he or she is gambling excessively. Second, and more importantly, it enables the individual to articulate and understand the underlying reasons why he or she gambles. The following are excerpts from their writings; the first one highlighting difficulties with interpersonal relationships and poor coping/adaptive skills, while the second example illustrates an individual's gambling to alleviate a depressed state and as a form of psychological escape

> I always had trouble making friends, and never had a girlfriend. Gambling has now become my best friend and my one true love. I can turn to her in good times and bad and she'll always be there for me. (Male, age 18)
> Gambling, well, it's strange to talk about the positive side because of how upside down it has turned my life, but I guess the pull of it is how it makes me feel so alive, so happy, and so much like I belong, but only when I am gambling. The low I feel after I realize what I did, and how much I have lost, is worse than anything I can explain. I guess I just need to feel good from time to time, it lets me escape the black hole that is my life. (Male, age 17)

Analysis of Gambling Episodes

Self-awareness is essential to the process of change. If individuals understand the underlying motivations prompting certain behaviors they begin to feel empowered to gain control and make change. Every person who repeatedly engages in a self-injurious pattern of excessive behavior can be guided through an analysis of his or her behavioral patterns. An awareness of their gambling triggers, their psychological and behavioral reactions to those triggers, as well as the consequences that ensue from this chain reaction is important to achieve. This type of analysis empowers the individual to make long-term successful changes to his or her behaviors. The following model provides an overview of the framework:

Triggers → Emotional Reactions and Rationalizations → Behavior
→ Consequences

Triggers

Triggers can consist of places, people, times of day, activities, particular situations, and/or emotions. While initially many individuals are unaware of their specific triggers, they can be identified through discussions of prior experiences, as well as by examining written journals (i.e., a component within the therapeutic process). Once identified, avoiding or effectively dealing with the triggers becomes possible. For example, one of the most common triggers for gamblers is the handling of large sums of money. We therefore help them adopt strategies to minimize the exposure to this trigger, such as arranging for payment of something to be made by a third party, or to have the money replaced by a check, and limiting access to cash withdrawals from bank machines. In one case, a parent who was financially supporting his son made daily deposits into his account rather than weekly deposits. Other examples of triggers include gambling advertisements or landmarks, personal anxiety or depressed feelings, interpersonal difficulties, enticement of peers, stressful situations (i.e., exams), the need to make money quickly, or quite simply daydreaming of engaging in gambling. Sometimes, just having the awareness of one's triggers provides a person with a better ability to deal with gambling urges. Additional research is needed to better understand the relationship between triggers and mechanisms of self-control.

Gambling-Free Times

It is also important to understand properly the times in a person's day when he or she does not seem to have the urge to gamble. Identifying the circumstances, time of day, whom the person is with, his or her emotional state, activity levels, physical location, etc. is essential. Understanding the circumstances in which the urge to gamble is less or absent provides a set of guidelines by which the therapist can help recreate similar situations at other times in the day. For example, we have noted that many of the young gamblers undergoing treatment often report that when actively engaged in playing sports with friends, bicycling, physical activity in gym, or rollerblading they felt better and had their minds clear of their gambling desires both during and after the activity. As a result, for these youth, when helping them to structure and organize their week, we attempt to include similar types of activities on a daily basis.

Establishing a Baseline of Gambling Behavior and Encouraging a Decrease in Gambling

Once the motivations for gambling are understood and an analysis of gambling patterns has been made, efforts focused on making changes to the adolescent's gambling behavior. To set goals and measure improvements, we find it useful and important to initially establish a baseline of gambling behavior. Adolescents are required to record their gambling behaviors in terms of frequency, duration, time of day, type of gambling activity, amount of money spent, losses, and wins. When establishing goals for a decrease in gambling participation, individuals are guided to establish *reasonable* goals for themselves. Some elect to target multiple factors such as frequency and duration and amount spent simultaneously, while others may focus on one form of behavior (e.g., frequency or duration). For these individuals we encourage a decrease in frequency or duration of each gambling episode versus initially focusing on amount wagered. Some meet their goals immediately, at which point we generally support decisions to maintain this decrease for several weeks while setting new goals immediately. Others struggle to meet their goals at which point goals are generally modified.

Addressing Cognitive Distortions

It has been well established that individuals with gambling problems experience multiple cognitive distortions (Ladouceur & Walker, 1998; Langer, 1975). They are prone to have an illusion of control and perceive that they can control the outcome of gambling events, they underestimate the amount of money lost and overestimate the amount won, they fail to utilize their understanding of the laws of independence of events, and they believe that if they persist at gambling they will likely win back all money lost (chasing behavior). Addressing these cognitive distortions remains an important treatment goal. Further, the analysis of their gambling behavior usually reveals the rationalizations they make to justify their gambling behavior, and these rationalizations need to be addressed, as they too represent distortions of reality. An example of a rationalization for gambling is, "If I gamble now, I will be in a good mood and I will be more able to have fun at my friend's party tonight," or "By gambling now, the urge will be out of my system and I'll be more able to focus on studying for my exam." The overarching goal would be to ensure the individual comprehends that the gambling episode will likely result in a bad mood if they were to lose money, thus a negative mood at their party; or an inability to focus on studying for their exam. Ultimately, the goal of addressing many of the cognitive distortions is to highlight how their thinking is self-deceptive, to provide pertinent information about randomness, to encourage a realization that they are incapable of controlling outcomes of random events and games, payout rates, etc.?

Establishing the Underlying Causes of Stress and Anxiety

In light of empirical research (Gupta & Derevensky, 1998a; Jacobs, 1998; Jacobs, Marsten, & Singer, 1985) and clinical findings, a primary treatment goal is to identify and treat any underlying problem that results in increased stress and/or anxiety. These in general include one or more of the following problems: personal (e.g., low self-esteem, depression, ADHD, oppositional defiant disorders), familial, peer, academic, vocational, and legal. Through traditional therapeutic techniques, these problems are addressed and alternative approaches to problem solving are supported while sublimation, projection, repression, and escape are discouraged. For example, Candice was initially struggling with chronic depression, a learning disability, and poor coping skills. The combination of these factors resulted in significant anxiety when faced with school assignments and exams; all of which resulted in a poor self-esteem affecting her ability to establish and maintain healthy peer relationships. As a result of a clinical evaluation, Candice's depression and learning problems were addressed. Candice gained insight as to the reasons she needed to escape through her excessive gambling. Ultimately, she was relieved to have her primary problems addressed, her self-esteem gradually improved, and she was encouraged to develop a healthier lifestyle and more effective coping skills. In time, Candice found developed a very good friendship with someone in whom she could confide about her struggles with gambling. This friend assisted her in overcoming her gambling urges, kept her occupied with healthy activities, and became a good study partner. This friendship also helped Candice develop a stronger sense of self-worth and she came to better understand her value and potential.

Evaluating and Improving Coping Abilities

The need to escape one's problems usually occurs more frequently among individuals who have poor coping and adaptive skills. Using gambling, or other addictive activities to deal with daily stressors, anxiety, or depression represents a form of maladaptive coping. Recent research efforts have confirmed these clinical observations, where adolescents who meet the criteria for pathological gambling demonstrated poor coping skills as compared to same age peers without a gambling problem (Gupta, Derevensky, & Marget, stay as in press; Marget, Gupta, & Derevensky, 1999; Nower, Gupta, & Derevensky, 2000). A primary therapeutic goal involves building and expanding the individual's repertoire of coping abilities. This happens best by using examples of situations in the individual's life that were dealt with inappropriately and suggesting more appropriate ways of handling them. As adolescents begin to comprehend the benefits of effective coping abilities and their repertoire of coping responses expands, they are more apt to apply these skills to their daily lives. Examples of healthy coping skills include honest communication with others, seeking social support, and learning to weigh the benefits or downfalls of potential behaviors. Also included in the discussions and role playing exercises are ways to improve social skills (e.g., learning to communicate with peers, developing healthy friendships, being considerate of others, and developing trust).

Rebuilding Healthy Interpersonal Relationships

Common consequences of a serious gambling problem involve impaired and severed relationships with friends and family members. Helping the adolescent rebuild these crucial relationships constitutes an important therapeutic goal. Often through lies and manipulative behaviors resulting from their gambling problem, friends and family members become alienated, leaving unresolved negative feelings. Once a youth has been identified as being a liar or a thief, it becomes difficult to earn back the trust of others and to resume healthy relationships. One needs to explain to family members and friends that these deceptive actions are part of the constellation of problematic behaviors exhibited by individuals who cannot control their gambling. Consequently, once the gambling is under control, family members and friends can anticipate being treated with more respect. Family members, peers, and significant others become important support personnel to help ensure abstinence and can take an active role in relapse prevention. We contend that youth with gambling problems will be happier and are more likely to abstain from gambling if they feel they belong to a peer group and are supported by family and friends. As a result, the occasional inclusion of family members and friends in therapy sessions can prove to be very beneficial.

As an example, Sonny, having stolen from his father's company, and having manipulated his mother with lies in order to obtain funds for gambling, faced a difficult challenge in regaining the trust of his parents. Both parents perceived him as being ruthless and were convinced that his antisocial criminal behaviors would not stop. Once he regained control of his gambling and was abstinent for several months, he came to understand how his behaviors were hurtful. As a result, he experienced significant remorse. Through inclusion of his parents in the therapeutic process, concomitant with improved communication skills and his willingness to accept responsibility for the emotional distress he caused his parents, he slowly regained the support and trust of his family members and peers. This process remains ongoing and often takes considerably longer than the client wants.

Restructuring Free Time

Adolescents struggling to overcome a gambling problem experience more positive outcomes when not faced with large amounts of unstructured time. Some adolescents in treatment are still in school and/or have a job, and as such their free time consists mainly of evenings and weekends. Others have dropped out of school and may have a part-time job while others are not working. For these youth, structuring their time becomes paramount as they initially find it exceedingly difficult to resist urges to gamble when they are bored. We frequently ask adolescents to carry an agenda with them where we have helped articulate ways of spending time with friends, family, or school- or work-related activities. Other activities can involve participating in organized sports, engaging in a hobby, and performing volunteer work. The *success* of their week is evaluated on how they achieve their weekly goals as agreed on, with their gambling-related goals (reduction or abstinence) being one part of the program. Thus, if individuals fail to meet their goals surrounding their gambling behavior, they still may achieve success in other areas. This approach tends to keep the young gamblers from being discouraged and motivates them to keep trying to attain a balanced lifestyle.

Fostering Effective Money Management Skills

Money management skills are typically lacking in adolescents who have a gambling problem. Therapeutic goals involve educating them as to the value of money (as they tend to lose perspective after gambling large sums), building money management skills, and helping them develop effective and reasonable debt repayment plans.

Relapse Prevention

Despite a lack of strong empirical evidence, our clinical work suggests that abstinence from gambling is necessary to prevent a relapse of pathological gambling behaviors. It should be noted that small, occasional relapses throughout the treatment process are to be expected. However, once gambling has ceased for an extended period of time (i.e., 4 to 6 months), an effective relapse prevention program should help these individuals remain free of gambling. Relapse prevention includes continued access to their primary therapist, the existence of a good social support network, engagement in either school or work, the practice of a healthy lifestyle, and avoidance of powerful triggers. Youth are contacted periodically via telephone for one year post-treatment to ensure they are maintaining their abstinence and doing well in general. Support is offered if required. Gamblers representative of Pathways 2 and 3 are more apt to need additional support after the termination of therapy.

Concluding Remarks

The authors acknowledge that the treatment program's efficacy has not been empirically validated using the standards necessary for a rigorous, scientifically controlled study (i.e., no random assignments to a control group matching for severity of gambling problems and other mental health disorders, controlling for age, socioeconomic status, frequency and type of gambling activity preferred, etc.). As such, more clinical research is necessary before definitive conclusions can be drawn. Nevertheless, based upon clinical criteria established for success (i.e., abstinence for 6 months post- treatment; return to school or work; not meeting the DSM criteria for pathological gambling; improved peer and family relationships; improved coping skills; and no marked signs of depressive symptomatology, delinquent behavior, or excessive use of alcohol or drugs), the McGill University treatment program appears to have reached its objectives in successfully working with youth with serious gambling problems.

The description of our treatment philosophy and approach were elaborated on to provide clinicians and treatment providers with a better understanding of the different components necessary when working with young problem gamblers. Treating youth with severe gambling problems requires clinical skills, a knowledge of adolescent development, an understanding of the risk factors associated with problem gambling, and a thorough grounding in the empirical work concerning the correlates associated with gambling problems. By no means should this chapter substitute for proper training.

While we did not elaborate on how to treat youth with multiple addictions in this chapter, it is clear that gamblers with concomitant substance abuse problems pose a greater challenge for treatment (Ladd & Petry, 2003). Youth with clinical levels of depression, high levels of impulsivity, and anxiety disorders are often referred to psychiatry to simultaneously undergo pharmacological treatment while undergoing our therapy. The use of serotonin reuptake inhibitors tend to be effective in helping these youth manage their depression and anxiety, and preliminary research suggests that they may be useful in lowering the levels of impulsivity that often underlie pathological gambling behavior (Grant, Chambers & Potenza, this volume; Grant et al., 2003).

The finding that several youth enter treatment immediately after stopping their gambling on their own, requesting assistance in maintaining abstinence and in dealing with the concomitant gambling-related problems and underlying issues, raises an interesting research and clinical question. Would these youth have maintained abstinence without intervention?

While the incidence of severe gambling problems among youth remains relatively small, the devastating short-term and long-term consequences to the individuals, their families, and friends are significant. One adolescent, when discussing the severity of his gambling problem responded, "It's an all-encompassing problem that invades every facet of my life. I wouldn't wish this problem on my worst enemy, for it's way too harsh a punishment."

The vast majority of the youth seen in our clinic have a wide array of problems. Merely treating the gambling problem without examining the individual's overall mental health functioning will likely have limited results. The following is a text written by a young pathological gambler we treated, 1 year post-treatment:

> Gambling is an extremely addictive activity which can get unbelievably out of control. It can lead to a very horrible reality, one in which just getting out of bed can seem unthinkable. Unfortunately, I have lived this reality. I was eighteen when I began to fight for my life back. My future did not look very good. I was severely depressed, anxious and overweight, I wanted to disappear. Thankfully, with the support of an amazing team I have managed to overcome my addiction, lose thirty pounds and continue my schooling. I feel like I am relearning how to live. This continues to be a very long and emotionally painful process, however it does get easier with time. My memories of the gambling, the lies and unhappiness are slowly fading away . . . becoming part of the past. However I will never forget my struggle or how easy it was to lose control. In my gambling years I have seen and experienced first hand an incredible amount of heartache. I hope to never witness such avoidable pain again. Now at twenty years old, I am beginning a journey which holds an endless amount of opportunity. My dream to be a health-care professional seems closer than ever. Please let my story be a source of hope for anyone in a similar situation. I understand how bad life can seem, I've been there, believe me. You are not alone. Get the help you need, be true to yourself and start your own journey.

While it appears as though large numbers of adolescents who gamble problematically appear to resolve their gambling problems without therapeutic intervention (natural recovery), providing support for those in need remains essential. Our governments, private corporations, and charitable organizations, recipients of the revenues generated from gambling, need to help address this issue by providing funding for the establishments of treatment centers and training of professionals. Problem gambling, even for adolescents, can have devastating short-term and long-term consequences.

The youth briefly described, Joe, Candice, and Sonny, are all doing relatively well and are living happy productive lives. Joe has channeled his energies into starting his own business, always taking significant but well reasoned risks. Candice has successfully returned to her studies, and although she was unable to enter into the health science university program (she always envisioned herself as attending medical school) as a result of academic failures during her excessive gambling days, she nevertheless is happily enrolled in an alternative, related program. She remains highly motivated and committed toward building her career. Sonny has learned to manage his ADHD and his depression and has integrated full time into the workforce. He has built a solid peer network of social support for himself and is working on repairing broken relationships with friends and family members.

In spite of gains in knowledge concerning the correlates and risk factors associated with severe gambling problems among youth during the past 10 years, a general lack of public and parental awareness exists. The fact that the prevalence rates for youth with severe gambling problems remain higher than that of adults is of significant concern. Whether maturation will result in individuals stopping their excessive gambling behavior by the time they become adults with additional responsibilities still remains an unanswered question (the issue of natural recovery remains a highly important issue in need of considerable research). As we have argued elsewhere, independent of whether or not individuals with severe gambling during adolescence become more responsible "social gamblers" as adults, the personal costs and consequences incurred along the way often remain with them.

Gambling problems among youth will raise important public health and social policy issues in the 21st century. Greater emphasis on outreach and prevention programs is absolutely essential. Our governments must help fund more basic and applied research and be responsible for supporting and developing effective and scientifically validated prevention and treatment programs. The treatment of young problem gamblers is a complex, multimodal process. While such an approach can take months or longer, the benefits to the individual and society outweigh the costs of funding such programs.

Chapter 17
The Evolution of Problem Gambling Helplines

Gary Clifford

Background

In this chapter, we look at the role of Helplines in adding value to the process of minimizing the harm caused by problem gambling. Helplines do this in their own right, but increasingly also by developing partnerships with callers/clients; therapists and other helping agencies; governments/funders; the gambling industry; providers of training; and media. We outline briefly the evolution of helplines as well as looking at the nature of potential "team approaches." We include case studies of both "traditional" and leading edge helplines. We look at examples of client/therapist/helpline and industry/training organization/helpline partnerships to illustrate how collaboration can work to provide prevention, intervention and ongoing support for harm minimization strategies. Specifically, these partnerships involve effective information-sharing, case management, and ongoing support to help gamblers and families cope with gambling problems. They also include providing support for gambling venue staff in identifying and intervening with problem gambling.

A large proportion of problem gamblers recycle through the standard addictions process of contemplation/action/maintenance/relapse but often with a greater sense of denial than, say, alcohol. Part of this seems to stem from a lack of society acceptance of gambling as an addiction but a large part may be due to the lack of ongoing brief intervention and support mechanisms available. Helplines can offer support and motivation from precontemplation through treatment and beyond.

The next phase of development is already seeing the harnessing of technology, professionalism, and humanity to provide structured help from (self) screening through self-managed care to integrated case management and to long-term follow-up and support. A variety of routes can be offered through the change process involving collaboration among therapists, medical professionals, financial advisers, and spiritual support as well as helplines.

Gary Clifford

Consultant, Responsible Gambling Consulting International, New Zealand, and private training practice

M. Zangeneh, A. Blaszczynski, N. Turner (eds.), *In the Pursuit of Winning.*
© Springer 2008

This integrated approach can also facilitate longitudinal studies of presenting populations. We comment on the lessons learned to date, both positive and negative, and possible directions for future development. Finally, we put forward a model that is proposed for testing and evaluation of helplines' ability to add value to the problem gambling prevention and treatment sector.

First Contact for the Problem Gambler

"Hello, this is the Problem Gambling Helpline; how may I help you?" These words, or something like them, are heard around the world, every hour of every day in the 50 or so dedicated helplines for problem gambling. And for many people they represent the first steps on the road to getting help with a gambling problem. The problem may be their own or someone else's. The problem may be a full on, debilitating demon that has brought the caller to the point of crisis, even suicide; it may be just the early arousing of suspicion that gambling is getting out of control. For all these people, the Problem Gambling Helpline is the gateway to building a potentially brighter future.

Just as the types and impact of gambling have changed over time, so the role of helpline services is evolving, from simple enquiry taking and information provision through to full involvement in the clinical management and support of clients. Traditionally helplines have been at best information and referral agencies. However, some, such as the helplines in New Zealand, Finland, and Vermont have extended their range to offer more in terms of distance counseling and motivation and in gathering a wide range of data about the trends and treatment results in problem gambling. This has been available both by phone and e-mail and, more recently in New Zealand through a forum on their Web site. Already they are seeing a noticeable improvement in client outcomes as the NZ Helpline undertakes follow up screening. In addition, the NZ Helpline and some others have begun trialing dedicated employee support programs for staff working in the gambling industry to assist them in identifying and caring for (potential) problem gamblers, as well as addressing their own gambling issues.

The growth in data collection is helping to profile the help seeking population and to focus additional service needs for both the individual and for broader groups. Data have often been the missing link in deciding policy and funding priorities in problem gambling services. Helplines can often be the best placed agencies for collecting long-term data.

The Operating Environment

Helplines operate in a variety of environments, from goodwill-based volunteerism, usually with uncertain funding, through to a professional and comprehensive sociolegal environment that emphasizes a public health approach. One of the

Table 17.1 Helpline calls

Region	Total Contacts 2005	% Hoax
Nova Scotia, CAN	5410	1
South Africa	66,054	60
Massachusetts, USA	1591	36
Louisiana, USA	68,662	96
Ontario, CAN	14,000	45
Vermont, USA	873	0
Sweden	5594	56.9
Oregon, USA	5028	34.6
Finland	1361	16
New Zealand	18,372	0
UK	22,589	1.4
Quebec, CAN	13,728	19

criticisms often raised about helplines is that they cannot prove their value. They frequently do not have data on their callers and are unable even to report on the real number of callers seeking help. Many are overburdened with calls that are not relevant to their core business (e.g., requests for information on winning lottery numbers). An international survey led by the New Zealand Helpline in 2006 showed significant numbers of and variations in non-productive calls (an extract is shown in Table 17.1 courtesy of the NZ Gambling Helpline).

Few helplines keep details of callers and their demographics; fewer still are able to identify whether a caller subsequently seeks more specialized help; and virtually none has information on caller outcomes. Notable exceptions are GamCare in the United Kingdom, which is an integrated service, and the New Zealand Helpline. Both of these are discussed later.

Some have begun to recognize that frequent brief interventions throughout a period of change and ongoing recovery are important in the sustainability of that recovery. Funders, too, are beginning to question old models, partly as a consequence of potential cost blowouts in traditional treatment models, and partly in acceptance that a client centered approach can operate at many levels.

A helpline is potentially more than just a brief telephone call center; when well run it is a first contact service opening the way to beating a problem. But it can also be more than a first contact service; it can provide the glue that makes long term success stick.

A Snapshot of the Helpline Scene

Rarely have Helplines featured strongly at international gambling and problem conferences. This has begun to change over the past few years. One of the big steps forward was the one-day workshop for Helplines at the (US) National Council on Problem Gambling (NCPG) Conference in Phoenix during 2004. Keith Whyte, the

Executive Director of NCPG, conducted a brief survey of helplines as a lead up to the workshop. Some of the key findings were:

Operating history: when did the helpline start?

New Jersey, US	1983
Florida, US	1988
New Zealand	1992
Quebec, Canada	1993
Wisconsin, US	1993
Arizona, US	1994
Connecticut, US	1994
Bensinger, DuPont, Assoc. US	1994
Delaware, US	1996
United Kingdom	1997
Ontario, Canada	1997
Vermont, US	1998
Michigan, US	1999
Louisiana, US	1999
Sweden	1999
West Virginia, US	2000
Oregon, US	2001
Norway	2003
Finland	2004

How many people do you employ?
>   In the survey group, there were on average 5.3 full-time staff:
>>   Highest: 19 Lowest: 1
>   And an average 8.7 part-time staff and volunteers:
>>   Highest: 40 Lowest: 1

How many hours do you operate each day?

Most respondents (13) offer services 24 hours a day, 7 days a week. Six offered partial days, ranging from 5 hours daily to 14 hours daily. Of those who were not available 24 hours, many had answering services that covered the time they were not available.

How many calls do you receive?

In the 18 helpline centers reporting, 372,836 calls were taken in 2003. The number of calls ranged from 398 to 175,000. The call center reporting 175,000 used "total calls," but indicated only 3% or 5250 calls were for gambling assistance. Many other helplines were unable to say how many of their calls were related to help with gambling problems (many Canadian helplines report that a large proportion of their calls are for information on lottery results!). The percentages of pranks/wrong numbers/non-problem-related calls varied widely, ranging from "almost none" to 93%. The average was 40%. Most of the helplines reported receiving fewer than 10 "real" calls a day on average, though some were much busier. A typical call probably lasts between 10 and 20 minutes. Around 60% of callers are gamblers and the remainder are families or other interested people.

How much funding ($US) do you receive and where does it come from?

$50,000–100,000:   3
$100,000–250,000:   5
$250,000 and above: 10

By far, the largest source of funding was government (13). Several helplines receive funding from both government and industry (4). Three respondents said they had other sources of revenue, including one (New Zealand) which received funds from a charitable trust set up by the gaming industry (though this has now changed).

What is the nature of calls?

Every helpline surveyed reported that it provided information and referral services to the caller. Clearly, it would be difficult to be defined as a helpline if this were not so. Virtually all respondents provide crisis counseling or other crisis stabilization methods to callers. Some helplines offer scheduled telephone counseling, but the majority do not. Many helplines are precluded from offering counseling.

What use is made of the Internet?

More than half of the helplines provide agency information, etc. on a Web site. Some also offer e-mail counseling and advice. New Zealand also has a Web-based chat room.

What literature do you provide?

More than half offer self help booklets and workbooks. Most have a range of information leaflets.

Conclusions were drawn on the inadequacy and inconsistency of funding for most helplines. Many have no idea from one year to the next whether they will receive any funding at all, far less what it will be. This makes service planning and staff development a nightmare. Sometimes, this is due to entrenched (and outdated) ideas on what a helpline can achieve; sometimes it is due to the helplines' own shortcomings in identifying and claiming their niche as the front line (and rarely glamorous) service for addressing problem gambling. The 2006 survey mentioned above updated the services offered by helplines, some examples of which are shown in Table 17.2.

Case Studies

Canada

A prime example of a well funded, traditional (i.e., information and referral) helpline is the *Ontario Problem Gambling Helpline (OPGH),* which opened in 1997. The OPGH is designed to link callers with problem gambling treatment resources within the province of Ontario. As a dedicated, toll-free, 1-888 province-wide telephone service, the OPGH provides immediate access to information about problem gambling treatment services, credit and debt counseling services, family services, self-help groups, and other resources related to problem gambling. Anyone concerned about their own or another person's gambling is welcome to call OPGH.

The OPGH maintains a comprehensive database includes problem gambling treatment services in Ontario that:

- receive funding from the Ministry of Health and Long-Term Care;
- offer specialized treatment service(s) for individuals having gambling problems; and
- accept referrals from the community.

OPGH also provides brochures, posters, and wallet cards describing the services of the Helpline. These may be ordered by e-mail or by calling a toll-free number. They are provided free of charge and are available in both English and French.

In addition to straightforward information and referrals, OPGH carries out a province-wide promotional strategy to inform problem gamblers, their family mem-

Table 17.2 Services offered by Helpline

Region	Information Provision	Phone Counseling	Referrals	Crisis Interventions	Self-Help Workbooks	Internet Help	Other
Nova Scotia, CAN	□	□	□	□	–	–	–
South Africa	□	□	□	□	□	□	–
Massachusetts, USA	□	□	□	□	□	□	–
Louisiana, USA	□	□	□	□	–	□	–
Ontario, CAN	□	□	□	□	□	□	□
Vermont, USA	□	□	□	□	□	□	□
Sweden	□	□	□	□	□	□	–
Oregon, USA	□	□	□	□	□	–	–
Finland	□	□	□	□	□	□	□
New Zealand	□	□	□	□	□	□	□
UK	□	□	□	□	–	□	–
Quebec, CAN	□	□	□	□	□	□	–

bers, co-workers, friends, and involved professionals about the services of the Helpline. Various materials are available on request and distributed in gaming venues such as casinos, raceways, bingo halls, and break-open and lottery ticket kiosks. OPGH promotional materials are also distributed to social service and health sector organizations.

In addition, the Ontario Lottery and Gaming Corporation (OLGC) provides support for the OPGH by including the toll-free Helpline telephone number on its communication vehicles, underneath the responsible gaming message "Know your limit, play within it!" The OPGH Helpline number appears as an electronic message (screen scrawl) on the slot machines, automated banking machines at gaming sites, gaming and lottery marketing and advertising material, lottery tickets, and *Lotto Post* (a magazine distributed to 10,000 retailers). The Ontario Problem Gambling Helpline 1-888 telephone service is open 24 hours per day, 7 days a week; free, confidential, and anonymous; available on a province-wide basis; and accessible by all (interpretation is available in more than 140 languages).

OPGH is an efficient, effective, and well run organization within the limitations placed on it. It maintains a range of statistics showing trends in calls but is unable to provide details of callers and what happens to them after they make contact with the Helpline.

United Kingdom

The GamCare Helpline is a confidential counseling, advice, and information service for anyone affected by a gambling dependency. It combines telephone counseling, crisis intervention, information delivery, referrals, and professional consultancy. The staff at the helpline are professionally trained and receive clinical supervision.

The GamCare Helpline was launched in 1997 at a time when gambling was being repositioned in the United Kingdom as a mainstream leisure activity, particularly through the hugely successful introduction of the National Lottery. Before the launch of the GamCare Helpline, the primary support for problem gamblers seeking help was the Gamblers Anonymous (GA) 24-hour helpline. However, this was allowed to offer support only within the standard format of GA. The British Amusement Catering Trades Association (BACTA) also funded a private service for young problem gamblers. A few other local helplines included gambling, but none of these were able to provide a depth of understanding to adequately address the high level of specialist needs and demands of the problem gambler. Since then, the impact of the growing gambling market and the implications of the liberalization of the UK gaming regime have made the need for a national helpline even more imperative.

The Helpline Target Population

The GamCare Helpline is "caller" (or client) centered. The premise upon which it is built is that the provision of help and support should be tailored to meet the demands of its caller population. The Helpline is specifically targeted to reach three main groups – the problem gambler; the partner, parent, or family member of a problem gambler; and professionals working in the field of gambling dependency or working with gambling-related issues.

The intensity of living with a problem gambler produces its own insecurities and fears every bit as profound, critical, and painful as that experienced by the gambler. GamCare has worked with many partners of problem gamblers and recognized that they, too, suffer feelings of desperation, guilt, anger, and depression, along with symptoms of physical illness such as headaches, stomach problems, breathing difficulties, and backaches. Parents face the distressing impact on the family and themselves of having a son or daughter with a gambling problem.

Some family members take considerable care to conceal their distress. Caught between their love and concern for their partner or child and the desperation of their situation, they have a deep-seated ambivalence about trying to get their own support. They fear that they will not be understood or listened to or that they will be dismissed as simply overreacting. They also fear that any help offered will be inadequate and insufficient or directed solely to the problem gambler. For some friends or family members, this ambivalence is compounded by fears of intimidation or physical violence. For others, it could mean the very real possibility of the break up of their relationship or family leaving them to face the world once again on their own.

Because gambling has become a mainstream leisure activity in the United Kingdom, healthcare professionals and other professional bodies have begun to see an increase in the number of people with gambling-related problems seeking their help. However, in many instances (as with most other jurisdictions), these professionals have been unable to fully assess gambling problems or intervene effectively. The lack of scientific data about gambling and the lack of funding for studies to investigate problem and pathological gambling have contributed to many professionals not having an adequate understanding of gambling related issues. GamCare, therefore, regards it as important that information and support is offered to professionals and to providers across the gambling spectrum in order that they may be made aware of the possible evidence of gambling problems, trained to identify their presence, and encouraged to make appropriate referrals.

What the GamCare Helpline claims as its point of uniqueness in the United Kingdom is its focus on counseling (i.e., not just information and referral). The Helpline's single most important feature is its capacity to offer immediate and either one-off or multisession counseling over the phone and deliver that counseling in such a way that it meets the conflicts and dilemmas of those who seek to use it. By so doing, it helps to attract many who would not normally engage in the counseling process.

Providing the Immediate Response

GamCare has analyzed its "market" and concluded that most problem gamblers who call the Helpline are seeking support in much the same way that they gamble. They are often impulsive and have a propensity to act when they find themselves in a crisis situation but then not follow through once the pressure of that crisis is relieved (a situation familiar throughout the mental health field). Their energy and motivation may often be tentative, short term, focused on finding a quick-fix solution or a way to modify their gambling but with little willingness to contemplate moving beyond the immediate stimulus to action.

The opportunity to access immediate support and have a one-stop resource at the point of call enables such callers to obtain the greatest amount of support with the minimum amount of frustration, confusion, and delay. If they are simply handed over to another agency or given a series of other numbers to contact when they do manage to call, it is very likely that their attempt to get support will end there and then. If, however, they are able to immediately receive counseling without having to make it to an on-site appointment and then go on to have a positive counseling experience, they are much more likely to sustain their motivation and be willing to receive further support. If immediacy is combined with the flexibility and anonymity of helpline counseling, this will help reduce the risk of personal exposure and social stigma that is often attached to seeking support and also widen the socio-economic group able to get help. Those problem gamblers, for example, without transport (and/or situated away from main centres), with limited mobility or with disability can access counseling when they may not be able to otherwise. Equally, those in high-profile positions or those from the ethnic communities, who would not necessarily encounter face-to-face counseling "cold," may use helpline counseling more readily.

Building a Bridge

Many problem gamblers, however, find it very difficult to ask for help, even when they are quite desperate to do so. The crisis they may find themselves in leaves them feeling unsafe and out of control. When they do call the helpline, they often use a practical or information request or the starting point of "someone else's problem" as the only acceptable way they can find of asking for help for themselves. Others may use the helpline to air their ideas; to check if their feelings are "normal," or just to check out what is involved. Here, the counselor's primary aim is to build a bridge between the place of crisis and danger to the place of safety and opportunity to move forward.

Holding the Ambivalence

Once that bridge has been made, the helpline can become for many gamblers a holding mechanism enabling them to contain and clarify issues they are struggling with until they are ready to move forward. Beneath the problem gambler's layer of impulsiveness lie particular insecurities and fears. Shame is known to be a strong factor among problem gamblers. A fragile or damaged person fears being found out and judged. Some seek help only when they are coerced or blackmailed into doing so. Others, although propelled by the pain or sheer desperation of their situation, may find themselves having second thoughts immediately after they have asked for help. They may feel guilty, angry, and trapped, and although they are often very good at concealing their emotions the very fact that they need help only serves to highlight their humiliation. Many people with a gambling problem talk of their loss of control; for some this sense is also present when they feel they "have to" ask for help.

All of this heightens the problem gambler's high degree of ambivalence about seeking out help. On the one hand, they fear failure—that in the end nothing will change and this will be added to all the other failures in their life. At the same time, they fear success—that changes will need to be made but at the cost of giving up the one comfort they have, namely their gambling.

Contracting for Counseling

Some problem gamblers do, however, want to work on a regular or weekly basis with the same counselor. When this is possible, the balance of control is altered. A contract is agreed between the caller and the helpline counselor, and although the caller continues to make the calls it is the counselor who sets the objectives of counseling and makes sure they are maintained. "Soft" contracts allow call times to be more open and flexible but where a "hard" contract is agreed, sessions are fixed in terms of date, length, and number.

The Importance of Training and Supervision

In the end, however, it is the sensitivity and skills of the helpline counselor and his or her ability to establish a good working relationship or alliance with the caller that will determine the effectiveness and quality of the service. The skills needed to be an effective helpline counselor are considerable. When working on the telephone active listening has to be more acute than in face-to-face counseling. However, when working with gambling issues, skills in the area of assessment making and particularly in managing the issue of control are especially needed. Control is very important for the problem gambler who may be reluctant to make a long-term commitment to resolving their situation. He or she may only call once, which will inevitably mean that the helpline counselor will have less time to build up a relationship. During that one call, the gambler may bring a list of issues to the counselor but not allow him- or herself the opportunity of working with them (i.e., give permission for the counselor to explore them). The gambler may also carry unrealistic expectations of what can be achieved in the one call.

All this places heavy demands on the helpline counselor and highlights the fundamental importance of building in to the helpline a structure of ongoing training and clinical supervision.

GamCare developed its approach in response to the impact that the growing gambling market was having in the United Kingdom. Its importance and uniqueness lies in its strong emphasis on the provision of helpline counseling. It may be that callers will not resolve all their deep emotional issues and conflicts over the telephone. However, evidence from the first 7 years of operation does suggest that the helpline is being effective in meeting its fundamental aim of being a support for all those affected in one way or another by a gambling dependency.

GamCare is in the fortunate position of being able to offer both helpline and face-to-face services, so providing a seamless transition for clients; but it has also recognized that well trained and supported people on the phones provide the motivation to help callers on to the path of long-term, sustained change.

A number of gambling helplines, such as New Zealand Gambling Helpline and GamCare, are increasingly run on commercial lines, even when they are not for profit organizations. As a result, some of the language and attitudes are changing within those organizations; it is not uncommon to hear of "customer focus" rather than client- centered approaches. As a result, staff have to be equipped with good negotiating and selling skills; after all, those skills are essential in facilitating a change in basic behavior.

New Zealand: The Developing Role of the Helpline in an Integrated Care Approach

Background to the New Zealand Gambling Helpline

First established as a hotline in 1992, the Gambling Helpline was a pioneer in extending its work beyond the simple provision of information and passing on of contact details for therapists. From the start, there was an element of counseling and motivational enhancement involved in the interaction with callers. The hotline also gathered information about callers and began to build a database that would allow some analysis of the caller population.

In 1998, the current NZ Gambling Helpline was established and took over the systems and some staff of the hotline. It set out to overcome the criticisms of helplines concerning "proof of adding value" (i.e., caller records and outcomes). It immediately developed a computerized database that now has records of more than 25,000 callers and 200,000 calls. It also developed its "hard referral" system. This involves the NZ Gambling Helpline setting up three-way calls with callers and therapists to facilitate acceptance of, and need for, one on one appointments; providing written records to the therapist (with caller permission); offering an appointment reminder call to the caller on behalf of the therapist; checking whether the caller attended the appointment (and preparing to remotivate callers who are "no-shows"); and following up on caller progress over time (see the section on Integrated Care later in this chapter). The "conversion rate" of gamblers, that is, callers who move on to face–to-face appointments, is around 60%.

With its extensive records and involvement in the wider therapeutic process, the NZ Helpline has been recognized as having great potential value as a research tool in its own right. It is currently undertaking work with a number of academic institutions to go to the next stage of development.

The NZ Gambling Helpline is run on commercial lines but with a public good ethos that it derives from its owner, LifeLine (the New Zealand branch of Lifeline International, a leading crisis intervention and counseling service). It has a Board of Directors drawn from both the helping sector and (non-gambling) industry. Recently the Helpline, as part of its review of its 3-year strategy, changed its name from Problem Gambling Helpline Service to Gambling Helpline, to drop the emphasis on "problem" and to reduce the labeling that such a word implies. The NZ Gambling Helpline certainly sees itself as a customer-centric organization.

Volumes and Services

The NZ Helpline had contact with more than 4500 new people in the peak 2004 year and several thousand repeat callers. Gamblers represent around 60% of all callers; significant others (family members, etc.) a further 30%; and more general inquiries make up the remainder. Prank calls, inquiries about lottery winning numbers, and so forth h are not included in the following statistics.

Since the peak, two major factors have changed the New Zealand landscape. The Gambling Act 2003 came into force and the Ministry of Health took over purchasing and contractual arrangements from the private sector. This took away some freedom of action and expression from helping agencies and generated a degree of "big brother" apprehension. In addition, smoke-free legislation came into effect; the large dropoff in caller numbers coincided with (was caused by?) the legislation. It is not yet clear whether the smoke-free legislation in particular will be of lasting effect. A full range of statistics can be found on the NZ Helpline's Web site (www.gamblingproblem.co.nz).

New Services

Over the past 3 years, the NZ Helpline has introduced a range of new services, with a view to offering a greater level of customization to the needs of callers. It has introduced dedicated lines for Maori (First Nations), Pacific peoples, youth, and debt

Table 17.3 New Zealand Gambling Helpline Contacts

	1999	2000	2001	2002	2003	2004	2005	2006
New clients	3393	3595	3735	4594	4538	4300	2875	2661
Repeat clients	1836	2847	3096	5505	7973	9009	7537	5732
Total contacts	11,023	14149	13524	19151	20453	21396	18366	16062

Source: Gambling Helpline database.

management. It has trialed an initiative to support gay/lesbian/bisexual/transgender people with gambling issues (anecdotal evidence suggests that young people with sexual identity issues may turn to gambling as a form of escape). It has a Talking Point forum on its Web site where peer support is available. Also, importantly, it has staff dedicated to outcalls; calling the client to check on progress and motivation for as long as it takes the client to become comfortable with his or her progress.

The Web site and forum have increased in significance, and this may well also be an important factor in the decline in the number of callers. There are now hundreds of visits each day to the Helpline's two (general and youth-oriented) Web sites. Anecdotal evidence to the NZ Gambling Helpline suggests more and more people would like to try avenues such as self-help and peer support before embarking on counseling or other interventions.

Helping the Gaming Industry

The NZ Gambling Helpline, together with a gambling policy and training organization (Responsible Gambling Consulting International), developed and trialed a specialist service for parts of the gaming industry to offer dedicated support for staff (and patrons). The Gambling Act 2003 placed explicit demands on venue staff to identify and intervene with problem gamblers but little training or support was available for frontline staff. The trial was discontinued because of lack of agreement on funding and a low level of promotion and demand. However, in its short life the dedicated helpline had a key role in preventing several potential suicides.

Integrated Care

Since 2004, the NZ Gambling Helpline has been working in collaboration with face to face therapists to offer what is termed the Integrated Care program for clients. Under this scheme, clients are referred from the therapist to the Helpline for ongoing support and monitoring over a period of 18 months to 2 years (or longer at the client's request). This involves regular checks on progress (including South Oaks Gambling Screen (SOGS) and spend levels) as well as motivational interviewing and, where appropriate, referral back to the therapist. This process is beginning to demonstrate both the difficulty in keeping contact with gamblers and the success of treatment to a level that was not previously possible.

The Importance of Standards

As with GamCare in the United Kingdom, the importance of training, supervision, and support has been recognized by the NZ Gambling Helpline. All recruits to the Helpline's telephone staff have to undergo a rigorous standard orientation and training course, irrespective of past experience or qualifications. This introduction typically requires more than 100 hours of training and is followed by mandatory, ongoing training and personal supervision as well as quality monitoring. Progress through various grades depends on satisfactory performance over sustained periods. This is made easier by two key factors:

- All telephone counselors are paid.
- There is a two-volume Operations and Administration Manual available for reference. This manual is maintained in consultation with the staff who use it. It includes sections covering:

    - Strategy, goals, and values of the Helpline
    - Services provided
    - Agency advice, referrals, and directory
    - Gambling venue support
    - Clients' and stakeholders' interests
    - Quality control
    - Client surveys, feedback, and complaint procedures
    - Staff training
    - Assessment, early identification, and screening
    - Case management and ongoing support
    - Key workers assigned to callers
    - Web site and talking point forum
    - Information packs
    - Referral and service handover
    - Culture and community
    - E-mail counseling
    - Taping/listening to calls
    - Documenting client contact
    - Client safety and confidentiality
    - Staff safety and support
    - Debriefing and supervision
    - Performance management and career development
    - Information systems and policies

Looking Forward

Useful as the first stage of Integrated Care has been, it is only a start. The NZ Gambling Helpline's view is that longer term support and motivation are essential elements of recovery from a gambling problem. And such support needs to be placed in a structured environment, not least to be able to assess the efficacy of the various approaches to treatment that are currently employed.

In addition, the whole environment is changing as technology and demand increase on an international scale. In New Zealand, in particular, the regulatory/

legislative environment has been altered by the introduction of the Gambling Act 2003, which places gambling and problem gambling firmly in the public health arena. Looking forward, the NZ Helpline faces some key assumptions about this changing environment:

- Gambling spend will continue to increase.
- New technologies will increase gambling penetration (today's slot or poker machines will be superseded).
- Presentations for help are likely to increase substantially as gambling issues gain more public attention.
- There will be a broader mix of presenting needs (including the so-called "worried well" or early-onset problems).
- Family doctors are likely to be involved (but may lack both time and expertise).
- Some populations will be at particular risk (e.g., youth, older people).
- Demand for longer term support will grow.
- Demand for information about gambling in general and problem gambling in particular will increase.
- The current model (where face-to-face therapy is offered to all) will be unaffordable with major growth (no one will fund a large increase in expensive therapy).
- Alternative support mechanisms will be required (including the use of technology and self-help programs).

Carlo DeClemente has pointed out that there is a major relapse rate for people with gambling problems. But he added that this relapse tendency is just as evident in other fields, and not just addictions. One hour of therapy every week for 6 weeks leaves more than 1000 hours without intervention. Yet frequent brief interventions could potentially reduce the relapse rate dramatically. This is a role the Helpline is ideally placed to fulfill, in collaboration with other agencies (not just therapists but also doctors, financial advisers, spiritual advisers, etc.).

The Helpline in New Zealand sees itself as a first and last contact service, supplementing other specialist services across a wide spectrum. In addition, it is well placed to use technology as a medium for help; this is covered in the next section.

Where next?

A number of agencies are already working on the next generation of Helplines. These move beyond traditional models of referral and information and even beyond the standard telephone as sole or prime communication tool. Hybrid models of support and therapy are being developed and tested around the world; these will result in the traditional view of the helpline becoming obsolete. The result should provide a truly "customer focused" and customized approach being available to help the real people who are caught up in problem gambling.

The following examples from Canada, the United Kingdom, and New Zealand represent some of the creative and leading edge thinking coming out of the helpline environment.

Canada—Centre for Addictions and Mental Health (CAMH)

CAMH embarked on a project in Ontario to develop and test a telephone-based treatment program and delivery model for problem gamblers. It is estimated that 340,000 adults (18 years and older) in Ontario are experiencing gambling problems of moderate to high severity but the treatment take-up rate is extremely low. As a result, the sector has been operating well below capacity.

Cognitive–behavioral therapies (CBTs) are being developed to deliver and evaluate a telephone-based program, with a carefully constructed manual for therapists and clients to use. The program is founded on advanced clinical design, coupled with a flexible and customer-oriented[1] delivery model. It is intended to increase help-seeking rates and to be available for everyone in the province.

The program as envisioned includes three formats: self-directed (workbook and online versions), low-intensity counseling (face-to-face and telephone-based versions), and high intensity counseling (face-to-face and telephone-based). The self-directed format is intended for clients who prefer to work independently, and have a history of completing undertakings on their own (i.e., higher self-efficacy). The low-intensity counseling format offers the same client handbook as the self-directed version, but provides four to six sessions, each of approximately 15 minutes' duration, with a counselor who "coaches" with problems and confirms that the client is on track. This format increases confidence levels among those who choose it, and provides a safety net in the event of difficulties. The high-intensity format increases counselor contact to approximately 4 hours, and provides direct assistance in developing skills, providing support, and solving problems. It is intended for people who anticipate considerable difficulty in successfully changing their behavior, and who have high needs for support and assistance (i.e., lower self-efficacy). Two additional features are designed to enhance completion and success rates. First, clients are permitted to switch formats/versions should their initial selection prove unsatisfactory. Such flexibility introduces alternatives to dropping out. Second, clients are given control over the pace of program delivery (i.e., faster or slower). This feature increases confidence levels by giving control over the rate at which new skills are learned and adopted.

Finally, in recognizing that people differ in how quickly they learn and master new skills, innovative CBTs include the option of client-initiated booster sessions. These sessions provide extra help with problems that remain after program

---

[1] Note the increasing trend to move away from the "patient" or "problem gambler" labels to think of callers as customers and the consequent mind shift that implies for counselors, etc.

completion. The program model incorporates booster sessions delivered by trained Helpline staff (complementing the after-hour crisis counseling services already provided).

A central telephone-based registration system is the entry point for the new treatment program. Located within the existing Problem Gambling Helpline infrastructure, this entry point can be accessed through the current toll-free number. Helpline staff are trained to answer questions about treatment options and to help callers select a preferred format and version (self-assessment questions/protocols will be developed for this purpose). In addition, staff are able to register callers who wish to sign up, making the inquiry/registration process truly a one-stop experience.

Use of the Helpline to keep records, including the provision of treatment information, client registration, counselor/agency assignment, and post-treatment follow-up, allows for the incorporation of a sophisticated monitoring and evaluation component. Registration information, entered directly on a computer database by Helpline staff, also serves as baseline data for ongoing evaluation of completions and outcome status.

CAMH has set targets for take up of the program and aims to reach 10,000 clients in year 5 (about 3% of the problem gambling population). However, recruitment of clients into the trial program was slow and the critical mass had not been achieved for completing the research.

United Kingdom—The Gambling Therapy Project

The Gambling Therapy project "ehelpline" was run from November 2004 to March 2005 by the Gordon House Association, a charity specializing since 1971 in the treatment of gambling addicts. The project's objective was to provide a pilot online support platform on which to trial, analyzes, and develop online support services for problem gamblers and those affected by them. It used standard commercial Internet products and servers.

Background

The nature of the ways in which gambling is promoted and experienced has changed radically as a result of the very effective ways in which gambling has exploited the new communication technologies. In addition, there has been a change in the way that many, especially the younger generations, now choose to communicate via the Internet, or by texting, rather by traditional methods. Gordon House Association wanted to respond to these changes and provide a service that allowed individuals to access support and help using whatever communication channel they were most able and comfortable with. This project set out to identify and assess the feasibility of such a service.

Basis

The pilot project was hosted by the Web site: www.gamblingtherapy.org. Here Gordon House Association offered live referral advice by way of customized Internet services—a chatroom, e-mail, sms messaging, and telephone call-back service, based on the new online assessment and counseling tools provided by www.DistanceTherapy.com. These tools were designed specifically to enforce security levels for therapeutic work far in excess of conventional Internet "security," without creating barriers to client access.

Visitors found the service by way of the Gordon House Web site, by Internet search, and by way of the GamCare link found on some Internet gambling sites. It was not advertised or promoted.

Key Features

The Adviser/Assessor

The chatroom, which featured a live cam picture of an assessor, was operated for 7 to 8 hours a day by adviser/assessors observed and supervised by a professional counselor. The adviser/assessors were recovering problem gamblers giving their own time voluntarily to help others in the situation they once found themselves to be in. The adviser/assessor assesses the needs of the caller and sends appropriate links (client options) to other local and Internet support service providers best suited to the caller's needs. The assessor will also be able to use some of his or her own experiences (without self-disclosures to the caller) to make any suggestions that may help the caller put coping techniques in place. The pilot operated a two-tiered system to ensure the maximum number of service users were able to connect immediately to an assessor, while only appropriate calls were allowed to book the more expensive and limited time of a counselor.

The Observer/Supervisor

The observer's role was to give guidance and support to the adviser/assessor when he or she was online to the caller. For example, the adviser/assessor might have been unsure of a response to a particular question asked by the caller. The observer was also able to recognize if or when the adviser/assessor may be getting out of his or her depth or becoming personally affected by the caller's issues.

The Counselor

The role of the counselor in Gambling Therapy was to work with the caller on a one-to-one basis in a confidential online counseling room that was developed as closely as possible to echo the dynamics of face-to-face counseling. This included the option of the client seeing the counselor and the counselor seeing the client via web cams (allowing the reading of body language), the option of either party using voice rather than text, art and drawing white board options, and the use of a unique text system that the counselor could use to "interrupt" the client and prevent the client from deleting those words or phrases the client may inadvertently use that can provide the counselor with valuable clues as to how the client is really feeling when in denial or avoidance.

E-mail

The e-mail facility was a 24-hour option for the person with a gambling problem and for family and friends affected by a gambling problem. They could write down their thoughts and feelings at any time day or night. Once they had a reply, they could then make their own choices as to either continue to communicate in this way, connect to the adviser/assessor, or book a counseling session. These e-mails could be sent using Gordon House's server, allowing individuals who do not have an Internet account of their own, and those who are accessing the service from a location where they cannot use their account, e.g., public library or Internet café, to send secure and confidential e-mails asking for help.

Therapeutic Conclusions

The pilot grew to deal with over a thousand visitors a week to the site (without promoting the service nor with direct links from online gambling sites). Feedback from users indicated that the service was highly effective, both in moving clients on to full counseling and in providing timely support for action by the friends and families of potential clients.

Much has been learned from the pilot. For example:

- Callers engage more rapidly and with greater intensity than in face-to-face or telephone services.
- Although technology allows it, an assessor/adviser cannot work with more than one client at a time.
- Training is essential in many practical aspects of working online (e.g., how to ensure the cam picture of the adviser does not show the adviser speaking to the supervisor).
- The service is valuable in helping recovered addicts consolidate their own resolve.
- The need for this service has been proved and quantified.
- How best to deliver the service.

It is well established that people say and do things in cyberspace that they might not ordinarily say or do in the face-to-face world. They feel more uninhibited and express themselves more openly. As a consequence, online callers appear to require shorter sessions than equivalent telephone callers. This effect allows friends and family to seek help on behalf of those with problems more easily, without feelings of disloyalty. More than half the calls to the helpline were of this type. Following such approaches there was the chance to engage with the problem gambler him- or herself, being able to engage earlier in the development of a problem, finding distressing stories and difficult circumstances that further emphasized the benefit of the online service.

As with many other initiatives, particularly in the rapidly changing (especially with new legislation to come into force in late 2007) and tightly funded UK problem gambling sector, ongoing funding is a major issue.

New Zealand—Extending the Integrated Care Approach and the Use of Technology

As with the Canadian and British examples above, the New Zealand approach blurs the boundaries between the Helpline and the face-to-face therapist. The first step in providing help is to gather information for screening purposes. The Helpline can, and often does, do the initial screen, using, for example, the Canadian Problem Gambling Severity Index (CPGSI) or SOGS. This can now be done either on the Web (where an interactive CPGSI-based screen is available) or over the phone or a combination of both. In discussion with the caller, on the phone or via e-mail, decisions can be made about the best form of help. This might include therapy, other specialist advice, or simply an ongoing maintenance program via the Helpline. The philosophy underpinning the concept is one of helping the client/caller (customer) to re-empower him- herself. Assuming a referral is made, information from the initial contact covering not just the CPGSI but all other relevant factors, for example, alcohol consumption, mental disorders, and family/social/economic issues can be passed on. A therapist might then undertake a fuller assessment/screen and decide a course of action. However, there is an additional advantage in the Helpline undertaking the initial screening: the client has some understanding of what information is needed and the first face-to-face encounter is not taken up by what is often perceived by clients as time-wasting administration.

The therapist also seeks assistance from the Gambling Helpline in supporting the client between sessions and this might involve specific exercises (e.g., CBT activities), or other activities such as ensuring financial or medical advice is obtained, through to simply making contact with the client to keep her or him motivated to follow through with a full program of help. The Helpline can report back to the therapist on what has transpired between sessions.

Over a period of weeks, this process can be recycled until the therapist is content to close the case. At this stage, on ongoing follow-up and support program can be agreed among client, therapist, and Helpline, through to reporting of long-term outcomes.

A truly seamless and customized service focused on the needs of the individual can be expected to be both effective and cost efficient, and initial experience is that clients do not object to agencies sharing information if it will help the process of overcoming gambling problems.

Implications and Issues

There are some implications in the variety of initiatives or programs being explored and these will need to be worked through. They include the following:

- How can therapists and other agencies be convinced to "share" clients?
- How can protocols be established to share case management?
- Who "owns" the case at any given point?
- What elements (e.g., CBT) should be in an integrated program?
- What needs to be done face-to-face, on the phone, or through other means, for example, the Internet?
- How can client agreement to a multiagency support program be obtained?
- What are the training implications for Gambling Helpline and other agency staff?
- Who will pay for shared case management and ongoing support?
- What measures will be put in place, over what period, to evaluate the effectiveness of such a program?

Sharing "Best Practice"/Performance Data

As helplines increasingly come into the mainstream of therapy and other forms of support, so they will need to conform to "best practice," not least in order to protect clients as well as ensure the agencies are adequately funded. To date there is no consensus on what best practice means. The first steps taken in Phoenix (as outlined in the preceding text) and the follow-up in 2006 are no more than the opening of dialogue among the "poor relations" of the problem gambling helping field. What is now needed is some measure of consistency; information share; and research and development. A first step that has been proposed is the agreement of a minimum data set. This in turn could include, for example, a Balanced Scorecard approach to operations and results, including, for example:

- Staffing:
  - Structure
  - Numbers of counselors/others (relative to market)
  - Training/development programs
  - Qualifications of staff
  - Turnover of staff
  - Hours worked by staff (shift length/frequency)
  - Supervision methods

- Clients

  - Numbers and trends
  - Call numbers (new v repeat) and trends
  - Satisfaction measures
  - Outcomes achieved
  - Referrals to other services (and show up rates)
  - Gambling modes/trends

- Financial

  - Cost per operating hour (normalized to local pricing)
  - Cost per call
  - Cost per client
  - Counselor pay rates (versus norms in the local market)

- Process

  - Counseling models
  - Information gathered/recorded
  - Information supplied
  - Call length

Reaching international consensus on these issues will undoubtedly be difficult. However, some agencies already have reasonably advanced understanding of their own sectors and would be willing to share experience and expertise. The challenge for Gambling Helplines and their funders now is to recognize the changing nature of the problem gambling market; the developing expectations of "customers"; the strides in technology development; and the need to adapt and evaluate responses to changes over time.

Acknowledgments The author thanks the following people for providing much of the detailed information on what is happening in different jurisdictions around the world: Keith Whyte, Executive Director, National Council on Problem Gambling, USA, especially for data from the first survey of gambling helplines; Adrian Scarfe, Clinical Manager, GamCare, UK, for general insights as well as information on the UK scene; Trixie Roberts and colleagues, Datasmith Director, Gambling Therapy, UK, especially for information on the online trial in the United Kingdom; Krista Ferguson, CEO, New Zealand Gambling Helpline, for New Zealand statistics and the updated Gambling Helpline survey; Tony Toneatto, Centre for Addiction and Mental Health, Toronto, in particular for sharing thoughts on the research basis for telephone counseling.

References

Abbot, M. W., Volberg, R. A., Bellringer, M., & Reith, G. (2004). *A review of research aspects of problem gambling: Summary, conclusions and recommendations*. Auckland: Auckland University of Technology.

Abbott, D. A., & Cramer, S. L. (1993). Gambling attitudes and participation: A Midwestern survey. *Journal of Gambling Studies, 9*(3), 247–263.

Abt, V., & McGurrin, M. C. (1991). The politics of problem gambling: Issues in the professionalization of addiction counseling. In Eadington, W. R., Cornelius, J. A. (Eds.), *Gambling and public policy: International perspectives* (pp. 657–659). Reno: University of Nevada Press.

Abt, V., McGurrin, M., & Smith, J. (1985). Toward a synoptic model of gambling behavior. *Journal of Gambling Behavior, 1*(2), 79–88.

Abt, V., Smith, J. F., & Christiansen, E. M. (1985). *The business of risk: Commercial gambling in mainstream America*. Lawrence, KA: University Press of Kansas.

Ackerman, P. T., Dykman, R. A., & Peters, J. E. (1977). Teenage Status of Hyperactive and Non-Hyperactive Learning Disabled Boys. *American Journal of Orthopsychiatry, 47*, 577–596.

Adlaf, E. M., & Ialomiteanu, A. (2000). Prevalence of problem gambling in adolescents: Findings from the 1999 Ontario Student Drug Use Survey. *Canadian Journal of Psychiatry, 45*, 752–755.

Alberta Alcohol & Drug Abuse Commission. (1994). *Impacts of problem gambling*. Edmonton: AADAC.

Alcoholics Anonymous World Services (AAWS), Inc. (1976). *Alcoholics Anonymous: The story of how many thousands of men and women have recovered from alcoholism*. New York: Alcoholics Anonymous World Services.

Alexander, B. K. (2001). The roots of addiction in free market society. Retrieved August 27, 2007 from http://www.policyalternatives.ca/bc/rootsofaddiction.html

Allock, C. C. (1986). Pathological gambling. *Australian and New Zealand Journal of Psychiatry, 20*, 259–265.

Allock, C. C., & Grace, D. M. (1988.) Pathological gamblers are neither impulsive nor sensation-seekers. *Australian and New Zealand Journal of Psychiatry, 22*, 307–311.

Almaas, A. (1996). *The point of existence: Transformations of narcissism in self-realization*. Berkeley, CA: Diamond Books.

American Psychiatric Association. (1994). *Diagnostic and statistical manual of mental disorders* (4th ed.). Washington, DC: American Psychiatric Association.

Anders, G. C. (1998). Indian gaming: Financial and regulatory issues. *Annals of the American Academy of Political and Social Science, 556*, 98–108.

Anderson, G., & Brown, R. I. F. (1984). Real and laboratory gambling, sensation-seeking and arousal. *British Journal of Psychology, 75*, 401–410.

Andrews, D. L., & Jackson, S. J. (Ed). (2001). *Sport stars: The cultural politics of sporting celebrity*. New York: Routledge.

Anjoul, F. (1999, November). *A revised history of gambling*. Paper presented at Culture and the Gambling Phenomenon, the Eleventh Conference of the National Association for Gambling Studies, Sydney.

Anjoul, F. (2003). An empirical investigation of cognitive process in problem gamblers. PhD Thesis. University of Sydney.

Annis, H. M., Herie, M. A., & Watkin-Merek, L. (1996). *Structured relapse prevention*. Addiction Research Foundation: Toronto.

Anton, R. F., Pettinati, H., Zweben, A., Kranzler, H. R., Johnson, B., Bohn, M. J., et al.(2004). A multi-site dose ranging study of nalmefene in the treatment of alcohol dependence. *Journal of Clinical Psychopharmacology, 24*, 421–428.

Antze, P. (1979). Role of ideologies in peer psychotherapy groups. In M. A. Lieberman & L.D. Borman (Eds.), *Self-help groups for coping with crisis: origins, members, processes, and impacts* (pp. 272–304). London: Jossey-Bass.

Antze, P. (1987). Symbolic action in Alcoholics Anonymous. In: M. Douglas (Ed.), *Constructive drinking: Perspectives on drink from anthropology*. New York: Cambridge University Press.

Argo, T. R., & Black, D. W. (2004). Clinical characteristics. In J. E. Grant & M. N. Potenza (Eds.), *Pathological gambling: A clinical guide to treatment* (pp. 39–53). Washington, DC: American Psychiatric Publishing.

Arkes, H. R., & Blumer, C. (1985). The psychology of sunk cost. *Organizational Behavior and Human Decision Processes, 35*, 124–140.

Arnold, L. (2000, May 5) Study examines gambling impact. *Newscan, 2*(18). Retrieved August 27, 2007 from http://www.cfcg.org/flash-newscan-newslink.html

Asbury, H. (1938). *Suckers' progress: An informal history of gambling in America*. New York: Thunder Mouth Press.

Assagiolo, R. (1971). *Psychosynthesis*. New York: Hobbs, Dorman.

Auckland Research Centre for Business Law. (1998). *Good faith in insurance law*. Auckland, New Zealand: University of Auckland.

Ausloos, G. (1995). *La compétence des familles*. France: Éditions Érès.

Avineri, S. (1968). *The social and political thought of Karl Marx*. New York: Cambridge University Press.

Azmier, J., Clemens, M., Dickey, M., Kelley, R., & Todosichuk, P. (2001). Gambling in Canada 2001: An overview. *Gambling in Canada Research Report, 13*, 1–17.

Babad, E., & Katz, Y. (1991). Wishful thinking–Against all odds. *Journal of Applied Social Psychology, 21*, 1921–1938.

Baron, R. (1995). *Psychology* (3rd ed.). Boston: Allyn & Bacon.

Batchelor, S. (2004). *Living with the devil: A meditation on good and evil*. New York: River Head Books.

Bateson, G. (1972). In *Steps Toward an Ecology of Mind*. New York: Ballantine.

Battersby, M. W., Ask, A., Reece, M. M., Markwick, M. J., & Collins, J. P. (2001). A case study using the "problems and goals approach" in a coordinated care trial: SA HealthPlus. *Australian Journal of Primary Health, 7*, 45–48.

Bayda, E. (2003). *At home in the muddy water: A guide to finding peace within the everyday chaos*. Boston: Shambhala.

Beaudoin, C. M., & Cox, B. J. (1999). Characteristics of problem gambling in a Canadian context: A preliminary study using a DSM–IV–based questionnaire. *Canadian Journal of Psychiatry, 44*, 483–486.

Bechara, A. (2003). Risky business: Emotion, decision-making, and addiction. *Journal of Gambling Studies, 19*, 23–51.

Beck, A. T. (1976). *Cognitive Therapy and the Emotional Disorders*. New York: Meridian.

Beck, A.T., Rush, A. J., Shaw, B. F. & Emery, G. (1979). *Cognitive Therapy of Depression*. New York: Guilford.

Beck, A. T., & Steer, R. A. (1990). *Beck anxiety inventory manual*. New York: Harcourt Brace Jovanovich.

Beck, A., Ward, C., Mendelson, M., Mock, J., & Erbaugh, J. (1961). An inventory for measuring depression. *Archives of General Psychiatry, 4*, 561–571.

Beck, D., & Cowan, C. (1996). *Spiral dynamics: Mastering values, leadership, and change*. Cambridge, MA: Blackwell.

Becona, E., Del-Carmen-Lorenzo, M., & Fuentes, M. (1996). Pathological gambling and depression. *Psychological Reports, 78*, 635–640.

Bem, D. (1972). Self-perception theory. In L. Berkowitz (Ed.), *Advances in experimental social psychology* (Vol. 6, pp. 1–62). New York: Academic Press.

Berger, H. L. (1988). Compulsive gamblers: Relationships between their games of choice and their personalities. In W. R. Eadington (Ed.), *Gambling research: Proceedings of the seventh international conference on gambling and risk taking* (5, pp. 159–179.9). Reno, University of Nevada.

Bergler, E. (1970). *The psychology of gambling.* New York: International Universities Press.

Bergler, E. (1957). *The psychology of gambling.* London: International Universities Press.

Berry, D. C., & Dienes, Z. (1993). *Implicit learning, theoretical, and empirical issues.* East Sussex: Lawrence Erlbaum Associates.

Bersabe, R., & Arias, R. M. (2000). Superstition in gambling. *Psychology in Spain, 4*(1), 28–34. Retrieved from http://www.psychologyinspain.com/content /full/2000/3.htm

Bilocq-Lebeau, L., Cantin, M., & Hamel, H. (2002). *Jeu : Aide et référence.* Rapport annuel 2001–2002. Montréal: Centre de Référence du grand Montréal.

Black, D. W. (2004). An open-label trial of bupropion in the treatment of pathologic gambling. *Journal of Clinical Psychopharmacology, 24*, 108–110 [letter].

Black, D. W., & Moyer, T. (1998a). Clinical features and psychiatric comorbidity of subjects with pathological gambling behavior. *Psychiatric Services, 49*(11), 1434–1439.

Black, D. W., & Moyer, T. (1998b). Clinical features and psychiatric comorbidity of subjects with pathological gambling behaviour. *Psychiatric Services, 49*(11), 1434–1439.

Blackmore, S. J. (1992). Psychic experiences: Psychic illusions, *Skeptical Inquirer 16*, 367–376. Retrieved from http://www.uwe.ac.uk/fas/staff/sb/si92.html

Blackwell, R. T., Galassi, M. D. & Watson, T. E. (1985). Are cognitive assessment methods equal? A comparison of think aloud and thought listing. *Cognitive Therapy and Research, 9*, 399–413.

Blackwell, T. (June 22, 2001). Provinces rake in 9 billion [sic] on gaming. *Newscan, 3*(25). Retrieved August 27, 2007 from http://www.cfcg.org/flash-newscan-newslink.html.

Blanck, R., & Blanck, G. (1979). *Ego psychology II : Psychoanalytic developmental psychology.* New York: Columbia University Press.

Blanco, C., Moreyra, P., Nunes, E. V., Saiz-Ruiz, S., & Ibanez, A. (2001). Pathological gambling: Addiction or compulsion? *Seminars in Clinical Neuropsychiatry, 6*, 167–176.

Blanco, C., Petkova, E., Ibanez, A., & Saiz-Ruiz, J. (2002). A pilot placebo-controlled study of fluvoxamine for pathological gambling. *Annals of Clinical Psychiatry, 14*, 9–15.

Bland, R., Newman, S., Orn, H., & Stebelsky, G. (1993). Epidemiology of pathological gambling in Edmonton. *Canadian Journal of Psychiatry, 38*(2), 108–112.

Blascovich, J., Ginsburg, G. P., & Howe, R. C. (1976). Blackjack choice shifts in the field. *Sociometry, 39*, 274–276.

Blascovich, J., Ginsburg, G. P., & Veach, T. L. (1975). A pluralistic explanation of choice shifts on the risk dimension. *Journal of Personality and Social Psychology, 31*, 422–429.

Blaszczynski, A. (1999). Pathological gambling and obsessive-compulsive disorders. *Psychological Reports, 84*, 107–133.

Blaszczynski, A. (March, 2000). Pathways to pathological gambling: Identifying typologies. *E-Gambling: The Electronic Journal of Gambling Issues, 4.* [Online serial]. Retrieved from http://www.camh.net/egambling/issue4/research/.

Blaszczynski, A. P., & Farrell, E. (1998). A case series of 44 completed gambling-related suicides. *Journal of Gambling Studies, 14*(2), 91–109.

Blaszczynski, A., Huynh, S., Dumlao, V. J., & Farrell, E. (1998). Problem gambling within a Chinese speaking community. *Journal of Gambling Studies, 14*(4), 359–380.

Blaszczynski, A., & Maccallum, F. (2003). Pathological gambling and suicidality: An analysis of severity and lethality. *Suicide and Life-Threatening Behavior, 33*(1), 88.

Blaszczynski, A. P., & McConaghy, N. (1988). Assessed psychopathology in pathological gamblers. *Psychological Reports, 62*, 547–552.

Blaszczynski, A. P., & McConaghy, N. (1989a). The medical model of pathological gambling: Current shortcomings. *Journal of Gambling Behavior, 5*(1), 42–52.

Blaszczynski, A., & McConaghy, N. (1989b). Anxiety and/or depression in the pathogenesis of addictive gambling. *The International Journal of the Addictions, 24*(4), 337–350.

Blaszczynski, A. P., & McConaghy, N. (1993). A two- to nine-year treatment follow-up study of pathological gambling. In W. Eadington & J. A. Cornelius (Eds.), *Gambling behavior and problem gambling.* Reno, NV: Institute for the Study of Gambling and Commercial Gambling.

Blaszczynski, A. P., McConaghy, N., & Frankova, A. (1989). Crime, antisocial personality and pathological gambling. *Journal of Gambling Behaviour, 5,* 137–152.

Blaszczynski, A., McConaghy, N., & Frankonova, A. (1991). Control versus abstinence in the treatment of pathological gambling: A two to nine year follow-up. *British Journal of Addiction, 86,* 299–306.

Blaszczynski, A. P., McConaghy, N., & Winters, S. W. (1986). Plasma endorphin levels in pathological gambling. *Journal of Gambling Studies, 2,* 3–14.

Blaszczynski, A., & Nower, L. (2002). A pathways model of problem and pathological gambling. *Addiction, 97*(5), 487–499.

Blaszczynski, A. P., & Silove, D. (1995). Cognitive and behavioral therapies for pathological gambling. *Journal of Gambling Studies, 11,* 195–220.

Blaszczynski, A., & Steel, Z. (1998). Personality disorders among pathological gamblers. *Journal of Gambling Studies, 14*(1), 51–71.

Blaszczynski, A. P., Wilson, A. C., & McConaghy, N. (1986). Sensation seeking and pathological gambling. *British Journal of Addiction, 81,* 113–117.

Bloch, H. A. (1951). The sociology of gambling. *American Journal of Sociology, 57,* 215–221.

Blum, K., Cull, J. G., Braverman, E. R., Chen, T. J. H., & Comings, D. E. (1996). Reward deficiency syndrome: Addictive, impulsive and compulsive disorders including alcoholism, attention-deficit disorder, drug abuse and food bingeing may have a common genetic basis. *American Scientist, 84,* 132–145.

Blume, S. B. (1986). Treatment for the addictions: Alcoholism, drug dependence and compulsive gambling in a psychiatric setting-South Oaks Hospital, Amityville, New York. *Journal of Substance Abuse Treatment, 3,* 131–133.

Blume, S. B. (1987). Compulsive gambling and the medical model. *Journal of Gambling Behavior, 3*(4), 237–247.

Bollas, C. (1987). *The shadow of the object.* London: Free Association Books.

Boorstin, D. J. (1992). *The image: A guide to pseudo-events in America.* New York: Random House.

Bostwick, J. M., & Pankratz, V. S. (2000). Affective disorders and suicide risk: A reexamination. *American Journal of Psychiatry, 157*(12), 1925–1932.

Bowen, J. T. (1996). Casino marketing. In William F. Harrah College of Hotel Administration International Gaming Institute (Eds.), *The gaming industry* (pp. 139–156). NewYork: John Wiley & Sons.

Boyd, W. H., & Bolen, D. W. (1970). The compulsive gambler and spouse in group psychotherapy. *International Journal of Group Psychotherapy, 20,* 77–90.

Brahen, L. S., Capone, T., Wiechert, V., & Desiderio, D. (1977). Naltrexone and cyclazocine. A controlled treatment study. *Archives of General Psychiatry, 34,* 1181–1184.

Brandt, J., Butters, N., Ryan, C., & Bayog, R. (1983). Cognitive loss and recovery in long-term alcohol abusers. *Archives of General Psychiatry, 40,* 435–442.

Brenner, R. (1990). *Gambling and speculation: A theory, a history, and a future of some Human decisions.* New York: Cambridge University Press.

Brenner, R., & Brenner, G. (1993). *Spéculation et jeux de hasard, une histoire de l'homme par le jeu.* Paris: Presses Universitaires de France.

Briggs, J. R., Goodin, B. J., & Nelson, T. (1996). Pathological gamblers and alcoholics: Do they share the same addictions? *Addictive Behaviors, 21*(4), 515–519.

Briley, D. A., & Wyer, R. S. (2001). Transitory determinants of values and decisions: The utility (or nonutility) of individualism and collectivism in understanding cultural differences. *Social Cognition, 19,* 197–227.

Broekkamp, C. L., & Phillips, A. G. (1979). Facilitation of self-stimulation behavior following intracerebral microinjections of opioids into the ventral tegmental area. *Pharmacology, Biochemistry, and Behavior, 11*, 289–295.

Brook, A. (1994). *Kant and the mind.* Cambridge: Cambridge University Press.

Brown, R. I. F. (1985). The effectiveness of gamblers anonymous. In W. R. Eadington (Ed.), *The gambling studies: Proceedings of the sixth national conference on gambling and risk taking* (5, 258–284). Reno: University of Nevada.

Brown, R. I. (1986a). Dropouts and continuers in gamblers anonymous: Life context and other factors. *Journal of Gambling Behavior, 2*, 130–140.

Brown, R. I. F. (1986b). Arousal and sensation-seeking components in the general explanation of gambling and gambling addictions. *The International Journal of the Addictions, 21*(9,10), 1001–1016.

Brown, R. I. F. (1987a). Dropouts and continuers in Gamblers Anonymous: Part 2. Analysis of free-style accounts of experiences with GA. *Journal of Gambling Behavior, 3*(1), 68–79.

Brown, R. I. F. (1987b). Dropouts and continuers in Gamblers Anonymous: Part 3: Some possible specific reasons for dropout. *Journal of Gambling Behavior, 3*(2),137–152.

Brown, R. I. (1987c). Dropouts and continuers in Gamblers Anonymous: Part 4. Evaluation and summary. *Journal of Gambling Behavior, 3*, 202–210.

Brown, R. I. F. (1987d). Pathological gambling and associated patterns of crime: Comparisons with alcohol and other drug addictions. *Journal of Gambling Behavior, 3*(2), 96–114.

Brown, R. I. F. (1987e). Classical and operant paradigms in the management of gambling addictions. *Behavioural Psychotherapy, 15*, 111–122.

Brown, R. I. F. (1987f). Models of gambling and gambling addictions as perceptual filters. *Journal of Gambling Behavior, 3*(4), 224–236.

Brown, R. I. F. (1988). Models of gambling and gambling addictions as perceptual filters. *Journal of Gambling Behavior, 4*, 224–236.

Brown, R. I. F. (1993). Some contributions of the study of gambling to the study of other addictions. In W. R. Eadington & J. A. Cornelius (Eds.), *Gambling behavior and problem gambling* (241–272). Reno: University of Nevada.

Browne, A., Salomon, A., & Bassuk, S. S. (1999). The impact of recent partner violence on poor women's capacity to maintain work. *Violence Against Women, 5*(4), 393–426.

Browne, B. R. (1989). Going on tilt: Frequent poker players and control. *Journal of Gambling Behavior, 5*(1), 3–21.

Browne, B. R. (1991). The selective adaptation of the Alcoholics Anonymous program by Gamblers Anonymous. *Journal of Studies on Gambling, 7*(3), 187–206.

Browne, B. R. (1994). Really not God: Secularization and pragmatism in Gamblers Anonymous. *Journal of Gambling Studies, 10*(3), 247–260.

Browne, B., & Brown, D. (1994). Predictors of lottery gambling among American college students. *Journal of Social Psychology, 134*(3), 339–345.

Buda, R., & Elsayed-Elkhouly, S.M. (1998). Culture differences between Arabs and Americans: Individualism-collectivism revisited. *Journal of Cross-Cultural Psychology, 29*, 487–492.

Bufe, C. (1991). *Alcoholics Anonymous: Cult or cure?* San Francisco: See Sharp Press.

Bujold, A., Ladouceur, R., Sylvain, C., & Boisvert, J. M. (1994). Treatment of pathological gamblers: An experimental study. *Journal of Behavioral Therapy and Experimental Psychiatry, 25*, 275–282.

Brunelle, C., Korman, L., Collins, J., & Cripps, E. (2005, June). *Anger, Gambling, and Substance Use: Is There a Functional Relationship?* Paper presented at Harvey Stancer Research Day, University of Toronto, Toronto, Ontario.

Bureau du coroner du Québec. (2004). *Relevé des sucides de joueurs compulsifs.* 25 Février.

Bush, G., Vogt, B. A., Holmes, J., Dale, A. M., Greve, D., Jenike, M. A., & Rosen, B. R. (2002). Dorsal anterior cingulate cortex: a role in reward-based decision making. *Proceedings of the National Academy of Science of the United States of America, 99*, 523–528.

Bybee, S. (1996). *Gaming regulation control.* Las Vegas: APS.

Caldwell, G. (1974). The gambling Australian. In Edgar, D. E. (Ed.), *Social Change in Australia* (pp. 12–28), Melbourne: Cheshire.

Camelot. (1995). *The National Lottery 1st Anniversary Press Pack.* Author: London.

Campbell, C. S. & Smith, G. J. (1998). Canadian gambling: Trends and public policy issues. *Annals of the American Academy of Political and Social Science, 556,* 22–35.

Campbell, J. (1968). *The hero with a thousand faces* (2nd ed.). Princeton, NJ: Princeton University Press.

Canadian Centre on Substance Abuse. (1996). http://www.ccsa.ca/gmbi.htm Ottawa: National Council of Welfare.

Canadian Foundation on Compulsive Gambling (Ontario). (1996). *Vision of and role in the Province of Ontario's comprehensive strategy for combating problem and compulsive gambling.* Ontario: Ontario Ministry of Health, Substance Abuse Bureau.

Canadian Foundation on Compulsive Gambling. (1999). Newlink Problem Gambling News & Information, Spring Issue, 12.

Carlton, P. L., & Goldstein, L. (1987). Physiological determinants of pathological gambling. In T. Galski (Ed.), *Handbook on pathological gambling.* Springfield, IL: Charles C Thomas.

Carlton, P. L., & Manowitz, P. (1994). Factors determining the severity of pathological gambling in males. *Journal of Gambling Studies, 10*(2), 147–157.

Carlton, P. L, Manowitz, P., McBride, H., Nora, R., Swartzburg, M., & Goldstein, L. (1987). Attention deficit disorder and pathological gambling. *Journal of Clinical Psychiatry, 48*(12), 487–488.

Carotenuto, A. (1985). *The vertical labyrinth.* Toronto, ON: Inner City Books.

Carotenuto, A. (1996). *To love to betray, life as betrayal.* Wilmette, IL: Chiron Publications.

Carrier, J., & Mitchell, N. (2007). Transpersonal theories. In D. Capuzzi & D. Gross (Eds.), *Counselling and psychotherapy: Theories and interventions* (4th ed.). Upper Saddle River, NJ: Pearson Prentice-Hall.

Carrig, H., Cheney, B., Philip-Harbutt, J., & Picone, W. (1996). *Coming to grief.* Towards 2000: The Future of Gambling. Seventh National Conference of the National Association for Gambling Studies, Adelaide, South Australia, pp. 271–277.

Carver, C. S., & Scheier, M. F. (1994). Situational coping and coping dispositions in a stressful transaction. *Journal of Personality and Social Psychology, 66,* 184–195.

Cassirer, E. (1955). *The philosophy of the enlightenment.* New Haven: Yale University Press.

Castellani, B. (2000). *Pathological gambling: The making of a medical problem.* New York: State University of New York Press.

Castellani, B., & Rugle, L. (1995). A comparison of pathological gamblers to alcoholics and cocaine misusers on impulsivity, sensation seeking, and craving. *International Journal of the Addictions, 30*(3), 275–289.

Castellani, B., Wootton, E., Rugle, L.,Wegeworth, R., Prabucki, K., & Olson, R. (1996). Homelessness, negative affect, and coping among veterans with gambling problems who misused substances. *Psychiatric Services, 47*(3), 298–299.

Castonguay, A (2004, April 10). Coût du jeu au Québec: 2.5 milliards de dollars. *Le Devoir.* Retrieved, from http://www.ledevoir.com

Cavedini, P., Riboldi, G., Keller R, D'Annucci, A., & Bellodi, L. (2002). Frontal lobe dysfunction in pathological gambling. *Biological Psychiatry, 51,* 334–341.

Chevalier, S., Geoffrion, C., Audet, C., Papineau, É., & Kimpton, M-A. (2003). *Évaluation du programme experimental sur le jeu pathologique. Rapport 8—Le point de vue des usagers.* Montréal : Institut nationale de sante publique du Québec.

Christiansen, E. M. (1998). Gambling and the American economy. *Annals of the American Academy of Political and Social Science, 556,* 36–52.

Clapson, M. (1992). *A bit of a flutter: Popular gambling and English society, c. 1823–1961.* Manchester: Manchester University Press.

Clotfelter, C. T., & Cook, P. (1989). *Selling hope: State lotteries in America.* London and Cambridge, MA: Harvard University Press.

Coccaro, E. F. (1996). Neurotransmitter correlates of impulsive aggression in humans. *Annals of the New York Academy of Science, 794,* 82–89.

Cochrane, R., & Stopes-Roe, M. (1977). Psychological and social re-adjustment of Asian immigrants to Britain: A community survey. *Social Psychiatry, 12*, 195–206.

Collins, J., Skinner, W., and Toneatto, T. (2005). Beyond Assessment: The Impact of Comorbidity of Pathological Gambling, Psychiatric Disorders and Substance Use Disorders on Treatment Course and Outcomes. Final report to the Ontario Problem Gambling Research Centre. http://www.gamblingresearch.org/contentdetail.sz?cid=145.

Coman, G., Burrows, G., & Evans, B. (1997). Stress and anxiety as factors in the onset of problem gambling: Implications for treatment. *Stress Medicine, 13*, 235–244.

Comings, D. (1998, June). The genetics of pathological gambling: The addictive effect of multiple genes. Paper presented at the National Conference on Problem Gambling, Las Vegas.

Comings, D. E., Rosenthal, R. J., Lesieur, H. R., Rugle, L. J., Muhleman, D., Chiu, C., Dietzand, G., & Gade, R. (1996). A study of the dopamine D_2 receptor gene in pathological gambling. *Pharmacogenetics, 6*, 223–234.

Condry, J., & Scheibe, C. (1989). Non program content of television: Mechanisms of persuasion. In J. Condry (Ed.), *The psychology of television* (pp. 217–219). London: Erlbaum.

Conventry, K. R., & Norman, A. (1998). Arousal, erroneous verbalizations and the illusion of control during a computer-generated gambling task. *British Journal of Psychology, 89*, 629–646.

Cook-Greuter, S. (1990). Maps for living: Ego development stages from symbiosis to conscious universal embeddedness. In M. Commons et al. (Eds.), *Adult development, Vol. 2: Models and methods in the study of adolescent and adult thought*. New York: Praeger.

Coram, A. T. (1997). Social class and luck: Some lessons from gambler's ruin and branching processes. *Political Studies, 45*(1), 66–77.

Corless, T., & Dickerson, M. G. (1989). Gamblers' self-perceptions of the determinants of impaired control. *British Journal of Addiction, 84*, 1527–1537.

Cornish, D. B. (1978). *Gambling: A review of the literature and its implications for policy and research*. London: HMSO.

Cortwright, B. (1997). *Psychotherapy and spirit: Theory and practice in transpersonal psychotherapy*. Albany, NY: State University of New York Press.

Costa, N. (1988). *Automatic pleasures: The history of the coin machine*. London: Kevin Francis.

Coulombe, A., Ladouceur, R., Desharnais, R., & Jobin, J. (1992). Erroneous perceptions and arousal among regular and occasional poker players. *Journal of Gambling Studies, 8*(3), 235–244.

Cox, B. J., Kwong, J., Michaud, V., & Enns, M. W. (2000). Problem and probable pathological gambling: Considerations from a community survey. *Canadian Journal of Psychiatry, 45*, 548–552.

Crisp, B. R., Thomas, S. A., Jackson, A. C., Thomason, N., Smith, S., Borrell, J., Ho, W., & Holt, T. A. (2000). Sex differences in the treatment needs and outcomes of problem gamblers. *Research on Social Work Practice, 10*(2), 229–242.

Crockford, D. N., & el-Guebaly, N. (1998a). Naltrexone in the treatment of pathological gambling and alcohol dependence. *Canadian Journal of Psychiatry, 43*, 86 [letter].

Crockford, D. N., & el-Guebaly, N. (1998b). Psychiatric comorbidity in pathological gambling: A critical review. *Canadian Journal of Psychiatry, 43*(1), 43–50.

Cromer, G. (1978). Gamblers Anonymous in Israel: A participant observation study of a self-help group. *The International Journal of the Addictions, 13*(7), 1069–1077.

Crosbie, P. (1996, January 6). So what's your chances of winning č40m? *The Daily Express*, pp. 27–29.

Cunningham-Williams, R. M., Cottler, L. B., Compton, W. M., & Spitznagel, E. L. (1998). Taking chances: Problem gamblers and mental health disorders-Results from the St. Louis Epidemiological Catchment Area Study. *American Journal of Public Health, 88*(7), 1093–1096.

Cunningham-Williams, R. M., Cottler, L. B., Compton, W. M., Spitznagel, E. L., & Ben-Abdallah, A. (2000). Problem gambling and comorbid psychiatric and substance use disorder among drug users recruited from drug treatment and community settings. *Journal of Gambling Studies, 16*(4), 347–376.

Cunningham, J. A., Sobell, L. C., & Sobell, M. B. (1998). Awareness of self-change as a pathway to recovery for alcohol abusers: Results from five different groups. *Addictive Behaviors, 23,* 399–404.

Custer, R. (1982a). Gambling and addiction. In R. J. Craig & S. L. Baker (Eds.), *Drug dependent patients: Treatment and research* (pp. 367–381). Springfield, IL: Charles C Thomas.

Custer, R. (1982b). An overview of compulsive gambling. In P. A. Carone, S. F. Yolles, S. N. Kieffer,& L. W. Krinsky (Eds.), *Addictive disorders update: Alcoholism/drug abuse/ gambling.* New York & London: Human Sciences Press.

Custer, R. L., & Milt, H. (1985). *When luck runs out.* New York: Warner Books.

Daghestani, A., Elenz, E. & Crayton, J. (1996). Pathological gambling in hospitalized substance abusing veterans. *Journal of Clinical Psychiatry, 57*(8), 360–362.

Dannon, P. N., Lowengrub, K., Gonopolski, Y., Musin, E., & Kotler, M. (2005). Topiramate versus fluvoxamine in the treatment of pathological gambling: a randomized, blind-rater comparison study. *Clinical Neuropharmacology, 28,* 6–10.

Darbyshire, P., Oster, C. & Carrig, H. (2001). The experience of pervasive loss: Children and young people living in a family where parental gambling is a problem. *Journal of Gambling Studies, 17*(1), 23–45.

David, F. (1962). *Games, gods, and gambling.* New York: Hafner Press.

Davison, K. P., Pennebacker. J. W., & Dickerson, S. S. (2000). Who talks? The social psychology of illness support groups. *American Psychologist, 55*(2), 205–217.

Dawes, R. M. (1988). *Rational choice in an uncertain world.* New York: Harcourt Brace College Publishers.

DeCaria, C., Hollander, E., & Wong, C. (August 27, 2007). Neuropsychiatric functioning in pathological gamblers. Paper presented at the National Conference on Problem Gambling, New Orleans.

de Champlain, P. (2004). *Mobsters, gangsters and men of honour: Cracking the mafia code.* Toronto: HarperCollins.

Deffenbacher J.L. (1995). Ideal treatment package for adults with anger disorders. In H Kassinove (Ed.), *Anger disorders: Definition, Diagnosis and Treatment* (pp. 151-172). Washington D.C.: Taylor & Francis.

Deffenbacher, J., & McKay, M. (2000). Overcoming Situational and General Anger: A Protocol for the Treatment of Anger Based on Relaxation, Cognitive Restructuring, and Coping Skills Training.

Delfabbro, P. (2005). *Gambling in South Australia: Trends and priorities.* Adelaide, Department of Psychology: University of Adelaide.

Delfabbro, P., & Winefield, A. (1999). Poker machine gambling: An analysis of within session characteristics. *British Journal of Psychology, 90,* 425–439.

Delfabbro, P., & Winefield, A. (2000). Predictors of irrational thinking in regular slot machine players. *Journal of Psychology, 134*(2), 117–128.

Derevensky, J. L., & Gupta, R. (2000). Prevalence estimates of adolescent gambling: A comparison of the SOGS-RA, DSM-IV-J, and the GA 20 Questions. *Journal of Gambling Studies, 16*(2/3), 227–251.

Derevensky, J., & Gupta, R. (2004). Adolescents with gambling problems: A review of our current knowledge. *The Electronic Journal of Gambling Issues, 10,* 119–140.

Derevensky, J., Gupta, R., & Winters, K. (2003). Prevalence rates of youth gambling problems: Are the current rates inflated? *Journal of Gambling Studies, 19,* 405–425.

Desai, R. A., Maciejewski, P. K., Dausey, D.J., Caldarone, B. J., & Potenza, M. N. (2004). Health correlates of recreational gambling in older adults. *American Journal of Psychiatry, 161*(9), 1672–1679.

Di Chiara, G., & North, R. A. (1992). Neurobiology of opiate abuse. *Trends in Pharmacological Science, 13,* 185–193.

Dickerson, M. (1979). FI schedules and persistence at gambling in the U.K. betting office. *Journal of Applied Behavioural Analysis, 12,* 315–323.

Dickerson, M. G. (1984). *Compulsive gamblers.* London: Longman.

Dickerson, M. G. (1993). Internal and external determinants of persistent gambling: Problems of generalizing from one form of gambling to another. *Journal of Gambling Studies, 9*(3), 225–245.

Dickerson, M. G. (1996). Why slots equals "grind" in any language: The cross-cultural popularity of the slot machine. In J. McMillen (Ed.), *Gambling cultures: Studies in history and interpretation* (pp. 152–166). London: Routledge.

Dickerson, M., & Adcock, S. (1987). Mood, arousal and cognitions in persistent gambling: Preliminary investigation of a theoretical model. *Journal of Gambling Behavior, 3*(1), 3–15.

Dickerson, M., Baron, E., Hong, S-M., & Cottrell, D. (1996). Estimating the extent and degree of gambling related problems in the Australian population: A national survey. *Journal of Gambling Studies, 12*(2), 161–178.

Dickerson, M., Hinchy, J., & Fabre, J. (1987). Chasing, arousal, and sensation seeking in off-course gamblers. *British Journal of Addiction, 82*, 673–680.

Dickerson, M. G., Hinchy, J., Legg-England, S., & Cunningham, R. (1992). On the operant determinants of persistent gambling behaviour. I. High-frequency poker machine players. *British Journal of Psychology, 83*, 237–248.

DiClemente, C. C., & Prochaska, J. O. (1998). Toward a comprehensive, transtheoretical model of change: Stages of change and addictive behaviors. In W. R. Miller & N. Heather, (Eds)., *Treating addictive behaviors* (2nd ed). New York: Plenum.

DiClemente, C. C., Prochaska, J. O., Fairhurst, S., Velicer, W. F., Rossi, J. S., & Velasquez, M. (1991). The process of smoking cessation: An analysis of precontemplation, contemplation and contemplation/action. *Journal of Consulting and Clinical Psychology, 59*, 295–304.

DiClemente C. C., Story, M., & Murray, K. (2000). On a roll: The process of initiation and cessation of problem gambling among adolescents. *Journal of Gambling Studies, 16*, 289–314.

Diskin, K. & Hodgins, D.C. (2001). Narrowed focus and dissociative experiences in a community sample of experienced video lottery gamblers. *Canadian Journal of Behavioural Science, 33*, 58–64.

Dorion, J. P., & Nicki, R. M. (2001). Epidemiology of problem gambling in Prince Edward Island: A Canadian microcosm. *Canadian Journal of Psychiatry, 46*, 413–417.

Dostoevsky, F. (1992). *The gambler.* Trans. J. Kentish. Oxford: Oxford University Press.

Douglas, A. (1995). *British charitable gambling 1956–1994: Towards a national lottery.* London: Athlone Press.

Douglas, V. I. (1984). The psychological processes implicated in ADD. In L. M. Bloomingdale (Ed.), *Attention deficit disorder: Diagnostic, cognitive, and therapeutic understanding* (pp. 147–162). New York: Spectrum.

Douglas, V. I., & Parry, P. A. (1983). Effects of reward on delayed reaction time task performance of hyperactive children. *Journal of Abnormal Child Psychology, 11*, 313–326.

Dryden, W. & Ellis, A. (1988). Rational-emotive therapy. In K. S. Dobson (Ed.), *Handbook of Cognitive-Behavioral Therapies.* (pp. 214–272). New York: Guilford.

Downes, D. M., Davies, B. P., David, M. E., & Stone, P. (1976). *Gambling, work and leisure: A study across three areas.* London: Routledge and Kegan Paul.

Dube, D., Freeston, M. H., & Ladouceur, R. (1996). Potential and probable pathological gamblers: Where do the differences lie? *Journal of Gambling Studies, 12*(4), 419–430.

Dutton, D.G., & Golant, S.K. (1995). *The Batterer: A Psychological Profile.* New York: Harper-Collins.

Duvarci, I., Varan, A., Coskumol, H. & Ersoy, M. A. (1997). DSM-IV and the South Oaks Gambling Screen: Diagnosing and assessing pathological gambling in Turkey. *Journal of Gambling Studies, 3*(3), 193–206.

Eade, V. H., & Eade, R. H. (1997). *Introduction to the casino entertainment industry.* Upper Saddle River, NJ: Prentice-Hall.

Eadington, W. (1995). Gambling: Philosophy and policy. *Journal of Gambling Studies, 11*(1), 9–13.

Eadington, W. R. (2003). Values and choices: The struggle to find balance with permitted gambling in modern society. In G. Reith (Ed.), *Gambling: Who wins? Who loses?* (pp. 31–48). Amherst, New York: Prometheus Books,

Edwards, G. (1990). *Dependence: uncertainties, mysteries and doubts.* In P.G. Erickson & H. Kalant (Eds.). Toronto: Addiction Research Foundation.

Eisler, H. (1990). *Gambling into the nineties: A guide to better odds.* Kenthurst, N.S.W.: Kangaroo Press.

Elia, C., & Jacobs, D. F. (1993). The incidence of pathological gambling among Native Americans treated for alcohol dependence. *International Journal of the Addictions, 28*(7), 659–666.

Ellis, A. (1989). Dangers of transpersonal psychology: A reply to Ken Wilber. *Journal of Counseling and Development, 65*, 146–150.

Ellis, A. & Tafrate, C. (1999). *How to Control Your Anger Before It Controls You.* Secaucus, N.J: Citadel Press.

Endler, N. S., & Parker, J. D. (1990). Stated trait anxiety, depression and coping styles. *Australian Journal of Psychology, 42*, 207–220.

Epstein, R. (1976). Theory of gambling and statistical logic (Rev. ed.). New York: Academic Press.

Faveri, A., & Gainer, L. (1996). *A report on gambling activities and related issues among clients of multicultural service providers in Ontario.* Toronto, ON: Addiction Research Foundation.

Feinstein, D., & Krippner, S. (1988). *Personal mythology: The psychology of your evolving self.* Los Angeles: Jeremy P. Tarcher.

Felton, B. J., & Revenson, T. A. (1984). Coping with chronic illness: A study of illness controllability and the influence of coping strategies on psychological adjustment. *Journal of Consulting and Clinical Psychology, 52*, 343–353.

Ferentzy, P., & Skinner, W. (2003). Gamblers Anonymous: A critical review of the literature. *Electronic Journal of Gambling Issues, Issue 9,* Retrieved August 27, 2007 from http://www.camh.net/egambling/.

FERNÁNDEZ-MONTALVO, J. & ECHEBURÚA, E. (2004). Pathological gambling and personality disorders: An exploratory study with the IPDE. *Journal of Personality Disorders, 18*, 500–505.

Ferris & Wynne (2001), predicted gambling problems as measured by the Canadian Problem Gambling Index of Severity, *Journal of Gambling Studies 2006 22*(1): 101–20

Festinger, L. (1957). *A theory of cognitive dissonance.* Stanford, CA: Stanford University Press.

Festinger, L. (1962). *A theory of cognitive dissonance.* Stanford: Stanford University Press.

Fiery, A. (1999). *The Book of Divination.* Chronicle Books. Hong Kong.

Fiorillo, C. D., Tobler, P. N., & Schultz, W. (2005). Adaptive coding of reward value by dopamine neurons. *Science, 307*, 1642–1645.

Fisher, S. E. (1992). Measuring pathological gambling in children: The case of fruit machines in the U.K. *Journal of Gambling Studies, 8*, 263–285.

Fisher, S. E. (1993a). Gambling and pathological gambling in adolescents. *Journal of Gambling Studies, 9*(3), 277–287.

Fisher, S. E. (1993b). The pull of the fruit machine: A sociological typology of young players. *Sociological Review, 41*(3), 446–475.

Fisher, S. E. (1999). A prevalence study of gambling and problem gambling in British adolescents. *Addiction Research, 7*(6), 509–538.

Fisher, S. E. (2000). Measuring the prevalence of sector-specific problem gambling: A study of casino patrons. *Journal of Gambling Studies, 16*(1), 25–51.

Flanagan, B. J. (1988). Alcohol and marijuana use among female adolescent incest victims. *Alcoholism Treatment Quarterly, 5*(1–2).

Flavin, M. (2003). *Gambling in the nineteenth-century English novel: "A leprosy is o'er the land."* Brighton, UK: Sussex Academic Press.

Flavin, D. K., & Morse, R. M. (1991). What is alcoholism? Current definitions and diagnostic criteria and their implications for treatment. *Alcohol Health & Research World, 15*(4), 266–271.

Flett, G., & Hewitt, P. (2002). *Personality factors and substance abuse in relationship violence and child abuse: A review and theoretical analysis.* Brunner-Routledge: New York.

Folkman, S. (1992). Making the case for coping. In B. N. Carpenter (Ed.), *Personal coping: Theory, research, and application* (pp. 31–46). Westport: Praeger.

Folkman, S., Chesney, M., Pollack, L., & Coates, T. (1993). Stress, control, coping and depressive mood in human immunodeficiency virus-positive and negative gay men in San Francisco. *The Journal of Nervous and Mental Disease, 181*, 409–416.

Folkman, S., Lazarus, R. S., Dunkel-Schetter, C., DeLongis, A., & Gruen, R. (1986). Dynamics of a stressful encounter: Cognitive appraisal, coping and encounter outcomes. *Journal of Personality and Social Psychology, 50*, 992–1003.

Foucault, M. (1975). *The birth of the clinic: An archaelolgy of medical perception.* New York: Vintage.

Frank, M., Lester, D., & Wexler, A. (1991). Suicidal behaviour among members of Gamblers Anonymous. *Journal of Gambling Studies, 7*, 249–254.

Frankl, V. (1965). *Man's search for meaning.* New York: Beacon.

Freedman, J., & Fraser, S. (1966). Compliance without pressure: The foot-in-the-door technique. *Journal of Personality and Social Psychology, 4*, 195–202.

Freeman, M. A., & Bordia, P. (2001). Assessing alternative models of individualism and collectivism: A confirmatory factor analysis. *European Journal of Personality, 15*, 105–121.

Freud, S. (1927). *The future of an illusion.* New York: W. W. Norton.

Freud, S. (1973). *Introductory lectures on psychoanalysis: Vol. 1.* London: Penguin Books.

Frijda, N. H. (1986). *The Emotions.* Cambridge: Cambridge University Press.

G. A. Publishing Company (GAPC). (1964a). *Gamblers Anonymous.* Los Angeles: GAPC.

G. A. Publishing Company (GAPC). (1964b). *The GA Group.* Los Angeles: GAPC.

Gaboury, A., & Ladouceur, R. (1989). Erroneous perceptions and gambling. *Journal of Social Behaviour and Personality, 4*, 411–420.

Gam-Anon International Service Office, Inc. (1986). *Gam-A-Teen.* Whitestone, New York: Gam-Anon International Service Office, Inc.

Gam-Anon International Service Office for Gam-Anon Family Groups. (1988). *The Gam-Anon way of life.* Whitestone, New York: Gam-Anon International Service Office.

Gamblers Anonymous International Service Office (GAISO). (1989). *GA: A new beginning.* Los Angeles: GAISO.

Gamblers Anonymous International Service Office (GAISO). (1999). *Gamblers Anonymous.* Los Angeles: GAISO.

Gamblers Anonymous National Service Office (GANSO). (1978). *The pressure group meeting handbook.* Los Angeles: GANSO.

Getty, H. A., Watson, J., & Frisch, G. R. (2000). A comparison of depression and styles of coping in male and female GA members and controls. *Journal of Gambling Studies, 16(4)*, 377–391.

Giacopassi, D. (1999). Attitudes of community leaders in new casino jurisdictions regarding casino gambling's effects on crime and quality of life. *Journal of Gambling Studies, 15(2)*, 123–147.

Giacopassi, D., Vandiver, M., & Stitt, B.G. (1997). College student perceptions of crime and casino gambling: A preliminary investigation. *Journal of Gambling Studies, 13(4)*, 353–361.

Gibson, M. (1998). Video lottery terminals: The government hype. Retrieved August 27, 2007 from http://www.telusplanet.net/public/gibson/hype.html.

Giddens, A. (1991). *Modernity and self-identity: self and society in late modern age.* Stanford: Stanford University Press.

Gilligan, C. (1982). *In a different voice: Psychological theory and women's development.* Cambridge, MA: Harvard University Press.

Gleick, J. (1987). *Chaos: Making a new science.* New York: Viking Penguin.

Goffman, E. (1967) *Interaction ritual: Essays in face to face behaviour.* New York: Anchor Books.

Goleman, D. (1988). *The meditative mind: Varieties of meditative experience.* Los Angeles: Jeremy P. Tarcher.

Gonzalez-Ibanez, A., Jimenez, S. & Aymami, M. N. (1999) Evaluacion y tratamiento cognitivo-conductual de jugadores patologicos de maquinas recreativas con premio [Evaluation of the cognitive-behavioural treatment of pathological poker machine gamblers]. *Anuario de Psicologia, 30*, 111–125.

Gottlieb, A., Todd, L., & Westlund, D. (1997). *Peyote and other psychoactive cacti*. New York: Ronin Publishing.

Govoni, R. (1998). Five years impact of casino gambling in a community. *Journal of Gambling Studies, 14*(4), 347–358.

Govoni, R., Rupcich, N., & Frisch, G. R. (1996). Gambling behaviour of adolescent gamblers. *Journal of Gambling Studies, 12*(3), 305–317.

Graham, J. R., & Lowenfeld, B. H. (1986). Personality dimensions of the pathological gambler. *Journal of Gambling Behaviour, 2*, 58–66.

Grant, I., Adams, K. M., Carlin, A. S., Rennick, P. M., Judd, L. L., Schooff, K., & Reed, R. (1978). Organic impairment in polydrug users: Risk factors. *American Journal of Psychiatry, 135*, 178–184.

Grant, J. E., Kim, S. W., & Potenza, M. N. (2003). Advances in the pharmacological treatment of pathological gambling. *Journal of Gambling Studies, 19*, 85–109.

Grant, J. E., Kim, S. W., Potenza, M. N., Blanco, C., Ibanez, A., Stevens, L. C., & Zaninelli, R. (2003). Paroxetine treatment of pathological gambling: A multi-center randomized controlled trial. *International Clinical Psychopharmacology, 18*, 243–249.

Grant, J. E., Potenza, M. N., Hollander, E., Cunningham-Williams, R., Nurminen, T., Smits, G., & Kallio, A. (2006). A multicenter investigation of the opioid antagonist nalmefene in the treatment of pathological gambling. *American Journal of Psychiatry, 163*, 303–312.

Greenberg, L.S., & Safran, J.D. (1987). Emotion in psychotherapy: *Affect, cognition and the process of change*. Guilford: New York

Greenlees, E. M. (1988). *Casino accounting and financial management*. Nevada: University of Nevada Press.

Griffiths, M. D. (1989). Gambling in children and adolescents. *Journal of Gambling Behaviour, 5*, 66–83.

Griffiths, M. D. (1990a). The acquisition, development and maintenance of fruit machine gambling in adolescence. *Journal of Gambling Studies, 6*(3), 193–204.

Griffiths, M. (1990b). The cognitive psychology of gambling. *Journal of Gambling Studies, 6*(1), 31–42.

Griffiths, M. D. (1991). The psychobiology of the near miss in fruit machine gambling. *Journal of Psychology, 125*, 347–357.

Griffiths, M. D. (1993). Fruit machine gambling: The importance of structural characteristics. *Journal of Gambling Studies, 9*, 101–120.

Griffiths, M. D. (1994a). The observational analysis of marketing methods in UK amusement arcades. *Society for the Study of Gambling Newsletter, 24*, 17–24.

Griffiths, M. D. (1994b). The role of cognitive bias and skill in fruit machine gambling. *British Journal of Psychology, 85*, 351–369.

Griffiths, M. (1996). *Adolescent gambling*. London: Routledge.

Griffiths, M. D. (1997). The national lottery and instant scratchcards: A psychological perspective. *The Psychologist: The Bulletin of the British Psychological Society, 10*, 26–29.

Griffiths, M. D. (1999a). Gambling technologies: Prospects for problem gambling. *Journal of Gambling Studies, 15*, 265–283.

Griffiths, M. D. (1999b). The psychology of the near miss (revisited): A comment on Delfabbro and Winefield. *British Journal of Psychology, 90*, 441–445.

Griffiths, M. D. (2001). Internet gambling: Preliminary results of the first UK prevalence study. *Journal of Gambling Issues, 5*. Retrieved August 27, 2007 from http://www.camh.net/egambling/issue5/research/griffiths_article.html.

Griffiths, M. D., & Dunbar, D. (1997). The role of familiarity in fruit machine gambling. *Society for the Study of Gambling Newsletter, 29*, 15–20.

Griffiths, M., & Minton, C. (1997). Arcade gambling: A research note. *Psychological Reports, 80*, 413–414.

Griffiths, M. D., & Parke, J. (2002). The environmental psychology of gambling. In G. Reith (Ed.), *Gambling for fun or profit: The controversies of the expansion of commercial gambling in America*. New York: Prometheus Books.

Griffiths, M. D., Parke, J., & Wood, R. T. A. (2002). Excessive gambling and substance abuse: Is there a relationship? *Journal of Substance Abuse, 7*, 187–190.

Griffiths, M. D., & Wood R. T. (2000). Risk factors in adolescence: The case of gambling, video-game playing, and the Internet. *Journal of Gambling Studies, 16,* 199–226.

Griffiths, M., & Wood R. (2001). The case of gambling, videogame playing, and the Internet. *Journal of Gambling Studies. Special Issue: Youth gambling, 16*(2–3), 199–225.

Grinols, E. L. (2003). Right thinking about gambling economics. In G. Reith (Ed.), *Gambling: Who wins? Who loses?* Amherst, NY: Prometheus Books, pp 67–87.

Grodsky, P. B., & Kogan, L. (1985). Does the client have a gambling problem? *Journal of Gambling Behaviour, 1*(1), 51–64.

Grof, C. (1993). *The thirst for wholeness.* New York: Harper Collins.

Grof, S. (1985). *Beyond the brain: Birth, death, and transcendence in psychotherapy.* Albany, NY: State University of New York Press.

Grof, S. (1988). *The adventure of self-discovery.* Albany, NY: State University of New York Press.

Grof, S. (2000). *Psychology of the future.* Albany, NY: State University of New York Press.

Guntrip, J. (1971) *Psychoanalytic theory, therapy, and the self.* New York: Basic Books.

Gupta, R., & Derevensky, J. L. (1997). Familial and social influences on juvenile gambling. *Journal of Gambling Studies, 13,* 179–192.

Gupta, R., & Derevensky, J. (1998a). Adolescent gambling behavior: A prevalence study and examination of the correlates associated with problem gambling. *Journal of Gambling Studies, 14*(4), 319–345.

Gupta, R., & Derevensky, J. (1998b). An empirical examination of Jacob's General Theory of Addictions: Do adolescent gamblers fit the theory? *Journal of Gambling Studies, 14,* 17–49.

Gupta, R., & Derevensky, J. (2001). *An examination of the differential coping styles of adolescents with gambling problems.* Report prepared for the Ontario Ministry of Health and Long-Term Care, Toronto.

Gupta, R., Derevensky, J., & Marget, N. (in press). Coping strategies employed by adolescents with gambling problems. *Child and Adolescent Mental Health.* In press.

Haller, R., & Hinterhuber, H. (1994). Treatment of pathological gambling with carbamazepine. *Pharmacopsychiatry, 27,* 129.

Halliday, J., & Fuller, P. (1974). *The psychology of gambling.* London: Allen Lane.

Hardoon, K., & Derevensky, J. (2002). Child and adolescent gambling behavior: Our current knowledge. *Clinical Child Psychology and Psychiatry, 7*(2), 263–281.

Hardoon, K., Gupta, R., & Derevensky, J. (in press). Psychosocial variables associated with adolescent gambling: A model for problem gambling. *Psychology of Addictive Behaviors.* In press

Harris, A. S. (1996). *Living with paradox: An introduction to Jungian psychology.* Pacific Grove, CA: Brooks/Cole.

Harroch, R. D., Krieger, L., & Reber, A. (2001). *Gambling for dummies.* New York: John Wiley & Sons.

Haw, J. E. (2000). *Gaming machine play.* PhD Thesis. University of Western Sydney.

Hayano, D. M. (1982). *Poker faces: The life and work of professional card players.* Berkeley: University of California Press.

Heakal, R. (2002). What is market efficiency? *Investopedia.* Retrieved March 10, 2006 from http://www.investopedia.com/articles/02/101502.asp.

Heidegger, M. 1968 *What is called thinking?* New York: Harper & Row.

Heineman, M. (1989). Parents of male compulsive gamblers: Clinical issues/treatment approaches. *Journal of Gambling Behaviour, 5*(4), 321–333.

Hendriks, V. M., Meerkerk, G., Van Oers, H. A. M., & Garretsen, H. F. L. (1997). The Dutch instant lottery: prevalence and correlates of at-risk playing. *Addiction, 92*(3), 335–346.

Henriot, C. (1999). Courtship, sex and money: The economics of courtesan houses in nineteenth- and twentieth-century Shanghai. *Women's History Review, 8*(3) 443–467.

Henslin, J. M. (1967). Craps and magic. *The American Journal of Sociology, 73,* 316–330.

Herscovitch, A. G (1999). *Alcoholism and pathological gambling: similarities and differences.* Florida: Learning Publications.

Hess, H. F., & Diller, J. V. (1969). Motivation for gambling as revealed in the marketing methods of the legitimate gambling industry. *Psychological Reports, 25*(1), 19–27.

Higgins, J. (2002). Exploring the relationship of lottery play and religiosity in a sample of western Massachusetts older adults. *Journal of Gambling Studies. 18*(2), 97–159.

Hilliker, G. (2001). *Liability insurance law in Canada* (3rd ed.). Toronto: Butterworths Canada.

Hing, N., & Breen, H. (2001). Profiling lady luck: An empirical study of gambling and problem gambling amongst female club members. *Journal of Gambling Studies, 17*(1), 47–69.

Hodgins, D., & el-Guebaly, N. (2004). Retrospective and Prospective Reports of Precipitants to Relapse in Pathological Gambling. *Journal of Consulting & Clinical Psychology, 72(1),* 72–80.

Hofstede, G. (1980). *Culture's consequences: International differences in work related values.* Beverly Hills, CA: Sage.

Hofstede, G. (1991). *Cultures and organizations: Software of the mind.* Berkshire, UK: McGraw-Hill.

Holahan, C. J., & Moos, R. J. (1987). Personal and contextual determinants of coping strategies. *Journal of Personality and Social Psychology, 52,* 946–955.

Holden, C. (2001). Behavioral addictions: Do they exist? *Science, 294,* 980–982.

Hollander, E., DeCaria, C. M., Finkell, J. N., Begaz, T., Wong, C. M., & Cartwright, C. (2000). A randomized double-blind fluvoxamine/placebo crossover trial in pathologic gambling. *Biological Psychiatry, 47,* 813–817.

Hollander, E., DeCaria, C. M., Mari, E., Wong, C. M., Mosovich, S., Grossman, R., & Begaz, T. (1998). Short-term single-blind fluvoxamine treatment of pathological gambling. *American Journal of Psychiatry 155,* 1781–1783.

Hollander, E., Frenkel, M., DeCaria, C., Trungold, S., & Stein, D. (1992). Treatment of pathological gambling with chlomipramine. *American Journal of Psychiatry, 149,* 710–711.

Hollander, E., Kaplan, A., & Pallanti, S. (2004). Pharmacological treatments. In J. E. Grant & M. N. Potenza (Eds.), *Pathological gambling: A clinical guide to treatment* (pp. 189–205). Washington, DC: American Psychiatric Publishing.

Hollander, E., Pallanti, S., Allen, A., Sood, E., & Baldini Rossi, N. (2005). Does sustained-release lithium reduce impulsive gambling and affective instability versus placebo in pathological gamblers with bipolar spectrum disorders? *American Journal of Psychiatry, 162,* 137–145.

Hollander, E., & Wong, C. M. (1995). Body dismorphic disorder, pathological gambling, and sexual compulsions. *Journal of Clinical Psychiatry, 56,* 7–12.

Holtgraves, T. M. (1988). Gambling as self-presentation. *Journal of Gambling Behavior, 4*(2), 78–91.

Hraba, J., & Lee, G. (1996). Gender, gambling and problem gambling. *Journal of Gambling Studies, 12*(1), 83–101.

Hraba, J., Mok, W., & Huff, D. (1990). Lottery play and problem gambling. *Journal of Gambling Behaviour, 6*(4), 355–377.

Hsu, C. H. C. (1999). *Legalized casino gambling in the United States: The economic and social impact.* Binghamton: Haworth Press.

Hyman, S. E. (1993). Molecular and cell biology of addiction. *Current Opinions Neurology and Neurosurgery, 6,* 609–613.

Ibanez, A., Blanco, C., Donahue, E., Lesieur, H. R., Perez de Castro, I., Fernandez-Piqueras, J., & Saiz-Ruiz, J. (2001). Psychiatric comorbidity in pathological gamblers seeking treatment. *American Journal of Psychiatry, 158,* 1733–1735.

Ide-Smith, S. G., & Lea, S. E. (1988). Gambling in young adolescents. *Journal of Gambling Studies, 8*(2), 167–179.

Israel, J. (2002). *Radical enlightenment: philosophy and the making of modernity 1650–1750.* London: Oxford University Press.

Jackson, A. C., Thomas, S. A., & Blaszczynski, A. (2003). *Best practice in problem gambling services.* Melbourne: Gambling Research Panel.

Jackson, A. C., Thomas, S. A., Thomason, N., Smith, S., Crisp, B. R., Borrell, J., Ho, W. Y., & Holt, T. (1998). Evaluating Victoria's problem gambling services. In G. Coman, B. Evans & R. Wootton (Eds.), *Responsible gambling: A future winner* (pp. 195–203). Adelaide, S.A.: National Association for Gambling Studies.

Jacobi, J. (1959). *Complex, archetype, symbol: In the psychology of C. G. Jung.* New York: Pantheon Books, Bollingen Series 57.

Jacobi, J. (1973). *The psychology of C. G. Jung, an introduction with illustrations.* (R. Manheim.

Trans.). New Haven: Yale University Press.

Jacobs, D. F. (1987). A general theory of addictions: Application to treatment and rehabilitation planning for pathological gamblers. In Galski, T. (Ed.), *Handbook of pathological gambling* (pp. 169–194), Springfield, IL: Charles C Thomas.

Jacobs, D. F. (1988). Evidence for a common dissociative-like reaction among addicts. *Journal of Gambling Behavior, 4*, 27–37.

Jacobs, D. F. (1998). *An overarching theory of addictions: A new paradigm for understanding and treating addictive behaviors.* Paper presented at the National Academy of Sciences Meeting, Washington, D.C.

Jacobs, D. F. (2000). Juvenile gambling in North America: An analysis of long-term trends and future prospects. *Journal of Gambling Studies, 16*(2/3), 119–152.

Jacobs, D. F., Marsten, A. R., & Singer, R. D. (1985). Testing a general theory of addictions: Similarities and differences between alcoholics, pathological gamblers and compulsive overeaters. In J. J. Sanchez-Soza (Ed.), *Health and clinical psychology.* Amsterdam: Elsevier.

Jacobs, D. F., Marston, A., Singer, R., Widaman, L., Little, T., & Veizades, M. (1989). Children of problem gamblers. *Journal of Gambling Behaviour, 5*(4), 261–268.

Jacobs, D. F. (1986). A general theory of addictions: A new theoretical model. *Journal of Gambling Behavior, 2*, 15–31.

Jacoby, M. (1985). *Longing for paradise: Psychological perspectives on an archetype.* Boston, MA: Sigo Press.

Jacoby, M. (1990). *Individuation and narcissism: The psychology of the self in Jung and Kohut.* New York: Routledge.

Jacques, C., & Ladouceur, R. (2003). DSM-IV-J Criteria: A scoring error that may be modifying the estimates of pathological gambling amongst youth. *Journal of Gambling Studies, 19*, 427–432.

Jacques, C., Ladouceur, R., & Ferland, F. (2000). Impact of availability on gambling: A longitudinal study. *Canadian Journal of Psychiatry, 45*, 810–815.

Jahoda, G. (1969). *The psychology of superstition.* London: Allen Lane.

Jellinek, E (1960). *The disease concept of alcoholism.* New Haven: Hill Press.

Jenike, M. A. (1983). Obsessive-compulsive disorder. *Comprehensive Psychiatry, 24*(2), 99–115.

Jentsch, J. D., & Taylor, J. R. (1999). Impulsivity resulting from frontostriatal dysfunction in drug abuse: Implications for the control of behavior by reward-related stimuli. *Psychopharmacology, 146*, 373–390.

Jeu: Aide et reference. (2000). Annual report.Government of Quebec. jar@info-reference.qc.ca.

Johnson, B. A., Ait-Daoud, N., Bowden, C. L., DiClemente, C. C., Roache, J. D., Lawson, K., Javors, M. A., & Ma, J. Z. (2003). Oral topiramate for treatment of alcohol dependence: A randomised controlled trial. *Lancet, 361*, 1677–1685.

Johnson, E. E., & Nora, R. M. (1992). Does spousal participation in Gamblers Anonymous benefit compulsive gamblers? *Psychological Reports, 71*, 914.

Judith, A. (1996). *Eastern body western mind: Psychology and the Chakra system as a path to the self.* Berkeley, CA: Celestial Arts.

Jung, C. G. (1959). *The archetypes and the collective unconscious*, CW 9.I. Princeton, NJ: Princeton University Press.

Kagitcibasi, C., & Berry, J. (1989). Cross-cultural psychology: Current research trends. *Annual Review of Psychology 40*, 493–531.

Kahnemann, D. & Tversky, A. (1982). The psychology of preferences. *Scientific American*, 136–142.

Kalivas, P. W., & Barnes, C. D. (1993). *Limbic motor circuits and neuropsychiatry.* Boca Raton, FL: CRC Press.

Kalivas, P. W., & Volkow, N. D. (2005). The neural basis of addiction: A pathology of motivation and choice. *American Journal of Psychiatry, 162*, 1403–1413.

Kaplan, A., & Hollander, E. (2003). A review of pharmacologic treatments for obsessive-compulsive disorder. *Psychiatric Services, 54*, 1111–1118.

Kaplan, H. K. (1989). State lotteries: Should government be a player? In H. J. Shaffer, S. Stein, B. Gambino, & T. Cummings (Eds.), *Compulsive gambling theory, research and practice* (pp.

187–203). Lexington, MA: D. C. Heath.

Kasprow, M. C., & Scotton, B. W. (1999). A review of transpersonal theory and its application to the practice of psychotherapy. *Journal of Psychotherapy, Practice and Research, 8*, 12–23.

Katie, B. (2001). *Loving what is.* New York: Harmony.

Kazdin, A. (2001). Progress of therapy research and clinical application of treatment requires better understanding of the process. *Clinical Psychology: Science and Practice, 8*, 143–151.

Keene, J., & Rayner, P. (1993). Addiction as a "soul sickness": The influence of client and therapist beliefs. *Addiction Research, 1*, 77–87.

Kegan, R. (1982). *The evolving self: Problem and process in human development.* Cambridge, MA: Harvard University Press.

Khantzian, E. J.(1985). The self-medication hypothesis of addictive disorders: focus on heroin and cocaine dependence. *Am J Psychiatry, 142*(11):1259–64

Kim, S. W. (1998). Opioid antagonists in the treatment of impulse control disorders. *Journal of Clinical Psychiatry, 59*, 159–162.

Kim, S. W., Grant, J. E., Adson, D. E., & Remmel, R. P. (2001b). A preliminary report on possible naltrexone and nonsteroidal analgesic interactions. *Journal of Clinical Psychopharmacology 21*, 632–634 [letter].

Kim, S. W., Grant, J. E., Adson, D. E., & Shin, Y. C. (2001a). Double-blind naltrexone and placebo comparison study in the treatment of pathological gambling. *Biological Psychiatry 49*, 914–921.

Kim, S. W., Grant, J. E., Adson, D. E., Shin, Y. C., & Zaninelli, R. (2002). A double-blind placebo-controlled study of the efficacy and safety of paroxetine in the treatment of pathological gambling. *Journal of Clinical Psychiatry 63*, 501–507.

King, K. M. (1990). Neutralizing marginally deviant behaviour: Bingo players and superstition. *Journal of Gambling Studies, 6*(1), 43–61.

Knapp, T. J., & Lech, B. C. (1987). Pathological gambling: A review with recommendations. *Advances in Behavior Research and Therapy, 9*, 21–449. knowledge. *Clinical Child Psychology and Psychiatry, 7*, 263–281.

Kohlberg, L. (1981). *Essays on moral development: Vol. 1.* San Francisco: Harper & Row.

Kohut, H. (1977). *The restoration of the self.* New York: International University Press.

Koob, G. F. (1992). Drugs of abuse: Anatomy, pharmacology and function of reward pathways. *Trends in Pharmacological Science, 13*, 177–184.

Koob, G. F., & Bloom, F. E. (1988).Cellular and molecular mechanisms of drug dependence. *Science, 242*, 715–723.

Korman, H. (2005). Harry's magic square. *Journal of Family Psychotherapy, 16*(1-2), 89–90

Korman, L. (2005). Concurrent anger and addiction treatment. In *Treating Concurrent Disorders: A Guide for Counsellors* (pp. 215–233). Toronto, ON: Centre for Addiction and Mental Health.

Korman, L. M. & Greenberg, L. S. (1996). Emotion and therapeutic change. In J. Panksepp (Ed.), *Advances in Biological Psychiatry, Vol. II.* (pp. 1–22). Greenwich, CT: JAI Press

Kornfield, J. (1989). *A path with heart: A guide through the perils and promises of the spiritual life.* New York: Bantam Books.

Kramer, A. S. (1988). A preliminary report on the relapse phenomenon among male pathological gamblers. In W. R. Eadington (Ed.), *Gambling research: Proceedings of the seventh international conference on gambling and risk taking (5,* 26–31). Reno: University of Nevada.

Krishnamurti, J. (1954). *The first and last freedom.* New York: Harper and Row.

Kurtz, E. (1979). *Not-God: A history of Alcoholics Anonymous.* Center City, MN: Hazeldon Educational Materials.

Labouvie-Vief, G. (1994). *Psyche & eros.* Cambridge: Cambridge University Press.

Lang, A. (1994). Measuring Psychological Responses to Media Messages. Hillsdale, NJ: Lawrence Erlbaum Associates.

Ladd, G. T., & Petry, N. M. (2003). A comparison of pathological gamblers with and without substance abuse treatment histories. *Experimental & Clinical Psychopharmacology, 11*, 202–209.

Ladouceur, R. (1996a). Erroneous perceptions in generating sequences of random events. *Journal* of Applied Social Psychology, 26, 2157–2166.

Ladouceur, R. (1996b). The prevalence of pathological gambling in Canada. *Journal of Gambling Studies, 12,* 129–142.

Ladouceur, R. (2004). Perceptions among pathological and non-pathological gamblers. *Addictive Behaviors, 29,* 555–565.

Ladouceur, R., Arsenault, C., Dube, D., Freeston, M. H., & Jacques, C. (1997). Psychological characteristics of volunteers in studies on gambling. *Journal of Gambling Studies, 13*(1), 69–84.

Ladouceur, R., Boisvert, J. M., & Dumont, J. (1994). Cognitive-behavioral treatment for adolescent pathological gamblers. *Behavioral Modification, 18,* 230–242.

Ladouceur, R., Bouchard, C., Rhéaume, N., Jacques, C., Ferland, F., Leblond, J., & Walker, M. (2000). Is the SOGS an accurate measure of pathological gambling among children, adolescents and adults? *Journal of Gambling Studies, 16,* 1–24.

Ladouceur, R., Boudreault, N., Jacques, C., & Vitaro, F. (1999). Pathological gambling and related problems among adolescents. *Journal of Child and Adolescent Substance Abuse, 8*(4), 55–68.

Ladouceur, R., & Dube, D. (1997). Erroneous perceptions in generating random sequences: Identification and strength of a basic misconception in gambling behavior. *Swiss Journal of Psychology, 56,* 256–259.

Ladouceur, R., Dube, D., & Bujold, A. (1994a). Prevalence of pathological gambling and related problems among college students in the Quebec metropolitan area. *Canadian Journal of Psychiatry, 49,* 289–293.

Ladouceur, R., Dube, D., & Bujold, A. (1994b). Gambling among primary school. *Canadian Journal of Gambling Studies, 10,* 363–370.

Ladouceur, R., Dube, D., Giroux, I., Legendre, N., & Gaudet, C. (1995). Cognitive biases in gambling: American roulette and 6/49 lottery. *Journal of Social Behavior & Personality, 10*(2), 473–479.

Ladouceur, R., & Gaboury, A. (1988). Effects of limited and unlimited stakes on gambling behavior. *Journal of Gambling Behavior, 4*(2), 119–126.

Ladouceur, R., Jacques, C., Ferland, F., & Giroux, I. (1998). Parents' attitudes and knowledge regarding gambling among youths. *Journal of Gambling Studies, 14*(1), 83–90.

Ladouceur, R., Stinchfield, R., & Turner, N. (2001). *The Canadian Problem Gambling Index: Final report.* Ottawa, Canada: Canadian Centre on Substance Abuse.

Ladouceur R., Sylvian C., Boutin C., & Doucet C. (2002) *Understanding and treating pathological gamblers.* London: John Wiley & Sons.

Ladouceur, R., Sylvain, C., Letarte, H., Giroux, I., & Jacques, C. (1998). Cognitive treatment of pathological gamblers. *Behaviour Research and Therapy, 36,* 1111–1120.

Ladouceur, R., Vitaro, F., & Arsenault, L. (1998). *Consommation de psychotropes et jeux de hasard chez les jeunes: Prévalence, coexistence et conséquences.* Quebec City: Comité permanent de lutte à la toxicomanie.

Ladouceur, R., & Walker, M. B. (1996). A cognitive perspective on gambling. In Salkovskis, P. M. (Ed.), *Trends in cognitive and behavioural therapies* (pp. 89–120). Chichester, UK: John Wiley & Sons.

Ladouceur, R., & Walker, M. (1998). Cognitive approach to understanding and treating pathological gambling. In A. S. Bellack & M. Hersen (Eds.), *Comprehensive clinical psychology.* New York: Pergamon.

Lamberton, A., & Oei, T. P.S. (1997). Problem gambling in adults: An overview. *Clinical Psychology and Psychotherapy, 4*(2), 84–104.

Langer, E. J. (1975). The illusion of control. *Journal of Personality and Social Psychology, 32,* 311–321.

Langer, E. J., & Roth, J. (1975). Heads I win, tails it's chance: The illusion of control as a function of the sequenced outcomes in a purely chance task. *Journal of Personality and Social Psychology, 32,* 951–955.

Langhinrichsen-Rohling, J., Rhode, P., Seeley, J. R., & Rohling, M. L. (2004). Individual, family, and peer correlates of adolescent gambling. *Journal of Gambling Studies, 20,* 23–46.

Lau, R. R. & Russell, D. (1980). Attribution in the sports pages. *Journal of Personality and Social Psycho- logy, 39*, 29–38.

Lazarus, R. S., & Folkman, S. (1984). *Stress, appraisal, and coping.* New York: Springer.

Leary, K., & Dickerson, M. (1985). Levels of arousal in high- and low-frequency gamblers. *Behaviour Research and Therapy, 23*, 635–640.

Leith, K. P., & Baumeister, R. F. (1996). Why do bad moods increase self-defeating behavior? Emotion, risk-taking and self-regulation. *Journal of Personality and Social Psychology, 71*, 1250–1267.

Leonard, L. S. (1989). *Witness to the fire: Creativity and the veil of addiction.* Boston, MA: Shambhala.

Lepage, C., Ladouceur, R., & Jacques, C. (2000). Prevalence of problem gambling among community service users. *Community of Mental Health Journal, 36*(6), 597–601.

Lerner, J. S., & Keltner, D. (2000). Beyond valence: Toward a model of emotion-specific influences on judgment and choice. *Cognition and Emotion, 14*(4) 473–493.

Lesieur, H. R. (1979). The compulsive gambler's spiral of options and involvement. *Psychiatry, 42*, 79–87.

Lesieur, H. R. (1984). *The chase.* Cambridge, MA: Schenkman Books.

Lesieur, H. R. (1987). Gambling, pathological gambling and crime. In T. Galski (Ed.), *The handbook of pathological gambling* (pp. 89–110). Springfield, IL: Charles C Thomas.

Lesieur, H. R. (1988). The female pathological gambler. In W. R. Eadington (Ed.), *Gambling research: Proceedings of the seventh international conference on gambling and risk taking* (*5*, 230–258). Reno: University of Nevada.

Lesieur, H. R. (1990). Working with and understanding Gamblers Anonymous. In T. J. Powell (Ed.), *Working With Self-Help* (pp. 237–253). Silver Spring: NASW Press.

Lesieur, H. R. (1992). Compulsive gambling. *Social Science and Modern Society, 29*(4), 43–50.

Lesieur, H. R. (1994). Epidemiological surveys of pathological gambling: Critique and suggestions for modification. *Journal of Gambling Studies, 10*, 385–398.

Lesieur, H. (1998). Costs and treatment of pathological gambling. *The Annals of the American Academy of Social Science, 556*, 153–171.

Lesieur, H. R., & Blume, S. B. (1987). The South Oaks Gambling Screen (SOGS): A new instrument for the identification of pathological gamblers. *The American Journal of Psychiatry, 144*, 1184–1188.

Lesieur, H. R., & Blume, S. B. (1991a). Evaluation of patients treated for pathological gambling in a combined alcohol, substance abuse, and pathological gambling treatment unit using the Addiction Severity Index. *British Journal of Addictions, 86*, 1017–1028.

Lesieur, H. R., & Blume, S. B. (1991b). When lady luck loses: Women and compulsive gambling treatment. In N. Van Den Bergh (Ed.), *Feminist perspectives on addictions* (pp. 181–197). New York: Springer.

Lesieur, H. R., Blume, S. B., & Zoppa, R. M. (1986). Alcoholism, drug abuse, and gambling. *Alcoholism: Clinical and Experimental Research, 10*, 33–38.

Lesieur, H. R. & Blume. S. B. Characteristics of pathological gamblers identified among patients on a psychiatric admission service. *Hospital & Community Psychiatry. 1990;41:* 10009–12.

Lesieur, H. R., Cross, J., Frank M., Welch, M., White, C. M., Rubenstein, G., Moseley, K., & Mark, M. (1991). Gambling and pathological gambling among university students. *Addictive Behaviors, 16*, 517–527.

Lesieur, H. R., & Klein, R. (1987). Pathological gambling among high school students. *Addictive Behaviour, 12*, 129–135.

Lesieur, H., & Rosenthal, R. (1991). Pathological gambling: A review of the literature. *Journal of Gambling Studies, 7*, 5–40.

Lesieur, H. R., & Rothschild, J. (1989). Children of Gamblers Anonymous members. *Journal of Gambling Behaviour, 5*, 269–282.

Levin, J. S. (1994). Religion and health: Is there an association, is it valid, and is it causal? *Social Science & Medicine, 38*(11), 1475–1482.

Linden, R. D., Pope, H. G. Jr., & Jonas, J. M. (1986). Pathological gambling and major affective disorder: Preliminary findings. *Journal of Clinical Psychiatry, 47*, 201–203.

Lindgren, H. E., Youngs, G. A., McDonald, T. D., Klenow, D. J., & Schriner, E. C. (1987). The impact of gender on gambling attitudes and behaviour. *Journal of Gambling Behaviour, 3*, 155–167.

Linehan, M. (1993a). *Cognitive-behavioural treatment of borderline personality disorder.* Guilford Press: New York.

Linehan, M. (1993b). Skills training manual for treating borderline personality disorder. Guilford Press: New York.

Linnoila, M., Virkkunen, M., George, T., & Higley, D. (1993). Impulse control disorders. *International Clinical Psychopharmacology, 8* Suppl 1, 53–56.

Livingston, J. (1971). *Compulsive gamblers.* Lafayette, Indiana: Purdue University. *Lloyd's law reports: Insurance and reinsurance.* (1998). London: LLP.

Loevinger, T. (1976). *Ego development.* San Francisco: Jossey-Bass.

Lord, C. G., Ross, L., & Lepper, M. (1975). Perseverance in self perception and social perception. Biased attributional process in the debriefing paradigm. *Journal of Personality and Social Psychology, 32*, 880–892.

Lorenz, V. C. (1981). Differences found among Catholic, Protestant and Jewish Families of pathological gamblers. In W. R. Eadington (Ed.), *The gambling papers: Proceeding of the fifth national conference on gambling and risk taking* (pp. 123–135). Reno: University of Nevada press.

Lorenz, V. C. (1987). Family dynamics of pathological gamblers. In T. Galski (Ed.). *The handbook of pathological gambling* (pp. 71–88). Springfield, IL: Charles C Thomas.

Lorenz, V. C., & Shuttlesworth, D. (1983). The impact of pathological gambling on the spouse of the gambler. *Journal of Community Psychology, 11*, 67–76.

Lorenz, V. C., & Yaffe, R. A. (1986). Pathological gambling: Psychosomatic, emotional and marital difficulties as reported by the gambler. *Journal of Gambling Behavior, 2*(1), 40–49.

Lorenz, V. C., & Yaffee, R. A. (1988). Pathological gambling: Psychosomatic, emotional, and marital difficulties as reported by the spouse. *Journal of Gambling Behaviour, 4*, 13–26.

Los Angeles Times. (2000, January 21). Laws on personal 'vices' have changed greatly over the years. *Newscan, 2*(3). Retrieved August 27, 2007 from http://www.cfcg.org/flash-newscan-newslink.html.

Love, A. A. (1999, November 5). Many see lottery as way to wealth. *Newscan, 1*(34). Retrieved August 27, 2007 from http://www.cfcg.org/flash-newscan-newslink.html.

Lovibond, S. H. (1968). The aversiveness of uncertainty: An analysis in terms of activation and information theory. *Australian Journal of Psychology, 20*, 85–91.

MacMillan, G. E. (1985). People and gambling. In G. Caldwell, B. Haig, M. G. Dickerson, & L. Sylvan (Eds.), *Gambling in Australia* (pp. 253–260). Sydney: Croom Helm.

Malaby, T. (1999). Fateful misconceptions: Rethinking paradigms of chance among gamblers in Crete. *Social Analysis, 43*(1), 141–165.

Mandal, V. P., & Doelen, C. V. (1999). *Chasing lightning: Gambling in Canada.* Etobicoke: United Church Publishing House.

Mano, H. (1992). Judgments under distress: Assessing the role of unpleasantness and arousal in judgment formation. *Organizational Behavior and Human Decision Processes, 52*, 216–245.

Mano, H. (1994). Risk taking, framing effects, and affect. *Organizational Behavior and Human Decision Processes, 57*, 38–58.

Marget, N., Gupta, R., & Derevensky, J. (1999, August). *The psychosocial factors underlying adolescent problem gambling.* Poster presented at the annual meeting of the American Psychological Association, Boston.

Mark, M. E., & Lesieur, H. R. (1992). A feminist critique of problem gambling research. *British Journal of Addiction, 87*, 549–565.

Marks, I. M. (1986). *Behavioural psychotherapy Maudsly pocket book of clinical management.* Bristol, England: IOP Publishing.

Marks, I. M. (1987). *Fears, phobias and rituals.* London: Oxford University Press.

Marks, I. M., & Mathews, A. M. (1979). Brief standard self-rating for phobic patients. *Behavior Research and Therapy, 17*, 263–267.

Marlatt, G. A., & Gordon, J. R. (Ed.). (1985). *Relapse prevention: Maintenance strategies in the treatment of addictive behaviors*. New York: Guilford Press.

Marshall, K. (2000, March 24). Gambling: An update. *Newscan, 2*(12). Retrieved August 27, 2007, from http://www.cfcg.org/flash-newscan-newslink.html

Marshall, K. (2001, May 4). The gambling industry: Raising the stakes. *Newscan, 3*(18). Retrieved July 15, 2001 from http://www.cfcg.org/flash-newscan-newslink.html

Martinez, T. M. (1983). *The gambling scene: Why people gamble*. Springfield, IL: Thomas.

Maslow, A. (1968). *Toward a psychology of being*. New York: Van Nostrand Reinhold.

Maslow, A. (1971). *The farther reaches of human nature*. New York: The Viking Press.

Matthews, R. T., & German, D. C. (1984). Electrophysiological evidence for excitation of rat ventral tegmental area dopamine neurons by morphine. *Neuroscience, 11*, 617–625.

Maurer, C. D. (1985). An outpatient approach to the treatment of pathological gambling. In W. R. Eadington (Ed.), *The gambling studies: Proceedings of the sixth national conference on gambling and risk taking* (5, pp. 205–217). Reno: University of Nevada.

May, R. (1958). The origins and significance of the existential movement in psychology. In R. May, E. Angel, & H. Ellenberger (Eds.), *Existence: A new dimension in psychiatry and psychology* (pp. 1–37). New York: Basic Books.

May, R. (1991). *The cry for myth*. New York: W. W. Norton.

McAleavy, T. (1995, September 10). More women among problem gamblers. *The Bergen Record*, p. H3.

McClelland, J. L., & Rumelhart, D. E. (1985). Distributed memory and the representation of general and specific information. *Journal of Experimental Psychology, General, 114*, 159–188.

McConaghy, N. (1980). Behaviour completion mechanisms rather than primary drives maintain behavioural patterns. *Activas Nervosa Superior* (Prague), *22*, 138–151.

McConaghy, N., Armstrong, M., Blaszczynski, A., & Allcock, C. (1983). Controlled comparison of aversive therapy and imaginal desensitization in compulsive gambling. *British Journal of Psychiatry, 142*, 366–372.

McCormick, R. A. (1993). Disinhibition and negative affectivity in substance abusers with and without a gambling problem. *Addictive Behaviors, 18*, 331–336.

McCormick, R. A. (1994). The importance of coping skill enhancement in the treatment of the pathological gambler. *Journal of Gambling Studies, 10*, 77–86.

McCormick, R. A., Russo, A. M., Ramirez, L. F., & Taber, J. I. (1984). Affective–disorders among pathological gamblers seeking treatment. *American Journal of Psychiatry, 141*, 215–218.

McCormick, R. A., & Taber, J. I. (1988). Attributional style in pathological gamblers in treatment. *Journal of Abnormal Psychology, 97*, 368–370.

McCown, W. G., & Chamberlain, L. L. (2000). *Best possible odds: Contemporary treatment strategies for gambling disorders*. New York: John Wiley & Sons.

McCrae, R. R. (1984). Situational determinants of coping responses: Loss, threat, and challenge. *Journal of Personality and Social Psychology, 46*, 919–928.

McCrae, R. R., & Costa, P. T. (1986). Personality and coping effectiveness in an adult sample. *Journal of Personality, 54*, 385–405.

McDonald, B., & Steel, Z. (1997). Immigrants and mental health: An epidemiological analysis. *Culture and Mental Health: Current Issues in Transcultural Mental Health*. Sydney, AU: Transcultural Mental Health Centre.

McGowan, V., Droessler, J., Nixon, G., & Grimshaw, M. (2000). *Recent research in the sociocultural domain of gaming and gambling: An annotated bibliography and critical overview*. Edmonton: Alberta Gaming Research Institute.

McManus, J. (2003). *Positively Fifth Street: Murderers, cheetahs, and Binion's world series of poker*. New York: Farrar, Straus and Giroux.

McMillen, J. (1996). From glamour to grind: The globalisation of casinos. In McMillen, J. (Ed.), *Gambling cultures: Studies in history and interpretation* (pp. 263–287). London: Routledge.

McNeilly, D. P., & Burke, W. J. (2000). Late life gambling: The attitudes and behaviours of older adults. *Journal of Gambling Studies, 16*(4), 393–415.

McQueen, P. (1995). Worldwide lottery sales reach $95 billion in 1994. *International Gaming & Wagering Business, 18*, 1.

Mehlman, P. T., Higley, J. D., & Faucher, I. (1995). Low CFS 5-HIAA concentrations and severe aggressionand imparied impulse control in nonhuman primates. *American Journal of Psychiatry, 151*, 1485–1491.

Meichenbaum, D., & Novaco, R. (1985). Stress inoculation: A preventative approach. *Issues in Mental Health Nursing Special Issue: Stress and anxiety, 7*(1–4), 419–435. Retrieved September 5, 2007, from PsycINFO database.

Merton, R. K. (1938). Social structure and anomie. *American Sociological Review, 3*, 672–82.

Messer, K., Clark, K. A., & Martin, S. L. (1996). Characteristics associated with pregnant women's utilization of substance abuse treatment services. *American Journal of Drug Alcohol Abuse, 22*(3), 403–422.

Metzger, M. A. (1985). Biases in betting: An application of laboratory findings. *Psychological Reports, 56*, 883–888.

Miliora, M. (1997). A self–psychological study of a shared gambling fantasy in Eugene O'Neil's "Hughie." *Journal of Gambling Studies, 13*(2), 105–123.

Miller, W. (1986). Individual outpatient treatment of pathological gambling. *Journal of Gambling Behavior, 2*, 95–107.

Moore, R., & Gillette, D. (1990). *King, warrior, magician, lover: Rediscovering the archetypes of the mature masculine.* San Francisco: Harper.

Moore, S. M., & Ohtsuka, K. (1997). Gambling activities of young Australians: Developing a model of behaviour. *Journal of Gambling Studies, 13*(3), 207–236.

Moore, S. M., & Ohtsuka, K. (1999a). Beliefs about control over gambling among young people, and their relation to problem gambling. *Psychology of Addictive Behaviours, 13*(4), 339–347.

Moore, S. M., & Ohtsuka, K. (1999b). The prediction of gambling behavior and problem gambling from attitudes and perceived norms. *Social Behavior and Personality, 27*(5), 455–466.

Moran, E. (1969, Winter). Taking the final risk. *Mental Health,* 21–22.

Moran, E. (1970). Gambling as a form of dependence. *British Journal of Addiction, 64,* 419–428.

Moran, E. (1987). *Gambling among schoolchildren: The impact of the fruit machine.* London: National Council on Gambling.

Moreyra, P., Ibanez, A., Liebowitz, M. R., Saiz-Ruiz, J., & Blanco, C. (2002). Pathological gambling: Addiction or obsession? *Psychiatric Annals, 32*(3),161–166.

Morgan, D. R., & Anderson, S. K. (1991). Assessing the effects of political culture: Religious affiliation and county political behaviour. *Social Science Journal, 28*(2), 163–174.

Moskowitz, J. A. (1980). Lithium and lady luck; use of lithium carbonate in compulsive gambling. *New York State Journal of Medicine, 80*, 785–788.

Muellerman, R. L., DenOtter T, Wadman, M. C., Tran, T. P., Anderson, J. (2002) Problem gambling in the partner of the emergency department patient as a risk factor for intimate partner violence. *Journal of Emergency Medicine 23*(3):307–12.

Mundt, J. C., Marks, I. M., Shear, M. K., & Greist, J. H. (2002). The work and social adjustment scale: A simple measure of impairment in functioning. *British Journal of Psychiatry, 180*, 461–464.

Munting, R. (1996). *An economic and social history of gambling in Britain and the USA.* Manchester: Manchester University Press.

Murray, J. B. (1993). Review of research on pathological gambling. *Psychological Reports, 72*, 791–810.

Murray, R. D. (2001). *Helping the problem gambler.* Toronto: Centre for Addiction and Mental Health.

Nathan, P. (2001). *Best practices for the treatment of gambling disorders: Too soon?* Paper presented at the annual Harvard–National Center for Responsible Gaming Conference, Las Vegas.

National Council of Welfare. (1996). *Gambling in Canada.* Ottawa: Government of Canada.

National Gambling Impact Study Commission. (1999). *National gambling impact study commission: Final report.* U.S.: US Independent Agencies and Commissions.

National Opinion Research Centre (1999). Overview of the National Survey and Community database Research on Gambling Behaviour.

National Indian Gaming Association. (2001). Retrieved August 27, 2007 from http://www.indiangaming.org/

National Research Council. (1999). *Pathological gambling: A critical review*. Washington, D.C.: National Academy Press.

Neisser, U. (1988). Five kinds of self-knowledge. *Philosophical Psychology, 1*(1), 35–59.

Nibert, D. (2000). *Hitting the lottery jackpot: State governments and the taxing of dreams*. New York: Monthly Review Press.

Nisbett, R. E., & Wilson, T. D. (1977). Telling more than we can know: Verbal reports on mental processes. *Psychological Review, 84*, 231–259.

Nixon, G. (2001a). Using Wilber's transpersonal model of psychological and spiritual growth in alcoholism treatment. *Alcoholism Treatment Quarterly, 19*(1), 75–95.

Nixon, G. (2001b). The transformational opportunity of embracing the silence beyond hopelessness. *Voices: Journal of the American Academy of Psychotherapists, 37*(2), 56–66.

Nixon, G. (2003). Using a Wilber development approach in working with Mary. *eGambling: Electronic Journal of Gambling Issues, 8*. Retrieved August 27, 2007 from http://www.camh.net/egambling/issue8/case_conference/responses.html

Nixon, G. (2005). Beyond dry drunkness: Facilitating second stage recovery using Wilber's Spectrum of Consciousness developmental model. *Journal of Social Work Practice in the Addictions, 5*(3), 55–71.

Nixon, G., Solowoniuk, J., & McGowan, V. (2006). The counterfeit hero's journey of the pathological gambler: A phenomenological-hermeneutics investigation. *International Journal of Mental Health and Addiction, 4*(3), 217–232.

Novaco, R. W. (1975). *Anger* Control. Lexington, MA: D.C. Health.

Novaco, R. W. (1976). Treatment of chronic anger through cognitive and relaxation controls. *Journal of Consulting and Clinical Psychology, 4*, 681.

Nower, L., Gupta, R., & Derevensky, J. (2000, June). *Youth gamblers and substance abusers: A comparison of stress-coping styles and risk-taking behavior of two addicted adolescent populations*. Paper presented at the Eleventh International Conference on Gambling and Risk-Taking, Las Vegas.

Oakley-Browne, M., Adams, P., & Mobberley, P. (2005). Interventions for pathological gambling. *The Cochrane Collaboration, (2)*:CD001521.

Ocean, G., & Smith, G. (1993). Social reward, conflict, and commitment: A theoretical model of gambling behavior. *Journal of Gambling Studies, 9*(4), 321–339.

O'Connor, J., & Dickerson, M. G. (2003). Impaired control over gambling in gaming machine and off-course gamblers. *Addiction, 98*, 53–60.

Ogborne, A. C. (1978). *Patient characteristics as predictors of treatment outcomes for alcohol and drug abusers*. Toronto, ON: Evaluation Studies Department, Addiction Research Foundation.

Ogborne, A. C., & Glaser, F. B. (1981). Characteristics of affiliates of Alcoholics Anonymous: A review of the literature. *Journal of Studies on Alcohol, 42*, 661–675.

Ohtsuka, K., Bruton, E., DeLuca, L., & Borg, V. (1997). Sex differences in pathological gambling using gaming machines. *Psychological Reports, 80*, 1051–1057.

Oldman, D. J. (1974). Compulsive gamblers. *Sociological Review, 26*, 349–371.

O'Malley, S. S., Jaffe, A. J., Chang, G., Rode, S., Schottenfeld, R., Meyer, R. E., & Rounsaville, B. (1996). Six-month follow-up of naltrexone and psychotherapy for alcohol dependence. *Archives of General Psychiatry, 53*, 217–224.

Oman, C. (1912). *The text of the old betting book of All Souls College, 1815–1873*. Oxford: All Sould College.

Ontario Lottery and Gaming. (2006). About OLG: Who we are & Where the money goes. Retrieved August 27, 2007 from www.olgc.ca/about/who_we_are/index.jsp

Orford, J. (1985). *Excessive appetites: A psychological view of addictions*. Chichester: John Wiley & Sons.

Orford, J., Daniels, V., & Somers, M. (1996). Drinking and gambling: A comparison with implications for theories of addiction. *Drug & Alcohol Review, 15*, 47–56.

Orkin, S. H. (2000). Diversification of haematopoietic stem cells to specific lineages. *Nature Reviews Genetics, 1*: 57–67.

Ornstein, R. E. (1986). *The psychology of consciousness*. New York: Penguin Books.

Ortiz, D. (1986). *On casino gambling*. New York: Dodd, Mead & Company.

Owen, D., Birds, J., & Legh-Jones, N. (2004). *Macgillivray on Insurance Law* (10th ed.). London: Sweet & Maxwell.

Pallanti, S., Baldini Rossi, N., Sood, E., & Hollander, E. (2002). Nefazodone treatment of pathological gambling: a prospective open-label controlled trial. *Journal of Clinical Psychiatry, 63*, 1034–1039.

Pallanti, S., Quercioli, L., Sood, E., & Hollander, E. (2002). Lithium and valproate treatment of pathological gambling: A randomized single-blind study. *Journal of Clinical Psychiatry, 63*, 559–564.

Pallesen, S., Mitsem, M., Kvale, G., Johnsen, B.-H., & Molde, H. (2005) Outcome of psychological treatments of pathological gambling: A review and meta-analysis. *Addiction, 100*, 1412–1422.

Parke, J., Griffiths, M. D., & Parke, A. (2003, May). *A new typology of British slot machine players.* Paper presented at the Twelfth International Conference on Gambling & Risk-Taking, Vancouver.

Parke, J., Griffiths, M. D., & Turner, N. (2003, May). *International differences in slot machine gambling.* Paper presented at the Twelfth International Conference on Gambling & Risk-Taking, Vancouver.

Parkes, K. R. (1986). Coping in stressful episodes: The role of individual differences, environmental factors, and situational characteristics. *Journal of Personality and Social Psychology, 46*, 655–668.

Parsons, E. S., & Farr, S. D. (1981). The neuropsychology of alcohol and drug abuse. In S. B. Filskob & T. S. Boll (Eds.), *Handbook of clinical neuropsychology: Vol. 1.* New York: John Wiley & Sons.

Parsons, T. (1975). The sick role and the role of the physician reconsidered. *Milbank Quarterly. 53*, 257–277.

Pasternak, A. (1997). Pathological gambling: America's newest addiction? *American Family Physician, 56*, 1293–1296.

Peacock, R., Day, P., & Peacock, T. (1999a). Adolescent gambling on a Great Lakes Indian reservation. In Weaver, H. (Ed.), *Voices of first nations people.* New York: Haworth Press, 5–17.

Peacock, R. B., Day, P. A., & Peacock, T. D. (1999b). Adolescent gambling on a Great Lakes Indian Reservation. *Journal of Human Behaviour in the Social Environment, 2*(1–2), 5–17.

Pearce, J. M. (1997). *Animal learning and cognition: An introduction* (2nd ed.) East Sussex, UK: Psychology Press.

Pearson, C. S. (1989). *The hero within: Six archetypes we live by.* New York:Publishers.

Peele, S. (1989). *Diseasing of America: Addiction treatment out of control.* Boston: Houghton Milton.

Peele, S. (1991). *The truth about addiction and recovery.* New York: Simon & Schuster.

Peele, S. (2001). Is gambling an addiction like drug and alcohol addiction? Developing realistic and useful conceptions of compulsive gambling. *Electronic Journal of Gambling Issues: eGambling, 3.* Retrieved August 27, 2007 from http://www.camh.net/egambling/

Perls, F. (1969). *Gestalt therapy verbatim.* Moab, UT: Real People Press.

Petry, N. M. (2000). Gambling problems in substance abusers are associated with increased sexual risk behaviours. *Addiction, 95*(7), 1089–1100.

Petry, N. M. (2002). Psychosocial treatments for pathological gambling: Current status and future directions. *Psychiatric Annals, 32*(3), 192–196.

Pfhol, S. (1985). *Images of deviance and social control.* New York: McGraw-Hill.

Phillips, A. G., & LePiane, F. G. (1980). Reinforcing effects of morphine microinjection onto the ventral tegmental area. *Pharmacology, Biochemistry, and Behavior, 12*, 965–968.

Piaget, J. (1977). *The essential Piaget.* New York: Basic Books.

Politzer R. M., Yesalis C. E., & Hudak, C. J. (1992). The epidemiologic model and the risk of legalized gambling: Where are we headed? *Health Values, 6*(2), 20–27.

Posner, M. I., & Presti, D. (1987). Selective attention and cognitive control. *Trends in Neuroscience, 10*, 12–17.

Potenza, M. N. (2002). A perspective on future directions in the prevention, treatment, and research of pathological gambling. *Psychiatric Annals, 32*(3), 203–207.

Potenza., M. N., Leung, H. C., Blumberg, H. P., Peterson, B. S., Fulbright, R. K., Lacadie, C. M., et al. (2003a). An FMRI Stroop task study of ventromedial prefrontal cortical function in pathological gamblers. *American Journal of Psychiatry, 60*, 1990–1994.

Potenza, M. N., Steinberg, M. A., Skudlarski, P., Fulbright, R. K., Lacadie, C. M., Wilber, M. K., et al. (2003b). Gambling urges in pathological gambling: A functional magnetic resonance imaging study. *Archives of General Psychiatry, 60*, 828–836.

Potenza, M. N., Xian, H., Shah, K. R., Scherrer, J. F., & Eisen, S. A. (2005). Shared genetic contributions to pathological gambling and major depression in men. *Archives of General Psychiatry, 62*, 1015–1021.

Poulin, C. (2000). Problem gambling among adolescent students in the Atlantic Provinces of Canada. *Journal of Gambling Studies, 16*(1), 53–78.

Pratkanis, A. R. (1995). How to sell pseudoscience. *The Skeptical Enquirer, 19*(4), 19–25.

Preston, F. W., Bernhard, B. J., Hunter, R. E., & Bybee, S. L. (1998). Gambling as stigmatized behaviour: Regional relabeling and the law. *Annals of the American Academy of Political and Social Science, 556*, 186–196.

Preston, F. W., & Smith, R. W. (1985). Delabeling and relabeling in Gamblers Anonymous: Problems with transferring the Alcoholics Anonymous paradigm. *Journal of Gambling Behavior, 1*(2), 97–105.

Prochaska, J. (2002). *Stages of change in addictive behavior.* RGCO Discovery conference. Niagara Falls.

Productivity Commission. (1999). *Australia's Gambling Industries, Report No. 10.* Canberra: Ausinfo.

Purcell, C. (2000, April 21). Ethnic gambling addicts run risks of shame and fear. *Newscan, 2*(16). Retrieved August 27, 2007 from http://www.cfcg.org/flash-newscan-newslink.html

Raghunathan, R., & Pham, M. T. (1999). All negative moods are not equal: Motivational influences of anxiety and sadness on decision making. *Organizational Behavior and Human Decision Processes, 79*(1), 56–77.

Ramirez, L. F., McCormick, R. A., Russo, A. M., & Taber, J. I. (1983). Patterns of substance abuse in pathological gamblers undergoing treatment. *Addictive Behaviors, 8*, 425–428.

Rankin, H. (1982). Control rather than abstinence as a goal in the treatment of excessive gambling. *Behaviour Research and Therapy, 20,* 185–187.

Raviv, M. (1993). Personality characteristics of sexual addicts and pathological gamblers. *Journal of Gambling Studies, 9*, 17–30.

Reber, A. S. (1993). *Implicit learning and tacit knowledge.* New York: Oxford University Press.

Reber, A. S. (1996). *The new gambler's Bible: How to beat the casinos, the track, your bookie, and your buddies.* New York: Crown Publishers.

Reich, J., & Green, A. (1991). Effects of personality disorders on outcome of treatment. *Journal of Nervous and Mental Disease, 179*, 74–82.

Reid, R. L. (1985). The psychology of the near miss. In W. R. Eadington (Ed.), *The gambling studies: Proceedings of the sixth national conference on gambling and risk taking* (3, pp. 1–12). Reno: University of Nevada.

Reid, R. L. (1986). The psychology of the near miss. *Journal of Gambling Behavior, 2*, 32–39.

Reith, G. (1999). *The age of chance: gambling and western culture.* New York: Routledge.

Rescorla, R. A. (1968). Pavlovian conditioned fear in Sidman avoidance learning. *Journal of Comparative and Physiological Psychology, 65*, 55–60.

Reuter, J., Raedler, T., Rose, M., Hand, I., Glascher, J., & Buchel, C. (2005). Pathological gambling is linked to reduced activation of the mesolimbic reward system. *Nature Neuroscience, 8*, 147–148.

Reutter, M. (2003). *Gambling in America: Costs and benefits.* Business and Law Editor.

Ricketts, T., Macaskill, A., (2003). Gambling as Emotion Management: Developing a grounded theory of problem. *Addiction Research and Theory 11*(6): 383–400.

Riesman, D. (1954). *Individualism reconsidered.* IL: The Free Press.

Riutort, M., & Small, S. E. (1985). *Working with assaulted immigrant women: A handbook for lay counsellors.* Toronto, ON: Chicago Education Wife Assault.

Roehl, W. S. (1999). Quality of life issues in a casino destination. *Journal of Business Research. Special Issue: Tourism & Quality-of-Life Issues, 44*(3), 223–229.

Rogers, R. D., Everitt, B. J., Baldacchino, A., Blackshaw, A. J., Swainson, R., Wynne, K., et al. (1999). Dissociable deficits in the decision-making cognition of chronic amphetamine abusers, opiate abusers, patients with focal damage to prefrontal cortex, and tryptophan-depleted normal volunteers: evidence for monoaminergic mechanisms. *Neuropsychopharmacology, 20*, 322–339.

Room, R. (1995). Issues in the cross–cultural validity of dependence definitions. *Proceedings of the 37th ICAA International Congress* (pp. 1–11). San Diego: University of San Diego.

Room, R., Turner, N., & Ialomiteau, A. (1998). *Effects of the opening of the Niagara casino: A first report.* Toronto: Centre for Addictions and Mental Health.

Room, R., Turner, N. E., & Ialomiteanu, A. (1999). Community effects of the opening of the Niagara casino. *Research Report, 94*(10), 1449–1466.

Rose, I. N. (2003). Gambling and the law: The new millennium. In G. Reith (Ed.), *Gambling: Who wins? Who loses?* Amherst, NY: Prometheus Books, pp. 113–131.

Rosecrance, J. (1985). *The degenerates of Lake Tahoe.* New York: Peter Lang.

Rosecrance, J. (1988). *Gambling without guilt: The legitimation of an American pastime.* California: Brooks/Cole.

Rosecrance, J. (1989). Controlled gambling: A promising future. In H. J. Shaffer, S. A. Stein, B. Gambino, & T. N. Cummings (Eds.), *Compulsive gambling: Theory, research, and practice* (pp. 150–151). Lexington, MA: Lexington Books.

Rosenthal, R. J. (1987). The psychodynamics of pathological gambling: A review of the literature. In T. Galski (Ed.), *The handbook of pathological gambling.* Springfield, IL: Charles C Thomas.

Rosenthal, R. J. (1992). Pathological gambling. *Psychiatric Annals, 22(2),* 72–78.

Rosenthal, R., & Lesieur, H. (1992). Self-reported withdrawal symptoms and pathological gambling. *American Journal of Addictions, 1,* 150–154.

Rosenthal, R. J., & Rugle, L. J. (1994). A psychodynamic approach to the treatment of pathological gambling: Part 1. Achieving abstinence. *Journal of Gambling Studies, 10*(1), 21–42.

Ross, M. & Sicoly, F. (1979). Egocentric biases in availability and attribution. *Journal of Personality and Social Psychology, 37,* 322–336.

Rossman, N. (1991). *Consciousness: Separation and integration.* Albany: State University of New York Press.

Rozin, P., & Stoess, C. (1993a). Gambling problems in substance abusers are associated with increased sexual risk behaviors. *Addiction, 95*(7), 1089–1100.

Rozin, P., & Stoess, C. (1993b). Is there a general tendency to become addicted? *Addictive Behaviors, 18,* 81–87.

Rugle, L., Derevensky, J., Gupta, R., Winters, K., & Stinchfield, R. (2001). *The treatment of problem and pathological gamblers.* Report prepared for the National Council for Problem Gambling, Center for Mental Health Services (CMHS) and the Substance Abuse and Mental Health Services Administration (SAMHSA), Washington, D.C.

Rugle, L., & Melamed, L. (1993). Neuropsychological assessment of attention problems in pathological gamblers. *Journal of Nervous and Mental Disease, 181*(2), 107–112.

Rugle, L. J., & Rosenthal, R. J. (1994). Transference and countertransference in the psychotherapy of pathological gamblers. *Journal of Gambling Studies, 10,* 43–65.

Rush, B., Moxam Shaw, R., & Urbanoski, K. (2002). Characteristics of people seeking help from specialized programs for the treatment of problem gambling in Ontario. *Electronic Journal of Gambling Issues, 6, 32–54 [Online].* Available: http://www.camh.net/egambling/archive/pdf/EJGI–issue6/EJGI–issue6–complete.pdf

Ruskan, J. (2004). *Emotional clearing.* New York: Random House.

Ryan, M. L. (1997). Interactive drama: Narrativity in a highly interactive environment. *Modern Fiction Studies, 43* (3), 677–707.

Rychlak, R. (1992). Lotteries, revenues and social costs: A historical examination of state-sponsored gambling. *Boston College Law Review, 34,* 11–81.

Sagarin, E. (1969). *Odd man in: societies of deviants in America.* Chicago: Quadrangle Books.

Saiz, J. (1992). No hagen juego, senores (Don't begin the game). *Interviu, 829,* 24–28.

Saiz-Ruiz, J., Blanco, C., Ibanez, A., Masramon, X., Gomez, M. M., Madrigal, M., & Diez,

T. (2005). Sertraline treatment of pathological gambling: A pilot study. *Journal of Clinical Psychiatry 66*, 28–33.

Salzman, L., & Thaler, F. (1981). Obsessive–compulsive disorders: A review of the literature. *American Journal of Psychiatry, 138*(3), 286–296.

Sartin, H. G. (1988). Win therapy: An alternative diagnostic and treatment therapy for problem gamblers. In W. R. Eadington (Ed.), *Gambling research: Proceedings of the Seventh International Conference on Gambling and Risk Taking* (5, 365–391). Reno: University of Nevada.

Scannell, E. D., Quirk, M. M., Smith, K., Maddem, R., & Dickerson, M. (2000). Females' coping styles and control over poker machine gambling. *Journal of Gambling Studies, 16*(4), 417–432.

Scarne, J. (1986). *Scarne's new complete guide to gambling*. New York: Simon and Schuster.

Schellinck, T., & Schrans, T. (1998). *The 1998 Nova Scotia Video Lottery Survey*. Halifax, Canada: Nova Scotia Department of Health.

Schellinck, T., & Schrans, T. (2002). *Atlantic Lottery Corporation video lottery responsible gaming feature research—Final report*. Focal Research Consultants Ltd.

Schellinck, T., Schrans T., & Walsh G. (2003). The role of informal and formal information sources in helping problem gambler. Presented at the National Association Gambling Studies 2002 Conference, Melbourne, Australia.

Schultz, W. (2002). Getting formal with dopamine and reward. *Neuron, 36*, 241–263.

Schwartz, S. (2007). Jungian analytic theory. In D. Capuzzi & D. Gross (Eds.), *Counselling and psychotherapy: Theories and interventions* (4th ed.). Upper Saddle River, NJ: Pearson Prentice-Hall.

Scodel, A. (1964). Inspirational group therapy: A study of Gamblers Anonymous. *American Journal of Psychotherapy, 18*, 115–125.

Scott, J. E. (2001). Everything's bubbling, but we don't know what the ingredients are—casino politics and policy in the periphery. *The Electronic Journal of Gambling Issues, 4*. Retrieved from http://www.camh.net/egambling/issue4/research/

Shaffer, H. J., & Hall, M. N. (1996). Estimating prevalence of adolescent gambling disorders: A quantitative synthesis and guide toward standard gambling nomenclature. *Journal of Gambling Studies, 12*, 193–214.

Shaffer, H. J., Hall, M. N., & Vander Bilt, J. (1999). Estimating the prevalence of disordered gambling behavior in the United States and Canada: A research synthesis. *American Journal of Public Health, 89*, 1369–1376.

Shaffer, H. J., & Korn, D. (2002). Gambling and related mental disorders: A public health analysis. *Annual Review of Public Health, 23*, 171–212.

Shah, K. R., Potenza, M. N., & Eisen, S. A. (2004). Biological basis for pathological gambling. In J. E. Grant & M. N. Potenza (Eds.), *Pathological gambling: A clinical guide to treatment* (pp. 127–142). Washington, DC: American Psychiatric Publishing.

Shapira, Z., & Venezia, I. (1992). Size and frequency of prizes as determinants of the demand for lotteries. *Organizational Behavior and Human Decision Processes, 52*, 307–318.

Sharpe, L., & Terrier, N. (1993). Towards a cognitive–behavioural theory of problem gambling. *British Journal of Psychiatry, 162*, 407–412.

Shepherd, L., & Dickerson, M. (2001). Situational coping with loss and control over gambling in regular poker machine players. *Australian Journal of Psychology, 53*(3), 160–169.

Shewan, D., & Brown, R. I. F. (1993). The role of fixed interval conditioning in promoting involvement in off-course betting. In W. R. Eadington & J. A. Cornelius (Eds.), *Gambling behavior and problem gambling* (pp. 111–132). Reno: Institute for the Study of Gambling and Commercial Gaming.

Shubin, S. (1977). The compulsive gambler. *Today in Psychiatry, 3*, 1–3.

Singer, J. (1994). *Boundaries of the soul: The practice of Jung's psychology* (2nd ed.). New York: Anchor Books.

Skinner, B. F. (1948). "Superstition" in the pigeon. *Journal of Experimental Psychology, 38*, 168–172.

Skinner, B. F. (1953). *Science and human behaviour.* New York: Free Press.

Skinner, W. (2003). Best clinical practices in concurrent disorders. Paper presented at the coming of age conference, Alcohol and Drug Recovery Association of Toronto, Ontario.

Skolnick, A., & Dombrink, J. (1978). The legalization of deviance. *Criminology: An Interdisciplinary Journal, 16*(2), 193–208.

Skolnick, J. H. (2003). Regulating vice: America's struggle with wicked pleasure. In G. Reith (Ed.), *Gambling: Who wins? Who loses?* Amherst, NY: Prometheus Books, pp. 311–321.

Smith, G. (1997). *Gambling and the public interest?* Calgary: Canada West Foundation.

Sobell, L. C., Kwan, E., & Sobell, M. B. (1995). Reliability of a drug history questionnaire (DHQ). *Addictive Behaviours, 20*(2), 233–241.

Solomon, R. C., & Higgins, K. M. (2000). *What Nietzsche really said.* New York: Schocken Books.

Sommerhoff, G. (2000). *Understanding consciousness: Its function and brain processes.* London: Sage Publications.

Specker, S. M., Carlson, G. A., Christenson, G. A., & Marcotte, M. (1995). Impulse control disorders and attention deficit disorder in pathological gamblers. *Annals of Clinical Psychiatry, 7*(4), 175–179.

Specker, S. M., Carlson, G. A., Edmonson, K. M., Johnson, P. E., & Marcotte, M. (1996). Psychopathological in pathological gamblers seeking treatment. *Journal of Gambling Studies, 12,* 67–81.

Spielberger, C. (1988). State-Trait Anger Expression Inventory (1st ed). Psychological Assessment Resources, Inc.

Spielberger, C. (1999). State-Trait Anger Expression Inventory – 2. (2nd ed). Psychological Assessment Resources, Inc.

Spunt, B., Dupont, I., Lesieur, H., Liberty, H. J., & Hunt, D. (1998). Pathological gambling and substance misuse: A review of the literature. *Substance Use and Misuse, 33*(13), 2535–2560.

Steel, Z. & Blaszczynski, A. (1996). The factorial structure of pathological gambling. *Journal of Gambling Studies, 12,* 3–20.

Stein, D. J., & Grant, J. E. (2005). Betting on dopamine. *CNS Spectrums, 10,* 268–270.

Stein, S. A. (1993). The role of support in recovery from compulsive gambling. In W. R. Eadington & J. A. Cornelius (Eds.), *Gambling behavior and problem gambling* (pp. 627–637). Reno: University of Nevada.

Steinberg, M. A. (1993). Couples treatment issues for recovering male compulsive gamblers and their partners. *Journal of Gambling Studies, 9*(2),153–167.

Steinberg, M. A., Kosten, T. A., & Rounsaville, B. J. (1992). Cocaine abuse and pathological gambling. *American Journal of Addictions, 1,* 121–132.

Steinmetz, A. (1870). The gaming table: Its votaries and victims, in all times and countries, especially in England and in France. Retrieved February 23, 2007 from http://etext.virginia.edu/toc/modeng/public/SteGami.html

Stewart, I. (1996). It probably won't be you. *The Times Higher Educational Supplement, April 12,* p. 14.

Stewart, J. (1984). Reinstatement of heroin and cocaine self-administration behavior in the rat by intracerebral application of morphine in the ventral tegmental area. *Pharmacology, Biochemistry, and Behavior, 20,* 917–923.

Stewart, R. M., & Brown, R. I. F. (1988). An outcome study of Gamblers Anonymous. *British Journal of Psychiatry, 152,* 284–288.

Stinchfield, R. (2000). Gambling and correlates of gambling among Minnesota public school students. *Journal of Gambling Studies, 16*(2/3), 153–173.

Stinchfield, R., Cassuto, N., Winters, K., & Latimer, W. (1997). Prevalence of gambling among Minnesota public school students in 1992 and 1995. *Journal of Gambling Studies, 13,* 25–48.

Stirpe, T. (1995). *Review of the literature on problem and compulsive gambling.* Toronto: Addiction Research Foundation of Ontario, Problem and Compulsive Gambling Project.

Stitt, B. G., Nichols, M., & Giacopassi, D. (2000). Perceptions of the extent of problem gambling within new casino communities. *Journal of Gambling Studies, 16*(4), 433–451.

Stitt, B. G., Nichols, M., & Giacopassi, D. (2003). Community satisfaction with casino gambling: An assessment after the fact. In G. Reith (Ed.), *Gambling: Who wins? Who loses?* Amherst, NY: Prometheus Books, pp. 96–111.

Stone, M. (1993). Long term outcome in personality disorders. *British Journal of Psychiatry, 162*, 299–313.

Stoppard, J. M. (2000). *Understanding depression: Feminist social constructionist approaches.* New York: Routledge.

Strachan, M. L., & Custer, R. L. (1993). Female compulsive gamblers in Las Vegas. In W. R. Eadington & J. A. Cornelius (Eds), *Gambling behavior and problem gambling* (pp. 235–239). Reno: University of Nevada.

Strickland, L. H., & Grote, F. W. (1967). Temporal presentation of winning symbols and slot-machine playing. *Journal of Experimental Psychology, 74*, 10–13.

Stripe, T. (1994). *Review of the literature on problem and compulsive gambling.* Toronto: Addiction Research Foundation.

Suissa, J. A. (1998). *Pourquoi l'alcoolisme n'est pas une maladie.* Montreal: Éditions Fidès.

Suissa, J. A. (2001a). La construction d'un problème social en une maladie: le cas de l'alcoolisme en Amérique du Nord. In R. Mayer & H. Dorvil (Eds.), *Problèmes sociaux: Théories et méthodologies. Tome I* (pp. 132–152). Sainte-Foy: Presses de l'Universite du Quebec.

Suissa, J. A. (2001b). Cannabis, social control and exclusion: The importance of social ties. *International Journal of Drug Policy, 2*(5–6), 385–396.

Suissa, J. A. (2002). Alcoholism, controlled drinking and abstinence: Scientific markers and social issues. *Journal of Addictions Nursing. 13*(3/4), 149–162.

Suissa, J. A. (2004a). *Gambling et dépendances: Jouer sa vie.* Québec. Canada: Presses Universitaires du Québec. (in press).

Suissa, J. A. (2004b). Social practitioners and families: A systemic perspective. *Journal of Family Social Work. 8*(4), 1–28.

Suits, D. B. (1982). Gambling as a source of revenue. In H. E. Brazer (Ed.), *Michigan's fiscal and economic structure* (pp. 828–853). Ann Arbor, MI: University of Michigan Press.

Suls, J., & Fletcher, B. (1985). The relative efficacy of avoidant and nonavoidant coping strategies: A meta analysis. *Health Psychology, 4*, 249–288.

Sundquist, J. (1994). Refugees, labour migrants and psychological distress: A population-based study of 338 Latin-American refugees, 161 South European and 396 Finnish labour migrants, and 996 Swedish age-, sex- and education-matched controls. *Social Psychiatry & Psychiatric Epidemiology, 29*(1), 20–24.

Sutich, A. J. (1969). Some considerations regarding transpersonal psychology. *Journal of Transpersonal Psychology, 1*(1), 15–16.

Swanbrow, D. (1997). Study of worldwide rates of religiosity, church attendance. Retrieved from http://www.umich.edu/~newsinfo/Releases/1997/

Taber, J. I., Russo, A. M., Adkins, B. J., & McCormick, R. A. (1986). Ego strength and achievement motivation in pathological gamblers. *Journal of Gambling Behavior, 2*(2), 69–80.

Tavares, H., Zilberman, M. L., Beites, F. J., & Gentil, V. (2001). Gender differences in gambling progression. *Journal of Gambling Studies, 17*(2), 151–159.

The Ontario Coalition for Social Justice and The Ontario Federation of Labour. (1996). *Unfair shares: Corporations and taxation in Canada.* Toronto, ON: The Ontario Coalition for Social Justice and The Ontario Federation of Labour.

Thomas, W. I. (1901). The gambling instinct. *American Journal of Sociology, 6*, 750–763.

Thompson, W. N. (1997). *Legalized gambling.* Denver: ABC–Clio.

Thorndike, E. (1913). *Educational psychology: The psychology of learning.* New York: Teachers College Press.

Thorson, J., Powell, F., & Hilt, M. (1994). Epidemiology of gambling and depression in an adult sample. *Psychological Reports, 74*, 987–994.

Tobacyk, J. J., & Wilkinson, L. V. (1991). Paranormal beliefs and preference for games of chance. *Psychological Reports, 68*, 1088–1090.

Tolchard, B., & Battersby, M. W. (2000). Nurse behavioural psychotherapy and pathological gambling: An Australian perspective. *Journal of Psychiatric and Mental Health Nursing, 7*, 335–342.

Tolle, E. (1996). *The power of now.* Vancouver, B.C.: Namaste.

Tolle, E. (2003). *Stillness speaks.* Vancouver, B.C.: Namaste.

Toneatto, T. (1999). Cognitive psychopathology of problem gambling. *Substance Use and Misuse, 34*(11), 1593–1604.

Toneatto, T., Blitz-Miller, T., Calderwood, K., Dragonetti, R., & Tsanos, A. (1997). Cognitive distortions in heavy gambling. *Journal of Gambling Studies, 13*, 253–266.

Toneatto, T., Blitz-Miller, T., Calderwood, K., Dragonetti, R., & Tsanos, A. (1997). Brief report: Cognitive distortions in heavy gambling. *Journal of Gambling Studies, 13*(3), 253–266.

Toneatto, T., & Ladouceur, R. (2003). Treatment of pathological gambling: A critical review of the literature. *Psychology of Addictive Behaviors, 17*, 284–292.

Toneatto, T., & Skinner, W. (2000). Relationship between gender and substance use among treatment-seeking gamblers. *The Electronic Journal of Gambling Issues: eGambling, 1*, 1–11.

Toneatto, T., & Sobell, L. C. (1990). Pathological gambling treated with cognitive behavior therapy: A case report. *Addictive Behaviors, 15*, 497–501.

Topp, J., & Charpentier, G. (2000). Jeu pathologique et toxicomanie. In Brisson, P. (Ed.), *L'usage des drogues et les toxicomanies* (Vol. 3, pp. 201–225). Montreal: Éditions Gaëtan Morin.

Trafimow, D., & Borrie W. T. (1999). Why past predicts intension. *Leisure Sciences, 21*, 31–42.

Triandis, H. C., & Gelfand, M. (1998). Converging measurement of horizontal and vertical individualism and collectivism. *Journal of Personality and Social Psychology, 74*, 118–128.

Trungpa, C. (1973). *Cutting through spiritual materialism.* Berkeley, CA: Shambhala

Turner, D. N., & Saunders, D. (1990). Medical relabelling in Gamblers Anonymous: The construction of an ideal member. *Small Group Research, 21*(1), 59–78.

Turner, N. (1998). Doubling versus constant bets as strategies for gambling. *Journal of Gambling Studies, 14*(4), 413–429.

Turner, N., Ialomiteanu, A. & Room, R. (1999). Checkered expectations: Predictors of approval of opening a casino in the Niagara community. *Journal of Gambling Studies, 15*(1), 45–70.

Turner, N. (2000, August). Randomness: Does it matter? *The Electronic Journal of Gambling Issues,* Issue 2. Retrieved August 27, 2007 from www.camh.net/egambling/issue2/research/

Turner, N. E., & Fritz, B. (2001). The effect of skilled gamblers on the success of less skilled gamblers. *The Electronic Journal of Gambling Issues, Issue 5.* Retrieved August 27, 2007 from www.camh.net/egambling

Turner, N. E., Fritz, B., & Mackenzie, B. (2003). How to gamble: Information and misinformation in books and other media on gambling. *The Electronic Journal of Gambling.*

Turner, N. E., & Horbay, R. (2003). Doubling revisited: The mathematical and psychological effect of betting strategy. *Gambling Research, 15*, 16–34.

Turner, N., & Horbay, R. (2004). How do slot machines and other electronic gambling machines actually work? *Journal of Gambling Issues,* Issue 11. http://www.camh.net/egambling/issue11/index.html

Turner, N., Horton, K., & Fritz, B. (2004). Implicit learning and problem gambling: Is there a connection? Final report to the Ontario Problem Gambling Research Centre. http://www.gamblingresearch.org/contentdetail.sz?cid=210

Turner, N. E., Howard, M., & Spence, W. (2006). Faro: A 19th century gambling craze. *Journal of Gambling Issues, Issue 16.*

Turner, N., Ialomiteanu, A., & Room, R. (1999). Checkered expectations: Predictors of approval of opening a casino in the Niagara community. *Journal of Gambling Studies, 15*(1), 45–70.

Turner, N., & Liu, E. (1999). *The naive human concept of random events.* Paper presented at the 1999 conference of the American Psychological Association, Boston.

Turner, N. E., Wiebe, J., Falkowski-Ham, A., Kelly, J., & Skinner, W. (2005). Public awareness of responsible gambling and gambling behaviours in Ontario. *International Gambling Studies, 5*(1), 95–112.

Turner, N. E., Zangeneh, M., & Littman-Sharp, N. (2006). The experience of gambling and its role in problem gambling. *International Gambling Studies, 6*(2), 237–266.

Tversky, A., & Kahneman, D. (1990). Judgement under uncertainty: Heuristics and biases. In P. K. Moser (Ed.), *Rationality in action: Contemporary approach.* New York: Cambridge University Press.

Twain, M. (2004). The professor's yarn. In J. Stravinsky (Ed.), *Read 'em and weep: A bed-*

side poker companion. New York: HarperCollins. (Reprinted from *Life on the Mississippi*, 1882.)

U.S. Commission on the Review of the National Policy Toward Gambling (1976). *Gambling in America.* Washington, DC: United States Government Printing Office.

Ursua, M. P., & Uribelarrea, L. L. (1998). 20 Questions of Gamblers Anonymous: A psychometric study with population of Spain. *Journal of Gambling Studies, 14*(1), 3–15.

Valverde, M. (1998). *Diseases of the will: Alcohol and the dilemmas of freedom.* Cambridge: Cambridge University.

Vance, J. (1989). *An analysis of the costs and benefits of public lotteries: The Canadian experience.* Queenston: The Edwin Mellen Press.

van der Leeuw, G. (1986). *Religion in essence and manifestation.* Trans. J. E. Turner & H. H. Penner. Princeton, NJ: Princeton University Press.

van Wolfswinkel, L., & van Ree, J. M. (1985). Effects of morphine and naloxone on thresholds of ventral tegmental electrical self-stimulation. *Naunyn-Schmiedebergs Archives of Pharmacology, 330*, 84–92.

Viets, V. C. L., & Miller, W. R. (1997). Treatment approaches for pathological gambling. *Clinical Psychology Review, 17*(7), 689–702.

Virkkunen, M., Goldman, D., & Nielsen, D. A. (1995). Low brain serotonin turnover rate (low CSF 5-HIAA) and impulsive violence. *Journal of Psychiatry & Neuroscience, 20*, 271–275.

Vitaro, F., Ladouceur, R., & Bujold, A. (1996). Predictive and concurrent correlates of gambling in early adolescent boys. *Journal of Early Adolescence, 13*, 79–93.

Vitaro, F., Wanner, B., Ladouceur, R., Brendgen, M., & Trembay, R. E. (2004). Trajectories of gambling during adolescence. *Journal of Gambling Studies, 20*, 47–69.

Volberg, R. A. (1994). The prevalence and demographics of pathological gamblers: Implications for public health. *American Journal of Public Health, 84*, 237–241.

Volberg, R. (1996). Prevalence studies of problem gambling in the United States. *Journal of Gambling Studies, 12*(2), 111–128.

Volberg, R. (2006). Characteristics of "early onset" and "late onset" gamblers in a community sample. Paper presented at the 13th international conference on gambling and risk taking, Lake Tahoe, Nevada.

Volberg, R. A., & Steadman, H. J. (1988). Refining the prevalence estimates of pathological gambling. *American Journal of Psychiatry, 145*, 502–505.

Volberg, R. A., & Steadman, H. J. 1989. Prevalence Estimates of Pathological Gambling in New Jersey and Maryland. *American Journal of Psychiatry, 146*, 1618–1619.

Vollrath, M., Torgersen, S., & Alnaes, R. (1995). Personality as a long–term predictor of coping. *Personality and Individual Differences, 18*, 117–125.

Volpicelli, J. R., Alterman, A. I., Hayashida, M., & O'Brien, C. P. (1992). Naltrexone in the treatment of alcohol dependence. *Archives of General Psychiatry, 49*, 876–880.

von Franz, M. L. (1997). *Archetypal dimensions of the psyche.* Boston: Shambhala.

Wade, J. (1996). *Changes of mind: A holonomic theory of the evolution of consciousness.* Albany, NY: SUNY Press.

Wagenaar, W. A. (1988). *Paradoxes of gambling behaviour.* Mahwah, NJ: Lawrence Erlbaum Associates.

Walker, G. (1985). The brief therapy of a compulsive gambler. *Journal of Family Therapy, 7*(1), 1–8.

Walker, M. B. (1988). A comparison of gambling in TAB shops and clubs. In W. R. Eadington (Ed.), *Gambling research: Proceedings of the seventh international conference on gambling and risk taking* (Vol. 3, pp. 65–82). Reno: University of Nevada-Reno.

Walker, M. (1990). The presence of irrational thinking among poker machine players. In M. Dickerson (Ed.), *200-Up* (pp. 133–144). Canberra: National Association for Gambling Studies.

Walker, M. B. (1992a). *The psychology of gambling.* Oxford: Pergamon Press.

Walker, M. B. (1992b). Irrational thinking among slot machine players. *Journal of Gambling Studies, 8*(3): 245–261.

Walker, M. B. (1993). Treatment strategies for problem gambling: A review of effectiveness. In

W. Eadington & J. Cornelius (Eds.), *Gambling behavior and problem gambling* (533–536). Reno: Institute for the Study of Gambling and Commercial Gaming.

Walker, M. (2001). Strategies for winning on poker machines. In A. Blaszczynski (Ed.)., *Culture and the gambling phenomenon* (pp. 391–396). Melbourne: National Association for Gambling Studies.

Walker, M. B., Blaszczynski, A. P., Sharpe, L., & Enersen, K. (2003). *Problem gamblers receiving counselling or treatment in New South Wales: Sixth Survey, 2002.* Sydney: Report to the Casino Community Benefit Fund.

Walker, M. B., & Dickerson, M. G. (1996). The prevalence of problem and pathological gambling: A critical analysis. *Journal of Gambling Studies, 12,* 233–249.

Walker, M. B., & Schellink, T. (2003, May). Strategies for beating electronic gaming machines. Paper presented at the Twelfth International Conference on Gambling & Risk-Taking, Vancouver.

Walker, M. B., Sturevska, S., & Turpie, D. (2000). The quality of blackjack play in Australian casinos. In O. Vancura, J.A. Cornelius & W. R. Eadington (Eds.), *Finding the edge* (pp. 151–160). Reno: Institute for the Study of Gambling and Commercial Gaming.

Walker, S. (1975). *Learning and reinforcement.* London: Methuen.

Walsh, R., & Vaughan, F. (Eds.) (1980). *Beyond ego.* Los Angeles: Jeremy Tarcher.

Walsh, R., & Vaughan, F. (Eds.) (1993). *Paths beyond ego: The transpersonal vision.* New York: Tarcher/Putnam.

Warren, K. (1996). *A winner's guide to Texas hold'em poker.* New York: Cardoza Publishing.

Washburn, M. (1988). *The ego and the dynamic ground.* Albany, NY: State University of New York Press.

Washburn, M. (1994). *Transpersonal psychology in psychoanalytic perspective.* Albany, NY: State University of New York Press.

Weingartner, H., Rapoport, J. L., Buchcaum, M. S., Bunney, W. F., Jr., Ebert, M. H., Mikkelsen, F. J., & Caine, E. D. (1980). Cognitive processes in normal and hyperactive children and their response to amphetamine treatment. *Journal of Abnormal Psychology, 89,* 25–37.

Weiten, D. & McCann, D. (2007). *Psychology: Themes and variations* (1st Can. Ed.). Toronto: Thomson & Nelson.

White, S. (1989). Against the odds. *Young People Now,* April, 26–27.

Whitman-Raymond, R. G. (1988, Summer). Pathological gambling as a defense against loss. *Journal of Gambling Behavior, 4*(2), 99–109.

Wilber, K. (1977). *The spectrum of consciousness.* Wheaton, IL: Quest.

Wilber, K. (1986). The spectrum of development. In K. Wilber, J. Engler, & D. Brown (Eds.), *Transformations of Consciousness.* Boston: Shambhala.

Wilber, K. (1990). *Eye to eye: The quest for the new paradigm* (Rev. Ed.). Boston: Shambhala.

Wilber, K. (1995). *Sex, ecology, and spirituality: The spirit of evolution.* Boston: Shambhala.

Wilber, K. (1997). *The eye of spirit: An integral version for a world gone slightly mad.* Boston: Shambhala.

Wilber, K. (2000). *Integral psychology.* Boston: Shambhala.

Wilber, K. (2006). *Integral spirituality.* Boston: Integral Books, Shambhala.

Wildman, R. W. (1997). *Gambling: An attempt at an integration.* Edmonton, Alberta: Wynne Resources.

Williamson, A., & Walker, M. (2000). Strategies for solving the insoluble: Playing to win Queen of the Nile. In G. Coman (Ed.), *Lessons of the past* (pp. 218–226). Mildura: National Association for Gambling Studies.

Windows Casino. Retrieved August 27, 2007 from http://webmaster.windowscasino.com/affiliates/aiddownload.asp?affid=1753

Windross, A. J. (2003). The luck of the draw: Superstition in gambling. *Gambling Research, 15,* 63–77.

Winokur, G., Clayton, P. J., & Reich, T. (1969). *Manic–depressive illness.* St. Louis: C. V. Mosby.

Winston, S., & Harris, H. (1984). *Nation of gamblers: America's billion-dollar-a-day habit.* Englewood Cliffs, NJ: Prentice-Hall.

Winters, K. G., Stinchfield, R. D., & Fulkerson, J. (1993). Patterns and characteristics of adolescent gambling. *Journal of Gambling Studies, 9*(4), 371–386.

Wong, S., & Spector, S. (1996). *The complete idiot's guide to gambling like a pro.* New York: Alpha Books.

Woolley, L., & Moorey, P. (1982). *Ur of the chaldees.* London: Herbert.

Wynne, H., Smith, G., & Jacobs, D. (1996). *Adolescent gambling and problem gambling in Alberta: Final Report.* Edmonton: Alberta Alcohol & Drug Abuse Commission.

World Service Office, Inc. (1982). *Narcotics anonymous.* Van Nuys: World Service Office, Inc.

Yalom, I. (1980). *Existential psychotherapy.* New York: Basic Books.

Youngman, B. (1999). Summary report: The impact of gaming upon Canadian non–profits: A 1999 survey of gaming grant recipients. Retrieved August 27, 2007 from http://www.cwf.ca/publications.html

Zangeneh, M. (2005). Suicide and gambling. *Australian e-Journal for the Advancement of Mental Health, 4*(1). Retrieved August 27, 2007 from www.auseinet.com/journal/vol4iss1/zangeneheditorial.pdf

Zimmerman, M., Breen, R. B., & Posternak, M. A. (2002). An open-label study of citalopram in the treatment of pathological gambling. *Journal of Clinical Psychiatry, 63,* 44–48.

Zizek, S. (1989). *The sublime object of ideology.* New York: Verso Books.

Zuckerman, M. (1979). *Sensation seeking: Beyond the optimal level of arousal.* Mahwah, NJ: Lawrence Erlbaum Associates.

Zweig, C., & Wolfe, S. (1997). *Romancing the shadow: Illuminating the dark side of the soul.*New York: Ballantine Books.

Subject Index

Author Index

Printed in the United States of America.